Stefan Dübel, Stefan Heuser (Hrsg.)
How Metaphors shape Biotechnology

Health Academy

Herausgegeben von
Arne Manzeschke und Thomas Wittenberg

Band 4

How Metaphors shape Biotechnology

Interdisziplinäre Perspektiven

Herausgegeben von
Stefan Dübel, Stefan Heuser

DE GRUYTER

Herausgeber
Prof. Dr. Stefan Dübel
Technische Universität Braunschweig
Inst. für Biochemie, Biotechnologie und Bioinformatik
Spielmannstr. 7
D-38106 Braunschweig

Prof. Dr. Stefan Heuser
Technische Universität Braunschweig
Institut für Evangelische Theologie und Religionspädagogik
Bienroder Weg 97
D-38106 Braunschweig

Funding was provided by the Program "Interdisciplinary Collaboration" of Braunschweig University of Technology.

ISBN 978-3-11-914512-1
e-ISBN (PDF) 978-3-11-221568-5
e-ISBN (EPUB) 978-3-11-221589-0
ISSN 1617-8874
DOI https://doi.org/10.1515/9783112215685

Library of Congress Control Number: 2025942161

Bibliografische Information der Deutschen Nationalbibliothek
Die Deutsche Nationalbibliothek verzeichnet diese Publikation in der Deutschen Nationalbibliografie; detaillierte bibliografische Daten sind im internet über http://dnb.dnb.de abrufbar.

Einbandabbildung: Stefan Dübel
Satz: Integra Software Services Pvt. Ltd.

www.degruyterbrill.com
Fragen zur allgemeinen Produktsicherheit:
productsafety@degruyterbrill.com

Vorwort / Preface

Die Beiträge dieses Bandes dokumentieren die Ergebnisse eines interdisziplinären Workshops mit dem Titel *„How Metaphors Shape Biotechnology“, der vom 23.–24.* November 2023 an der Technischen Universität Braunschweig stattfand. Wissenschaftlerinnen und Wissenschaftler aus den Bereichen Biologie, Biotechnologie, Philosophie, Ethik, Theologie, Bildungswissenschaften und Wissenschaftskommunikation trafen sich im Haus der Wissenschaft in Braunschweig, um über den Einfluss von Metaphern auf die Lebenswissenschaften zu diskutieren. Wir danken allen, die zu diesem Workshop beigetragen haben sowie den Autorinnen und Autoren dieses Tagungsbandes. Ebenso danken wir dem Forschungsservice der Technischen Universität Braunschweig für die finanzielle Unterstützung des Workshops durch Mittel aus dem Seedfunding Programm „Interdisciplinary Collaboration“.

Ein Hinweis noch zur Sprache dieses Tagungsbands: Die Vorträge und Diskussionen auf dem Workshop waren in deutscher Sprache. Da die Beiträge zu diesem Tagungsband überwiegend mit Ausnahme der englischsprachigen Originalbeiträge von Jonathan Benecke und Stefan Heuser darauf aufbauen und die jeweilige Sprache beim Thema „Metapher“ eine zentrale Rolle spielt, haben wir darauf verzichtet, diese Beiträge zu übersetzen. Um englischsprachigen Leserinnen und Lesern einen Einblick in den hier dokumentierten deutschsprachigen Diskurs zu geben, haben wir die Einleitung auf Englisch geschrieben und mit englischen Abstracts der einzelnen Beiträge versehen.

--

The contributions in this volume document the results of an interdisciplinary workshop entitled “How Metaphors Shape Biotechnology”, which took place at Technische Universität Braunschweig from November 23–24, 2023. Scholars from the fields of biology, biotechnology, philosophy, ethics, theology, educational sciences, and science communication gathered at Braunschweig’s Haus der Wissenschaft to discuss the influence of metaphors on the life sciences. We would like to thank everyone who contributed to this workshop, as well as the authors of this conference volume. Our gratitude also goes to the Research Service of Technische Universität Braunschweig for financially supporting the workshop through funding from the Seed-Funding Program “Interdisciplinary Collaboration.”

A brief note on the language used in this volume: The presentations and discussions at the workshop took place in German. Since most of the contributions to this conference volume (with the exception of the English-language original contributions by Jonathan Benecke and Stefan Heuser) build upon these interactions – and given that language itself plays a key role in the topic of metaphor – we have refrained

https://doi.org/10.1515/9783112215685-202

from translating them. To offer English-speaking readers an insight into the German-language discourse documented here, however, we have written the introduction in English and included English abstracts for the individual contributions.

Braunschweig, Juni 2025
Stefan Dübel und Stefan Heuser

Inhaltsverzeichnis

Autorenliste

Chapter 1, 9
Prof. Dr. Stefan Dübel
Technische Universität Braunschweig
Inst. für Biochemie, Biotechnologie und Bioinformatik
Spielmannstr. 7
D- 38106 Braunschweig
s.duebel@tu-braunschweig.de

Chapter 1, 7, 9, 10
Prof. Dr. Stefan Heuser
Technische Universität Braunschweig
Institut für Evangelische Theologie und Religionspädagogik
Bienroder Weg 97
D- 38106 Braunschweig
s.heuser@tu-braunschweig.de

Chapter 6
Jonathan Benecke
Geysostraße 3a
38106 Braunschweig
jo.benecke@ostfalia.de; jonathan.benecke23@googlemail.com

Chapter 5
PD Dr. phil. Joachim Boldt
Albert-Ludwigs-Universität Freiburg
Institut für Ethik und Geschichte der Medizin
Stefan-Meier-Str. 26
79104 Freiburg
boldt@egm.uni-freiburg.de

Chapter 10
PD Dr. Bruno Gransche
Karlsruher Institut für Technologie KIT
Institut für Technikzukünfte ITZ
Douglasstr. 24
76133 Karlsruhe
bruno.gransche@kit.edu

Chapter 2, 11
Prof. Dr. Nicole Karafyllis
Universität Braunschweig
Institut für Philosophie
Bienroder Weg 80
38106 Braunschweig
n.karafyllis@tu-braunschweig.de

Chapter 8
Daniel Keck
Karl-Finkelnburg-Str. 9
53173 Bonn
d.keck78@googlemail.com

Chapter 10
Prof. Dr. theol. habil. Arne Manzeschke
Evangelische Hochschule Nürnberg
Institut für Pflegeforschung, Gerontologie und Ethik (IPGE)
Bärenschanzstr. 4
90429 Nürnberg
arne.manzeschke@evhn.de

Chapter 4
Dr. Dipl-Math. Domenico Schneider
Rathenower Str. 35
10559 Berlin
domenico.schneider@tu-braunschweig.de

Chapter 3, 9
Prof. Dr. Hans G. Ulrich
Coburger Straße 49a
91056 Erlangen
Hansg.ulrich@t-online.de
Chapter 3,9

https://doi.org/10.1515/9783112215685-204

Stefan Dübel & Stefan Heuser

1 How metaphors shape biotechnology. An introduction

1.1 The research questions of this volume

This volume is based on a scoping workshop funded by Technische Universität Braunschweig's Seed Funding Programme "Interdisciplinary Collaboration". During this workshop, Stefan Dübel and Stefan Heuser brought together leading experts in metaphor research and early career scientists to examine and collaboratively explore metaphors in scientific language. The participants, drawn from various academic fields – including biology, biotechnology, philosophy, theology, ethics, education, and social sciences – discussed the use of conceptual metaphors in biotechnological research (for instance, "genetic scissors" for CRISPR/Cas-9 or "patch" for mRNA therapies). They also examined "absolute" metaphors (such as "life" and "world") and "hidden" metaphors, exemplified by the imagery of "reading" and "writing" in molecular structures. This workshop started from the insight that scientific research uses metaphors

a. to describe previously unknown biological phenomena, processes and interventions as essential part of adequate hypotheses,
b. to facilitate the identification of novel problems, topics and uncharted fields or aims of research and
c. to convey fundamental aspects of research to a wider public.

In a) or b), metaphors are essential to grasp and map molecular life processes as they lend themselves to scientific exploration and to understanding, both in research and in academic education. In c), the use of metaphors in science communication is a very important factor that shapes the public perception of such technologies, and may yield their acceptance or repudiation. All aspects of the use of metaphors in scientific language – their epistemological power to guide the perception of research itself and their discursive power to frame public science communication – call for interdisciplinary approaches to collaborative work on metaphors.

This leads to the following set of research questions:

- What is the epistemic contribution of metaphors to the genesis und shape of scientific knowledge in the fields of molecular biology and biotechnology?
- How do metaphors in molecular biology and biotechnology guide and direct the perception of the contours of human life? Which (set of) metaphors may promote a richer understanding of the conditio humana, and of related questions such as the understanding of health, of disease, and of therapy?

https://doi.org/10.1515/9783112215685-001

- How can new scientific insights contribute to the transformation of metaphors, and to the renewal of scientific language, and vice versa: how can the renewal of metaphors inspire new scientific insights and biotechnological innovation?
- What can metaphors that are rooted in the human lifeworld (e.g. reading, writing, understanding) contribute to the identification of common objectives of research, such as methods and therapies that follow the logics of "communication"?
- Which metaphors prove functional or dysfunctional for scientific exploration processes – and for public science communication?
- How do metaphors in scientific language contribute to the public acceptability of the methods and results of biotechnological research and of biotechnological innovations, and in how far do metaphors entail and yield moral evaluations?
- Practical consequences: What follows from the answers to these questions for the use, critique and active transformation of metaphors in scientific language?

The methods of approaching these questions were presentations and plenary discussions, followed by intense exchange on the drafts of the papers. Some of this exchange, and further work on the conference topic is documented in two writing conversations that were conducted with collaborative real-time text editors. All of these discussions set out from the following state of research.

1.2 State of research

In the wake of Max Black's seminal interaction theory of metaphors [1] and of Hans Blumenberg's reconstruction of the importance of metaphors for scientific discoveries [2; 3], there have been various attempts to re-evaluate the contribution of metaphors for epistemology in general [4; 5; 6; 7; 8; 9; 10; 11; 12; 13; 14; 15; 16; 17; 18; 19; 20]. Attention has specifically been drawn to the role of metaphors in science language and science communication [21; 22; 23; 24; 25; 26], particularly in the fields of genetics and synthetic biology [27; 28; 29; 30; 31; 32; 33; 34; 35; 36; 37]. Furthermore, outlines of a philosophy of genetics have been developed that pay specific attention to the functionality of metaphors [38; 39; 40; 41; 42; 43; 44; 45]. It has been shown that metaphors in science fulfil different functions, or context specific "roles".

According to Reynolds [45, p. 7], metaphors have 1) a heuristic role by suggesting analogical models or hypotheses to be explored in order to discover important unifying similarities or patterns in nature (context of discovery), 2) a cognitive role in the development of explanations that increase our understanding of nature and its mechanisms (context of justification), and 3) metaphors are a pedagogical or rhetorical device in the communication between scientists and non-scientists and students.

While we agree on this account of epistemological, heuristic, rhetoric functions that the use of metaphors in biosciences fulfil, we would like to add and emphasize two interwoven aspects. First, metaphors *have* a function, e.g. a rhetoric and/or a heuristic function. Second, and in line of its heuristic function, metaphors *indicate* a function. They let us see something *as something*, above all, in its functionality. Metaphors let us see the target domain in the light of a particular function suggested by the source domain, e.g. the metaphor of "life" as a "journey" suggests that life has functions similar to the functions of a journey. To capture such functions may even entail to attribute and to discuss a certain meaning to the target domain, or at least to locate it meaningfully in our world of understanding. This may also include to view, attribute and discuss functions to single parts, aspects or processes of the whole target domain, e.g. the metaphors of life as a journey suggests that certain phenomena of life can be regarded as functions (e.g. stages) of a journey, with the living entity being a traveller or hiker.

However, there is only minimal awareness within the biotech community for the role of metaphors, as it has not been any systematic collaborative work on the topic in the fields of Ethics and of Biosciences that would sufficiently answer to the research questions mentioned above, particularly to the problem of the contribution of metaphors to a common understanding of reality and to the formation of collaborative objectives of research.

1.3 Outline of this volume

Building on these findings, our project started with the identification and analysis of crucial metaphors in genetics and biotechnology, leading to the interdisciplinary workshop documented in this volume. In this two-day workshop, methods of systematic metaphor analysis [46] and insights of science ethics, epistemology and of the philosophy of genetics were applied to the use and logics of metaphors in biotechnological and other research, education and science communication. Not all of the delivered papers could eventually be included in this volume. Those aspects of our discussion that deemed us central to answer our research questions, are taken up in two writing conversations.

This volume sets off with **Nicole Karafyllis**' article "Lesen biotechnologisch". In this work, Karafyllis investigates the challenges and assumptions surrounding readability in the life sciences, highlighting the complex relationship between metaphors of readability and biological information. She argues that "reading" DNA and genetic information cannot simply be equated with reading traditional texts, thereby calling for a reevaluation of this relationship. Through a critical examination of the various presuppositions, implications and expectations of readability, Karafyllis demonstrates that they open up new hermeneutic and practical dimensions that extend far beyond the mere provision of information. Drawing on Hans Blumenberg, Karafyllis explores tensions between the closedness of canonical texts and the openness of the biological world, and she addresses the issue of different reductionist forms of biotechnological reading, particularly infrastructural reductionism, thereby focusing on the practice of collecting genetic material in biobanks, which carries fare-reaching cultural and technical implications. Read against this background, the „dead“ metaphor of „collecting“ (German: „Lesen“) seeds may be very much alive when applied to reading, because it generates productive inconsistencies. These inconsistencies shed light on the intricate relationship between nature, culture, and technology, as well as on the processes by which biology becomes a resource and the object of legal and economic interests. At the same time, the metaphor of readability is also profoundly linked to the reader's longing for meaning and need for intimacy, who seeks not merely to perceive or calculate the world, but to experience it in a meaning-generating way. Karafyllis concludes that the metaphor of readability in the life sciences serves not only as a tool for the dissemination of knowledge but also holds creative potential that addresses a wide range scientific, philosophical and cultural practices.

Hans G. Ulrich's contribution “Metaphern – ein Kapitel zur Forschungsethik” sheds light on the complex interplay between scientific knowledge, especially in molecular biology, and ethical reflection. Central to his discussion are metaphors such as “communication,” “program,” or “blueprint,” thereby revealing the tension between what can be scientifically grasped and what remains indefinable. Building on Hans Blumenberg's metaphorology, Ulrich demonstrates that metaphors are not merely tools for scientific description; they also serve as frameworks for orientation that touch upon ethical issues. A key motif is the metaphor of “communication,” which, on the one hand, captures internal exchange processes in the genome (including epigenetic interactions) and, on the other hand, points to the continuous focus on an “end product,” for instance an organ or an entire organism. This perspective — from the finished product back to its genesis — necessarily involves a chain of functional steps. Raised in this context are questions of teleology: Is the goal of genetic development understood solely as functional, or does it extend beyond purpose-driven reasoning to include dimensions of meaning? This tension is particularly evident in the case of humans, where there is a gap between functional and teleological metaphors. In this regard, Nietzsche's provocative question: “Wozu Mensch überhaupt?” takes center stage. Ulrich stresses that humans apprehend their world via metaphors, while never being entirely certain of what “true reality” might mean in its ultimate sense. This “intellectual-historical drama” is closely intertwined with the metaphors of molecular biology because it ultimately raises existential questions that exceed purely scientific explanatory models. Herein lies the value of an interdisciplinary engagement with metaphors: They keep present that dimension which cannot be fully captured by conceptual categories and thus invite us to further reflection. Ulrich concludes that metaphors act as bridges — between what is methodically comprehensible and an openness to that which lies beyond definitive ends and purposes in the process of scientific exploration.

In his article “Eine wissenschafts- und verkörperungsphilosophische Betrachtung der Metapher in wissenschaftlicher Praxis”, **Domenico Schneider** addresses two key aspects: First, drawing on George Lakoff and Mark Johnson, he highlights the embodied and intermodal nature of metaphor, illustrating its importance both in everyday language use and in the formation of scientific theories. Second, he explores the dynamics of how metaphors emerge, referring to Max Black’s description of the diverse processes involved in the emergence of metaphors. From this, he posits that metaphors in an increasingly technologized world are substantially shaped by technology, instruments, and the related thinking in models and theories. Schneider initially rivisits the debate between Max Black and Daniel Davidson, focusing on the necessity of a dynamic perspective on metaphor production. Here, particular attention is paid to the lack of embodiment in classical theories of metaphor. In the next step, Schneider integrates this viewpoint with an embodiment-based approach, underscoring the influence of bodily experience on metaphor usage. Subsequently, he demonstrates how the ergonomics of scientific instruments affects imaging techniques and their metaphorical dimensions. The technical instruments themselves even define the research paradigms and their accompanying metaphors. Building on Ian Hacking’s concept of “instrumental intervention”, Schneider argues that the development of scientific metaphors is significantly driven by a technologically shaped relation between humans and their environment. Since the metaphors used in the natural sciences employ a researcher-specific language, Schneider concludes that this technological prestructuring gives rise to a specific “technoimagination” (Flusser), which transforms researchers’ relationship with the world and ultimately leads to communication and comprehension difficulties in the public sphere. With reference to science communication, Schneider thus shows that it remains unclear how technologically mediated metaphors can be meaningfully introduced into a sensus communis, or into public debates on development paths in the biotechnologies.

In his article “Maschinenmetaphern und Ethik in der Synthetischen Biologie”, **Joachim Boldt** explores how machine metaphors — such as “genetically engineered machine,” “genetic circuit,” or “platform organism” — shape both the self-conception and practical work in this field of research. Borrowed from electronics, automotive engineering, and information technology, these metaphors act as a conceptual lens that highlights the targeted modifiability of genetic elements and their functions. At the same time, however, they sideline aspects such as evolutionary development, ecological interdependencies, and long-term environmental impacts, potentially leading to an underestimation of related risks. Boldt shows that this one-sided view not only complicates the assessment of hazards and environmental effects but also presents ethical challenges: attributing moral status to living beings – including humans – becomes problematic if organisms are primarily regarded as machines. Furthermore, from a machine-focused perspective, simply producing slightly modified natural organisms falls short of realizing the full potential of synthetic biology – such as through the development of entirely novel organisms partially comprised of synthetic DNA.

Boldt contents that the question of how to adequately assess the side effects of such organisms on the environment and ecosystems remains both open and pressing. Boldt also illustrates that the machine metaphor implies a certain concept of progress, portraying synthetic biology as the spearhead of scientific and technological innovation and potentially overstating its ability to solve societal and ecological problems. Drawing on concrete examples, he demonstrates how this narrowed perspective shapes both scientific discourse and public debate. In conclusion, Boldt calls for critical reflection on the ethical and epistemological implications of machine-driven metaphors: strengthening multidisciplinary risk assessment, addressing the moral status of organisms beyond the machine paradigm, and giving due consideration to alternative solutions in science, society, and policymaking.

In „On the Problem of Epistemic Metaphor", **Jonathan Benecke** examines the elusive nature of metaphoricity by challenging the traditional view of metaphor as a mere transfer of meaning from one domain to another. Departing from an Aristotelian approach that seeks a fixed concept of metaphor in strictly defined categories, Benecke shows how such an "essentialist" perspective either trivializes metaphor – by reducing it to a reversible substitution – or renders it unrepresentable, in line with Nietzsche's insistence on the perpetual displacement inherent in metaphorical processes. Drawing on Deleuze and Guattari's notion of shifting meanings, he argues that metaphors are neither static nor incidental, but rather historically and contextually constructed. They possess a "(meta)stability" that allows for communication while simultaneously fostering conceptual innovation and transformation. Reconceptualized as experiments in language, metaphors refuse any strict priority of fixed concepts; instead, they function as self-subducting processes in which meaning-making unfolds dynamically. By foregrounding their experimental and constructive role, Benecke illustrates how epistemic metaphors contribute to modern scientific inquiry — not merely by dressing up pre-formed ideas in figurative language, but by generating new pathways of thinking and reinforcing the recursive relationship between thought and the world.

In his article "Metaphors in ELSA Research: Bridging the Gap Between the Laboratory and the Life-World," **Stefan Heuser** examines how metaphors influence the development of biotechnology and biomedicine in the context of ELSA (ethical, legal, and social aspects) research. Since the launch of the Human Genome Project, interdisciplinary discussions between the natural and social sciences have often been framed as ELSI (in the United States) or ELSA (in Europe), referring to the ethical, legal, and social aspects or implications of life science research. Over time, these ELSA/I programs have expanded to encompass emerging technological fields, from biotechnology to AI. Although designed to improve the acceptability of biomedical and biotechnological innovations and to strengthen the trustworthiness of science, ELSA research has faced criticism over its close integration with science policy and bio-industry funding. Critics argue that it risks becoming a mere tool of legitimization or "fig leaf" for otherwise unchecked scientific and commercial interests. Despite these concerns, it is evident that ELSA research remains vital for ensuring that scientific developments are aligned with societal values and needs, mitigating potential harms, and fostering trust between the public and innovators. Ongoing critiques and resulting reforms have spurred new, more collaborative modes of inquiry, including "post-ELSI" and "integrated" research frameworks, which seek to involve stakeholders earlier ("upstream") in decision-making processes. This article explores one such collaborative approach, focusing on the central role of metaphors in shaping both research agendas and public perceptions. Drawing on conceptual metaphor theory and underscoring the importance of collective, interdisciplinary, and participatory engagement, it demonstrates how metaphorical language can help embed ethical, social, and cultural considerations into biotechnological research from the outset. By highlighting metaphors as potent "bridges" between laboratory work and the life-world, the article offers insights into how these tools can facilitate stakeholder involvement and guide scientific innovation toward genuinely shared objectives. Heuser concludes that a conscientious and critical integration of conceptual metaphors into scientific discourse, policymaking, and public engagement can inspire new insights and promote a more inclusive, collaborative approach to biotechnological innovation.

In his article „Das bedrohte Gleichgewicht. Der Begriff der Krankheit in Pflege und Medizin. Eine historisch-vergleichende Metaphernanalyse", **Daniel Keck** introduces a metaphorological perspective to the longstanding debate on the concept of illness. Central to his investigation is how medical and nursing textbooks employ particular metaphors, and how these metaphors influence healthcare professionals' conceptualization and practice. Although health and illness have taken center stage in social discourse – especially during and after recent pandemic years – public debates often reduce these complex issues to questions of cost and resource allocation, overlooking the conceptual nuances of "health" and "illness." Since the 1970s, medical philosophy has wrestled with devising a comprehensive concept of illness, but these attempts have largely stalled amid tensions between naturalistic and normativistic theoretical approaches. Naturalistic theories, such as Christopher Boorse's biostatistical account, insist on defining illness through biological and functional deviations from a statistical norm. By contrast, normativistic theories assert that the notions of health and illness intrinsically incorporate value judgments and social norms. Building on these contrasting perspectives, Keck's study employs a metaphorological lens to illuminate how different metaphors – drawn from domains as varied as war, technology, and the idea of equilibrium – shape professional understandings of illness. Drawing on Susan Sontag's insight that diseases carry narrative and often moral dimensions beyond their biological reality, he reveals the ways in which metaphorical language informs the thinking and actions of healthcare practitioners. Keck analyzes eleven medical and nursing textbooks, published from the 1950s to 2015, alongside trivial comparison texts, to identify how metaphors construct representations of illness. His methodology combines Lakoff and Johnson's cognitive theory of metaphor with Schmitt et al.'s systematic metaphor analysis framework, which provides a structured procedure for uncovering underlying metaphorical concepts and examining their shifts over time. Keck's analysis shows that textbooks from the 1950s rely heavily on vivid metaphors stemming from spatial perception, mechanical imagery, and warfare. In these early texts, the human body is likened to a machine that must stand guard against external and internal threats, fighting to preserve its fragile balance. By contrast, more recent textbooks show a marked decline in warlike and technological metaphors and increasingly revolve around the equilibrium metaphor, underscoring a move toward a holistic, systems-based view of illness in which maintaining balance supersedes a narrative of relentless defense. To conclude, Keck's historical-comparative examination of metaphors across five decades of medical and nursing literature reveals significant shifts in how illness is conceptualized. These findings underscore the need for critical engagement with metaphorical language in healthcare education, as the metaphors embedded within educational materials profoundly shape how practitioners diagnose and treat illness.

The written conversation, titled "Metaphern in den Wissenschaften: Ein Gespräch zwischen Biotechnologie und Ethik", stems from discussions held at the workshop "How Metaphors Shape Biotechnology" (November 23–24, 2023, at the Technical University of Braunschweig). Building on the idea that metaphors inform both scientific inquiry and ethical reflection, the authors **Stefan Dübel**, **Hans G. Ulrich** and **Stefan Heuser** explore multiple facets of biotechnological innovations and the ways they are interpreted. They illustrate how metaphorical language can guide research and public perception by emphasizing certain understandings while sidelining others. Concurrently, they consider how theological and ethical viewpoints can enrich collective deliberation on the objectives and boundaries of biotechnological endeavors. The conversation between biotechnology, theology, and ethics highlights two central themes: (1) the generative power of figurative language in formulating fresh scientific hypotheses and conceptual frameworks, and (2) the importance of ongoing critical examination to ensure that metaphors are continually adapted to evolving scientific and ethical contexts.

In a subsequent written dialogue, which builds on two lectures delivered by **Bruno Gransche** and **Arne Manzeschke** at the Braunschweig workshop, the two authors, together with **Stefan Heuser** as moderator, discuss the knowledge-guiding, orientational, and structuring functions of metaphors within contemporary scientific and technological cultures. This chapter, "Anthropomorphisierungen. Ein Gespräch über Metapherntechnik und Technikmetaphern," is grounded in Gransche's reflections on metaphor as a fundamental structure of thought – which allows us to grasp the new through the lens of the familiar – and in Manzeschke's anthropological insight that both our self-understanding and our worldview are constantly mediated and developed through metaphors. Gransche and Manzeschke emphasize that metaphors are not merely rhetorical devices but are, in fact, genuine cognitive tools that shape understanding, especially in encounters with novel phenomena such as biotechnology or artificial intelligence (AI). While metaphors offer orientation, their selective nature can also have limiting or even problematic effects: they prompt certain actions, structure research agendas, and influence societal communication. To systematically analyze the relationships between the source and target domains of metaphors, Gransche and Manzeschke introduce a metaphorological matrix. This matrix enables differentiation among physiomorphic (nature-shaped), biomorphic (life-shaped), anthropomorphic (human-shaped), and technomorphic (technology-shaped) forms of conceptual transfer. Through numerous examples – from biomorphic architectural metaphors to technicized conceptions of humanity, and from the "gene scissors" and evolution as a programming concept to mythological figures such as Prometheus – Gransche and Manzeschke demonstrate how clusters and trends of metaphorization can be mapped using the matrix. Special attention is given to the dynamics emerging at the intersections of these fields: for example, the tendency toward the biologization and psychologization of technology (as in the case of AI), and conversely, the technicization of psychic, organic, or even divine phenomena (such as cloning, technological enhancement, and Intelligent Design). The matrix reveals that, in modern discourse, technological concepts are frequently anthropomorphized and attributed vitality, while humans, nature, and even the divine are increasingly conceptualized through technological metaphors. This has profound implications for research, ethics, science communication, and broader societal reflection. The authors argue that the receptive and productive variability of metaphorizations necessitates a targeted critique of metaphors – one that addresses not only ideological implications but also questions of epistemic adequacy and practical orientation to reality. The systematic, matrix-guided analysis and reflection on metaphorical constructions is described as a "task of cultivation." The goal is to promote metaphor literacy: the ability to recognize the orientational power of metaphors, to use them competently, and to critically reflect on their knowledge-guiding, limiting, and ethically significant consequences. The authors advocate for institutionalized spaces for reflection and for an open, systematic engagement with metaphors in order to ensure and enhance their orientational and communicative function in the face of an increasingly complex and ever-changing reality.

In her obituary for Evelyn Fox Keller (1936–2023), **Nicole Karafyllis** offers a nuanced portrait of a scholar who blazed new trails in molecular biology, philosophy, and the history of science. Born in New York to Russian-Jewish immigrants, Keller completed her doctorate under Matthew Meselson in 1963 and actively participated in the "Golden Age" of molecular biology. At the same time, she was influenced by the linguistic turn in the humanities and the second wave of the women's movement – factors that led to her becoming one of the founders of feminist epistemology. Keller placed particular emphasis on the concept of the "gene" and its evolution from a simple code to a complex network. In *The Century of the Gene*, she criticized the widespread essentialism that ascribes excessive causal power to genes regarding behavior or disease, and instead advocated for a relational, epigenetically informed understanding of heredity. Through her historical case studies and biomathematical research, she also highlighted how scientific practice is deeply shaped by cultural metaphors and modes of thought. Alongside her critical perspective on knowledge, Keller laid the groundwork for feminist epistemology, emphasizing that science becomes more robust when it embraces diverse voices. Although some poststructuralist thinkers deemed Keller's commitment to objectivity and truth conservative, she insisted that while theories may be constructed, they remain tied to a real foundation. Karafyllis concludes that Evelyn Fox Keller's call for a broadened conception of science that transcends gender boundaries and flourishes through openness and diversity leaves a legacy that points the way to the future.

The editors thank all authors for their contributions and wish every reader a stimulating reading experience.

References

[1] Black M. Models and metaphors. Studies in language and philosophy. Ithaca: Cornell University Press, 1962.

[2] Blumenberg H. Die Lesbarkeit der Welt, Frankfurt/Main: Suhrkamp (2. Auflage), 1983.

[3] Blumenberg H. Paradigmen zu einer Metaphorologie, Frankfurt/Main: Suhrkamp, 1997.

[4] Ricoeur P. Die lebendige Metapher, Rainer Rochlitz (Üb.), München: Fink, 1986.

[5] Kuhn T S. Metaphor in science. In: Metaphor and thought. Ortony, A (Ed.). (2. Aufl.) Cambridge: Cambridge Univ. Press, 1993: 409–419.

[6] Hesse M B. Models, Metaphors and Truth. In: From a Metaphorical Point of View: A Multidisciplinary Approach to the Cognitive Content of Metaphor. Radman, Z (Ed.). Berlin: De Gruyter, 1995: 351–372. Doi: 10.1515/9783110867831-017.

[7] Hesse M B. Models and Analogies. In: A Companion to the Philosophy of Science. Newton-Smith, W H (Ed.), Oxford: Blackwell, 2000: 299–307.

[8] Radman Z (Ed.). From a Metaphorical Point of View: A Multidisciplinary Approach to the Cognitive Content of Metaphor. Philosophie und Wissenschaft 7. Berlin: De Gruyter, 1995.

[9] Schneider H J. Wittgensteins Begriff der Grammatik und das Phänomen der Metapher, in: ders. (Hg.), Metapher, Kognition, Künstliche Intelligenz, München: Fink, 1996.

[10] Hallyn F (Ed.). Metaphor and analogy in the sciences. Studies in the sources of scientific creativity Vol. 1. Dordrecht: Springer, 2000.

[11] Harré R. Modeling: gateway to the unknown. Daniel Rothbart (Ed.), Studies in multidisciplinarity Vol. 1. Amsterdam: Elsevier, 2004.

[12] Bailer-Jones D M. Scientific Models as Metaphors. In: Metaphor and Analogy in the Sciences, Hallyn, F (Ed.). Origins, Studies in the sources of scientific creativity Vol. 1. Dordrecht: Springer, 2000: 181–198.

[13] Bailer-Jones D M. Scientific models in philosophy of science. Pittsburgh: Pittsburgh University Press, 2009.

[14] Eckard R. Metaphertheorien. Typologie. Darstellung. Bibliographie. Berlin, New York: Walter de Gruyter, 2005.

[15] Rentetzi M. The Metaphorical Conception of Scientific Explanation: Rereading Mary Hesse. In: Journal for General Philosophy of Science / Zeitschrift Für Allgemeine Wissenschaftstheorie, 36/2, 2005: 377–391. http://www.jstor.org/stable/25171322

[16] Glucksberg S. Understanding Metaphors: The paradox of unlike things compared. In: Affective computing and sentiment analysis. Emotion, metaphor and terminology. Ahmad K (Ed.). Dordrecht: Springer, 2011: 1–12.
[17] Lakoff G; Johnson M. Leben in Metaphern. Konstruktion und Gebrauch von Sprachbildern. Hildenbrand A (Üb.). (8. Aufl.) Heidelberg: Carl-Auer, 2014.
[18] Taylor C, Dewsbury B M. On the Problem and Promise of Metaphor Use in Science and Science Communication. In: Journal of Microbiology and Biology Education 19/1, 2018: 46.
[19] Sullivan-Clarke A. Misled by metaphor: The problem of ingrained analogy. In: Perspectives on Science 27/2, 2019: 153–170.
[20] Thibodeau P H, Matlock T, Flusberg S J. The role of metaphor in communication and thought. In: Language and Linguistics Compass 13/5, 2019. https://doi.org/10.1111/lnc3.12327.
[21] Sontag S. Krankheit als Metapher. Aids und seine Metaphern. (4. Aufl.) Frankfurt: Fischer, 1977/2016.
[22] Bauer A W. Metaphern. Bildersprache und Selbstverständnis der Medizin. In: Anaesthesist 55, 2006: 1307–1314.
[23] Marron J M, Dizon D S; Symington B, Thompson M A, Rosenberg A R. Waging War on War Metaphors in Cancer and COVID-19. In: JCO Oncology Practice 624/14, 2020. Online: https://doi.org/10.1200/OP.20.00542.
[24] Becker R. Methodischer Mechanismus und instrumentelle Vernunft: Warum Lebewesen keine Organismen sind. In: Deutsche Zeitschrift für Philosophie, 68/5, 2020: 734–749. https://doi.org/10.1515/dzph-2020-0050.
[25] Pasler M. Zur Kriegsmetapher in der Corona-Krise, in: Arnold C, Flügel-Martinsen O, Mohammed S, Vasilache A (Ed.). Kritik in der Krise. Perspektiven politischer Theorie auf die Corona-Pandemie, Baden-Baden: Nomos, 2020: 49–60.
[26] Krug H. Mit den Augen Susan Sontags: Metaphern im Umgang mit COVID-19. In: Zeitschrift für Ethik und Moralphilosophie 4, 2021: 213–229. Online: https://doi.org/10.1007/s42048-021-00098-4.
[27] Blute M. If the Genome isn't a God-like Ghost in the Machine, then What is it? In: Biology & Philosophy 20/2–3, 2005: 401–407. Doi: 10.1007/s10539-004-0191-5.
[28] Boudry M, Pigliucci M. The mismeasure of machine: Synthetic biology and the trouble with engineering metaphors. In: Studies in history and philosophy of biological and biomedical sciences 44/4, 2013: 660–668. Doi: 10.1016/j.shpsc.2013.05.013.
[29] O'Keefe M, Perrault S, Halpern J, Ikemoto L, Yarborough M. "Editing" genes: A case study about how language matters in bioethics. American Journal of Bioethics 15/12, 2015: 3–10. Doi: 10.1080/15265161.2015.1103804.
[30] Nelson S C, Yu J-H, Ceccarelli L. How metaphors about the genome constrain CRISPR metaphors: Separating the "text" from its "editor". In: The American Journal of Bioethics, 15/12, 2015: 60–62. Doi: 10.1080/15265161.2015.
[31] Frezza G. Metaphors, Risk and Blind Spots in Health Communication: The Case of Gene-editing and CRISPR-Cas9 Technology. In: estetica. studi e ricerche 2/1, 2017: 105–120. Doi: 10.14648/86779.
[32] Braun M, Fernau S, Dabrock P. Images of synthetic life: Mapping the use and function of metaphors in the public discourse on synthetic biology. In: PloS One 13/6, 2018. Doi: 10.1371/journal.pone.0199597.
[33] Ceccarelli L. CRISPR as agent: A metaphor that rhetorically inhibits the prospects for responsible research. In: Genomics, Society and Policy 14/1, 2018. Doi: 10.1186/s40504-018-0088-8.
[34] Boldt J. Machine metaphors and ethics in synthetic biology. In: Genomics, Society and Policy 14/1, 2018. Doi: 10.1186/s40504-018-0077-y.
[35] Nicholson D J. Is the cell really a machine? In: Journal of theoretical biology 477, 2019: 108–126. Doi: 10.1016/j.jtbi.2019.06.002.
[36] Lee Y Y. Genome Editing or Genome Cutting? Communicating CRISPR in the British and German Press. In: Yearbook of the German Cognitive Linguistics Association 8/1, 2020: 45–66.

[37] Nerlich B, Stelmach, A. Gene drive communication. Exploring experts' lived experience of metaphor use. In: New genetics and society 45/4, 2022: 1–20. Doi: 10.1080/14636778.2021.2020633.
[38] Keller E F. Das Leben neu denken: Metaphern der Biologie im 20. Jahrhundert, München: Kunstmann, 1998.
[39] Oyama S. The Ontogeny of Information. Developmental Systems and Evolution, (2. Aufl.) Durham: Duke University Press, 2000.
[40] Griffiths P E. Genetic Information: A Metaphor in search of a theory. In: Philosophy of Science 68/3, 2001: 394–412. Doi: 10.1086/392891.
[41] Rehmann-Sutter C. Gene, Körperlichkeit und Identität, in: Zwischen den Molekülen. Beiträge zur Philosophie der Genetik, Tübingen: Francke, 2005: 135–174.
[42] Rehmann-Sutter C. Zur biophilosophischen Bedeutung der Epigenetik. In: Walter J, Hümpel A (Ed.). Epigenetik: Implikationen für die Lebens- und Geisteswissenschaften. Baden-Baden: Nomos, 2017: 115–133.
[43] Perrault S T, O'Keefe M. New Metaphors for New Understandings of Genomes. In: Perspectives in biology and medicine 62/1, 2019: 1–19. Doi: 10.1353/pbm.2019.0000.
[44] Zerbe M J. Toward a Rhetoric of DNA: The Advent of CRISPR. In: Poroi 14/2, 2019: 1–26. Doi: 10.13008/2151-2957.1276.
[45] Reynolds A S. Understanding metaphors in the life sciences. Cambridge/New York: Cambridge University Press, 2022.
[46] Schmitt R, Schröder J, Pfaller L. Systematische Metaphernanalyse. Eine Einführung. Wiesbaden, Springer VS, 2018.

Nicole C. Karafyllis

2 Lesen biotechnologisch

2.1 Einleitung: Problematiken der Lesbarkeit

In den Biowissenschaften wird viel gelesen. Dies immer weniger in Büchern und Zeitschriften als vielmehr in Molekülen und ihren Aggregaten, zuvorderst in der RNA[1] und DNA – auch wenn man „in der DNA" zu lesen nicht derart sinnvoll sagen kann, wie „in einem Text" oder „in den Wolken" zu lesen. Wer ist hier die Leserin und wo befindet sie sich beim Lesen? In die DNA kann man nicht metaphorisch eintauchen wie in eine Geschichte, die als Text vorliegen kann oder auch nicht. Man kann sie sich auch nicht zu Gemüte führen wie ein gutes Buch in einer Bibliothek. Die DNA spult sich auch nicht ab wie ein Film von einer Filmrolle,[2] projiziert auf eine Leinwand, wenngleich Film und Molekularbiologie das Wort „Sequenz" nutzen, um die Linearität, Kontinuität und Expressivität einer informativen Einheit zu adressieren.[3] Daraus ein „Gen" zu konzipieren geschieht biotechnologisch durch das Zusammenspiel von DNA-Sequenzierung und Sequenzanalyse, basierend auf der sinnhaften („logischen") Unterstellung, dass sich ein Gen wie ein Schnipsel eines informierenden Satzes, eines Codes, lesen lassen wird. Es handelt sich demnach um eine zukunftsverwiesene Lesetechnik, die, wie jede Technik, mit Funktionierbarkeitserwartungen handelt [1]. Und doch ist „die Vergleichswelt von Schrift und Buch" selbst keine mechanistische wie die von Uhr und Uhrwerk, die vor jener sich zur Erklärung des Lebens bewährt hatte, ihr aber in den Implikationen feindlich gegenübersteht [2, S. 375]. Eine Gensequenz ist die Abfolge einer Nukleotidsequenz, sie ‚erzeugt' Proteine und ist selbst erzeugt worden, philosophisch: sie ist *natura naturans* und *natura naturata*. In dieser Selbstbezüglichkeit steht sie dem Text und der Schrift nahe. Deshalb kann man beim genannten Zusammenspiel von biotechnischem Werkzeughandeln im Labor und den angenommenen logischen Verknüpfungen zwischen Syntax und Semantik eines Textes durchaus von „biotechnologischem Lesen" sprechen. Allerdings ist keine Metapher perfekt passend, sonst wäre sie keine Metapher. Metaphern können nur mehr oder weniger stimmig sein für denjenigen Zweck, der mit ihrem Einsatz verfolgt wird.

Dass die DNA in der Zeit ihrer Entdeckung und Analyse während des Kalten Kriegs als „genetischer Code" verstanden wurde (vgl. [3], [4]), plausibilisierte die Annahme, dass eine Biologin sie decodieren kann wie ein Kryptographie-Forscher. Dies

---

1 Hier ist zuvorderst an die messenger-RNA (mRNA) und die ribosomale RNA der kleinen Untereinheit des Ribosoms (16S rRNA) zu denken.

2 An die Verbindung zum Aufrollen einer Schriftrolle im Begriff „Evolution" erinnerte Blumenberg [2].

3 Bei der mittlerweile veralteten Sequenzierungsmethode nach Sanger spielte das Ablesen der Sequenz(schnipsel) auf einem Röntgenfilm eine zentrale Rolle.

https://doi.org/10.1515/9783112215685-002

ist eine reduzierte Form von „Lesen“ und auch von „Wissen“, weil es sich um Informationen handelt, d. h. um bereits zweckorientiertes und für einen bestimmten Empfänger codiertes Wissen. Dies veranschaulichend als „Lesen“ zu fassen, zog das *Metaphernfeld* nach sich: Sowohl in Lehrbüchern als auch in wissenschaftsjournalistischen Texten wird bis dato gerne von Organismen als Büchern mit Seiten (als Bild für die Quantität an Basenpaaren) und von Genomen als Enzyklopädien gesprochen (s. u.). Es gilt jedoch zu beachten, dass ein Buch mit seinem Inhalt ein Objekt ist und metaphorisch nicht das gleiche bedeutet wie die Handlung des Lesens.

Die an Text gekoppelte Lesemetapher soll bezüglich der Zugänglichkeit der Erbinformation überzeugen, dabei gehört es zu den Mythen des Lesens, dass man nur in Texten lesen könne [5]. Man fragt sich unweigerlich, wie ein Lesen aussähe, dass nicht textverwiesen ist, sondern etwa den Wolkenformationen oder Sternkonstellationen nicht nur Bild-, sondern auch Zeichencharakter entnimmt und diese Zeichen konsekutiv zu Bedeutungen verknüpft (vgl. die charakterologische Astrologie). Dass die Schrift- und Textmetapher der DNA zur Ergänzung der Film- und damit Bildmetapher bedarf, wenn es um die Erzeugung von Bedeutung und damit um die Medialität geht, ist ein erster Hinweis darauf, dass jedes für wissenschaftliche Entdeckungen genutzte Metaphernfeld eine Restbedeutung übriglässt, die mit ihr nicht ausgedrückt werden kann (s. u.).

Dieser Artikel versucht nach dem Aufriss der (1.) Problematiken der Lesbarkeit einen kurzen Überblick über (2.) die Präsuppositionen bzw. Vorannahmen des „biotechnologischen Lesens“ bzw. der „biotechnologischen Lesbarkeit“ zu geben. Dafür arbeitet er (3.) mit Bausteinen aus Theorien der Metapher (Max Black, Jörg Zimmer, Hans Blumenberg) im Allgemeinen und mit Blick auf die Molekularbiologie (Evelyn Fox Keller) im Speziellen. Evozierte *Reduktionismen* (4.) werden von bewusst in Kauf genommenen und für den wissenschaftlichen Fortschritt als potenziell kreativ erachteten (5.) *Unstimmigkeiten* unterschieden. Dem hier sog. infrastrukturellen Reduktionismus – d. h. der Ignoranz des Instandhaltens und Bevorratens von Genmaterial in Genombibliotheken bzw. Biobanken – kommt dabei eine wichtige Rolle zu, wie Nicole C. Karafyllis beforscht hat. (6.) Biobanken bilden zusammen mit Ganzheitsmetaphern wie der der Lesbarkeit einen ideell und materiell vorstellbaren Zugriff auf das Ganze der Welt.

2.2 Vorannahmen der Lesbarkeit

Im Kontext biochemisch-molekularbiologischer Techniken werden Annahmen zur *Lesbarkeit* gemacht, die zu hinterfragen sind, bevor man das Wagnis des Lesens unternimmt. So kann die Metapher der Lesbarkeit mit vielem, was daran hängt – die Vorstellungen von Text, Buch, Leser(n), Autor, Bibliothek u. a. – auf ihre Stimmigkeit hin befragt werden, was wichtig für ihre inner- und außerwissenschaftliche Verwendung ist. Einiges davon und Verwandtes wurde bereits durch Wissenschaftshistoriker:innen und Forschende im Bereich STS und ihren Arbeiten zur epistemologischen Funktion der Metapher für die Biowissenschaften geleistet (neben Fox Kellers Arbeiten u. a. die von Susan Sontag und Laura Otis, vgl. [6] und [7]). 2020 erschien ein dem Problemfeld Metapher gewidmetes Themenheft der Zeitschrift *Interdisciplinary Science Reviews* (Vol. 45, Heft 3). Eine übergreifende Darstellung oder Theorie des biotechnologischen Lesens gibt es jedoch nicht.

Wenn Sie den Artikel zu lesen begonnen haben, werden Sie von der Erwartung getragen, dass in dem Text (1.) *Informationen enthalten* sind, er (2.) einen Sinn, womöglich sogar einen tieferen *Sinn ergibt*. Dies sind bereits zwei Bedeutungsvarianten von „Lesbarkeit", die man als seine Innen- und seine Außenseite bezeichnen könnte. Ersteres dürfte hier der Fall sein, wenngleich die bereitgestellten Informationen für einen bestimmten, eher phänomenologischen Fragehorizont relevant sind. Vor diesem könnten sie auch einen tieferen Sinn ergeben, für einen anderen womöglich nicht; es sei denn, die Leserin ist sehr aufgeschlossen dahingehend, (3.) perspektivisch Neues zu lesen und zu lernen. Dies ist eine dritte Bedeutung von „Lesbarkeit", die über die Bereitstellung von Informationen und Sinnerwartung hinausgeht, weil eine *Perspektivenerweiterung* wenn nicht angestrebt, dann doch in Kauf genommen wird. Die Lesbarkeit wäre demnach eine Potenzialerwartung u. a. im Hinblick auf ein größeres Überblickswissen. Erst vor dieser Pluralisierung der Wissenshorizonte kann sich die Lesbarkeit auf ein Lesen beziehen, das auch Interpretieren einschließt und das Lesen zu einem hermeneutischen Projekt macht (vgl. [2], S. 21). Zum vierten kann „Lesbarkeit" auch *semiotisch* verstanden werden: ob eine (4.) Buchstabenfolge, selbst wenn sie etwas fehlerhaft geschrieben sein sollte, noch *funktional* sinnhaft gelesen werden kann (und von wem).[4] Hier besteht eine Verbindung zur Artikulation und zum Hörverstehen, und damit zur Vorlesbarkeit (alternativ auch zur gebärdensprachlichen Darstellbarkeit). (5.) Fünftens kann es bei der Lesbarkeit auch um die *Leserlichkeit* gehen, d. h. ob einzelne Buchstaben und Wörter als solche entzifferbar sind und der Text nicht, wie etwa bei handschriftlich verfassten Texten oder altem Schriftgut, kryptisch oder korrupt ist.

Aber auch bei derartigen Zuschreibungen ist Vorsicht geboten, denn sie hängen von einer bestimmten Lesbarkeitserwartung ab. Die ab den 1960ern bis weit in die 1990er Jahre standardmäßig in der Genetik zu findende Vorstellung von *junk DNA* (wörtlich: Müll-DNA), weil sie als ablesbarer Abschnitt auf einem Chromosom keine Codierungsfunktion für ein Gen zu haben schien, ist mittlerweile überholt (was auch an der Neumodellierung des Gen-Modells bzw. des Operon-Ansatzes und der Ein-Gen-ein-Protein-Hypothese liegt; vgl. [4]). Denn man hat sich vom Fokus auf die nukleare DNA und dem direkten Gen-Funktionalismus gelöst, der an das Modell des Codes und den Informationsbegriff von Sender/Empfänger (Shannon/Weaver) gekoppelt war.

---

4 Genauer anzuschauen wäre auch mit linguistischen Methoden, wie weit die Analogie Aminosäure/Code zu Phonem/Buchstabe wirklich trägt. Ich danke Philip Kraut, Berlin, für diesen Hinweis.

Stattdessen wurde genomisch auch das Erbgut in den Organellen (Mitochondrien, Ribosomen) einbezogen, zusätzlich das Metabolom. Denn die einst als *junk* titulierte, heute ncDNA (noncoding DNA) genannte DNA wirkt in der Zelle regulatorisch, v. a. über zahlreiche Zwischenstadien und Umschriftprodukte wie die m-RNA, die t-RNA und die RNAi. Dieses Problemfeld einer übergreifenden Semantik der DNA wird unter dem Schlagwort „Epigenetik“ behandelt. Man hat also gemäß (3.) die Perspektive auf Lesbarkeit im Kontext der Zelle erweitert und ihre Übersetzbarkeit in verwandte Sprachen und Textbestandteile (vgl. alternatives Spleißen) einbezogen, was mit dem vierten Lesbarkeitsverständnis oben korrespondiert. Das ENCODE-Projekt (**Enc**ylopedia **of** **D**NA **E**lements) konnte für das Humangenom ca. 80% funktionale Einheiten ausmachen [8]. Warum es aber im Sinne von oben (5.) bei Eukaryonten so viele repetitive Sequenzen gibt, die scheinbar keine Funktion haben (Pseudogene) oder eben nicht (richtig) lesbar sind, bleibt ein Rätsel. Die Aussage, dass etwas nicht lesbar ist, setzt die Lesbarkeit als begründete Erwartung voraus, weshalb es sich hier um gewusstes Nichtwissen unter Annahme der Funktionalität handelt (nonknowledge). Dagegen fiel die Zuschreibung von *junk DNA* unter *ignorance*. Das passende Bild dazu ist, beim Lesen die Lesebrille nicht aufgehabt zu haben: das extranukleare Erbgut in Mitochondrien und Ribosomen schlicht ‚übersehen‘ zu haben.

2.3 Theorie der Metapher und die Metapher der Lesbarkeit

Die Vorstellung einer eindeutig lesbaren Natur geht in der westlichen Geistesgeschichte zurück auf das Konzept des „Buchs der Natur“, das sich bereits bei frühchristlichen Autoren findet ([2], [9]). Hier besteht noch eine enge Verbindung zu vorwissenschaftlichen Praktiken. Lesen ist mit alten rituellen Praxen verbunden, die noch keine eindeutige Differenz von Natur und Kultur der Sprache und ihrer Zeichen erlauben, sondern die Bedingung ihrer Möglichkeit sind: „Dies Lesen ist das älteste: das Lesen vor aller Sprache, aus den Eingeweiden, den Sternen oder Tänzen“ ([10], S. 213). Lesen ist eingebunden in eine mediale Welt des Werdens und Vergehens mit einer eigenen Magie der Schöpfung. Diese sei vernichtet worden, so Walter Benjamin (ebd.). Es ist die Welt, in der Lesen und Leben noch untrennbar miteinander verbunden waren. In den Lebensmedien wie Urin und Blut wurde lange zum Gesundheitszustand gelesen (unter Einsatz von Sehen und Schmecken). Letzten Endes ist das Blutbild noch ein Relikt dieses symptomatischen Lesens, auch wenn es schon im Modus des Zählens und Rechnens operiert. Es verspricht, das Innere der Vitalität über Medien entäußern und lesbar machen zu können. Das biotechnologische Lesen aber bedient sich der Moleküle als toter Stoffe wie ein molekularanalytisches Lesegerät. Dem vorausgegangen ist eine Physikalisierung des Lebens im Rahmen der jungen Molekularbiologie, die in den 1950er und 1960er Jahren noch hauptsächlich von Chemiker:

innen und Physiker:innen betrieben wurde und den neuen Lebensbegriff von dem des Organismus abkoppelte ([11], S. 96–97).

Die metaphorische Verknüpfung von molekularen Vervielfältigungs- und Sequenzierungstechniken zu einem imaginären Lesegerät, das wiederum seinen Text als eine archäologische Urschrift zu verstehen erlaubt, gelang den Biochemikern Emile Zuckerkandl und Linus Pauling mit ihrer Publikation „Molecules as documents of evolutionary history“ (1965) [12].[5] Mit linguistischem Rückgriff auf die Schriftmetaphorik des Erbguts (vgl. [3]) zeigen die Autoren, dass man in Typen von Makromolekülen nun *lesen* könne nicht nur wie in einem Buch, sondern wie in Archivdokumenten. Dabei verweisen die Moleküle auf die Organismen, denen sie entnommen wurden; in dem Fall: Bakterien. So rückte sich die Mikrobiologie über das Methodenarsenal der Biochemie in die Nähe einer empiristischen Geisteswissenschaft.[6] Biochemiker sahen sich als „Molekular-Historiker“, im Hintergrund stand die Suche nach dem Baum des Lebens [13]. Nimmt man diesen Ausdruck ernst, dann geht es seitdem um nicht weniger als das Schreiben einer molekular-mikrobiellen *Weltgeschichte*. Denn die Frage nach einem Urahn aller Lebewesen (LUCA – Last Universal Common Ancestor) und seiner Entstehung hat bis heute Konjunktur und wird intensiv erforscht. Dazu gehört eine materialistische Weltvorstellung, die den Planeten mit seinen Elementen, Stoffwechselvorgängen und „Informationen“ als Totalität von Welt deutet wie auch im Anthropozän-Diskurs (kritisch etwa Karafyllis [15]). Diese Weltvorstellung wiederum wirkt auf die Frage der Relevanz von Organismen oder ganzen biologischen Reichen aufmerksamkeitsökonomisch zurück. Im Zeitungsartikel „Planet of the Bacteria“ von 1996 beschwor der durch die rasanten Fortschritte der molekularbiologisch arbeitenden Mikrobiologie inspirierte Paläontologe und Wissenschaftshistoriker Stephen Jay Gould (1941–2002) ein neues Zeitalter: ein Bakterien-Zeitalter gegen das naive wie kurzlebige „Age of Man“:

> We live now in the ‘Age of Bacteria.‘ Our planet has always been in the ‘Age of Bacteria,’ ever since the first fossils—bacteria, of course—were entombed in rocks more than 3 billion years ago. On any possible, reasonable or fair criterion, bacteria are—and always have been—the dominant forms of life on Earth. [16]

Das Bakterium ist sowohl epochemachend wie epochenvernichtend (gemeint sind die Eubacteria und das separate Reich der Archaea), denn sie waren fast immer „da“, wobei dieses Dasein im Modus der Rekonstruktion behauptet wird. Diese Sicht ist diametral entgegengesetzt zu der mit dem Wort „Anthropozän“ adressierten. Gemeint ist die bislang nicht offiziell als solche anerkannte Erdepoche mit dem erst sehr kurzen Auftreten der Hominiden, die sich aber – und das ist für den Erfolg des Begriffs ent-

5 Die Publikation wurde bereits 1963 angefertigt und erschien zuerst auf Russisch. Weitere Hintergründe bei Sapp [13].

6 Weiterführend in naturphilosophisch-mikrobiologischer Hinsicht Karafyllis [14].

scheidend – Möglichkeiten erschlossen, den ganzen Planeten zu besiedeln; und diese in wenigen Jahrhunderten wieder verschlossen, wie es scheint (Stichwort: anthropogener Klimawandel). Das „Age of Bacteria" mit seinen über 3 Mrd. Jahren Bewährung scheint hingegen ein Garant von immer neuen Möglichkeiten des Lebens zu sein.

Max Black klassifizierte drei Typen von Erklärungsmodellen zur Funktionsweise der Metapher, die er Substitutions-, Vergleichs- und Interaktionstheorie nannte [17]. Dahinter stehen unterschiedliche Vorstellungen der Relation von Sprache und Sprechhandeln, aber auch von Sprache und Begriffsbildung. Für die Funktion der Metapher in den Wissenschaften ist die *Interaktionstheorie* besonders relevant. Hier wird die Metapher nicht als wörtlicher Lückenfüller gesehen, sondern die beiden von einer Metapher angesprochenen Gebiete stehen in einem gegenseitigen Zusammenhang. Sie wirken so zusammen, dass eine neue Bedeutung als Resultat dieser Interaktion entsteht (Black erklärt die Interaktion am Beispiel des Satzes „Der Mensch ist ein Wolf"). Man könnte hier ergänzen, dass wenn Menschen jüngst über ihre Identität sprechen möchten, sie auch sagen: „Es ist Teil meiner DNA" oder kurz „es ist in meiner DNA". Kann man also *in* der DNA sein oder gar als DNA *sein*? Die DNA ist doch in einer Zelle. Selbst wenn wir uns als aggregierte Zellhaufen inklusive DNA verstehen würden, braucht es mehrere emergente Phänomene – v. a. Leib und Seele – um an das Konzept der Persönlichkeit aufzuschließen. Umgekehrt, also *top down* verstanden, zitiert der identitäre Hinweis auf die eigene DNA forensische Methoden aus entsprechenden Filmen; der Bedeutungshintergrund bestünde aus Straftat, Schuld und Überführung. Dem Kontext von Entstehung und Verwendung der Metapher kommt generell besondere Bedeutung zu, so auch hier bezüglich der Schriftlichkeit. Erinnert werden muss an die frühe Unstimmigkeit zwischen Code und Buch (der Natur). Die Metaphorik des Codes und der Schrift lässt an sich keine räumliche Deutung (Zelle, Körper/Leib) zu, wohl aber die Kompilation von Schriften in Form eines Buches und dessen Versammlung in einer Bibliothek.

Die Metapher ist mit Jörg Zimmer eine genuin dialektische Denkform, weil sie als Interaktion die übergreifende Einheit von Identität und Nicht-Identität als solche in sich zum Ausdruck bringen kann ([18], S. 7). Die Metapher wirkt interaktiv so, dass sie uns etwas durch den *Filter* von etwas anderem sehen lässt. So werden bestimmte Aspekte hervorgehoben, andere vernachlässigt, und die einzelnen Aspekte werden strukturell neu organisiert. Die Stimmigkeit und Treffsicherheit der Metapher bleibt als hermeneutisches Problem in Bezug auf ihren eigenen Realismus begründungsbedürftig ([18], S. 44).[7] Dies gilt umso mehr, wenn man die Biologie selbst als hermeneutische Wissenschaft begreift, die zum Verstehen des Lebens forscht und arbeitet. In dieser Hinsicht spielen sog. lebende Metaphern (im Gegensatz zu „toten") eine besondere Rolle, weil sie durch die offensichtliche Nicht-Identität der Bedeutung verstören

7 Die Passagen zur Metapherntheorie nach Black und Zimmer habe ich erstmals in meiner philosophischen Habilitationsschrift *Die Phänomenologie des Wachstums*, Universität Stuttgart, 2006, verwendet.

und in ihrer Unstimmigkeit ein kreatives Potenzial haben, durch das Wissenschaften voranschreiten können. Die naturwissenschaftlich ausgebildete Metaphern-Forscherin und Philosophin Evelyn Fox Keller fasst dies folgendermaßen:

> Indeed, the essence of a live metaphor is precisely the juxtaposition of similarity and difference, the manifest untruth of equating source and target. And what gives it its value in the logic of scientific discovery is precisely the instability it generates by virtue of its insistence on both similarity *and* difference, its insistence that, at one and the same time, man both *is* and *is not* a wolf. Lose this duality, and one loses the vitality of the metaphor. ([19], S. 250).

2.4 Verkürzungen

Beim biotechnologischen Lesen gibt es vier wesentliche Arten von Verkürzungen, die für die weitere Theorieentwicklung relevant sind. Im Gegensatz zu den für die Metapher typischen Unstimmigkeiten werden Reduktionismen als zwar pragmatisch dienlich, aber nicht als produktiv angesehen. Die ersten drei Reduktionismen sind aus der biophilosophischen und STS-Literatur gut bekannt. Sie werden zusammen mit einem vierten, um den es nachfolgend verstärkt gehen soll (infrastruktureller Reduktionismus), von mir hier mit je eigenen Differenzbezeichnungen benannt:

1. Die DNA wird als Code, der Code als Text, das Lesen als Decodieren von Informationen unterkomplex verstanden (s. o., enge Verbindung von Molekularbiologie zur frühen Kybernetik, vgl. [3]) (*semantischer Reduktionismus*).
2. Das Lebende wird durch Totes erklärt, was einen Reduktionismus der Genese und Teleologie hin auf den Organismus beschreibt (vgl. [20]). Es scheint dann so, als sei die DNA selbst der Organismus ([4], [19]). Auf das Phänomen „Leben“ bezogen handelt es sich um einen eliminativen Reduktionismus (*metaphysischer Reduktionismus*).
3. Dadurch ist der Schritt vom molekularbiologischen Analysieren zum bioinformatisch gestützten, gentechnischen Synthetisieren in greifbare Nähe gerückt, entsprechend auch die Vorstellung, die Leserichtung durch *reverse engineering* umzudrehen und den genetischen Code nun selbst schreiben zu können (von DNAread zu DNAwrite, vgl. [2], S. 398 mit Hinweis auf Hans Jonas) (*technischer Reduktionismus*).[8]
4. Die DNA lebt nur in Form eines Organismus, Gene stehen nicht als solche kontext- und medienfrei zur Verfügung. Die entsprechenden Organismen müssen in Biobanken gesammelt werden, um technisch zur Verfügung zu stehen (*infrastruktureller Reduktionismus*). Denn Lebendiges kann bislang nicht aus Totem erzeugt werden, sondern bedarf lebender Zellen als Voraussetzung.

8 Genaugenommen handelt es sich hier nicht um einen Reduktionismus, sondern um einen Metapherntransfer von der Lesbarkeit der Schrift zur Rechenbarkeit der Zahl (vgl. für die biochemischemolekularbiologische Modernisierung der Mikrobiologie die Fallstudie von Waszynski und Karafyllis [21]).

2.5 Das Sammeln als tote Metapher des Lesens (*Infrastruktureller Reduktionismus*)

Für Laien stellt sich meist nicht die Frage, woher diejenigen Gene zuletzt kommen, die gentechnisch verwendet werden. Denn in öffentlichen Gentechnikdebatten, in denen es um Biofakte ([22], [23]) geht, fokussiert man die Übertragung von Genen einer bestimmten Spezies auf andere, und der Speziesübergriff wird oft nach Maßgabe von Natürlichkeitsargumenten debattiert [15]. Dass bei derartigen biotechnologischen Praktiken stabilisierende Zwischenschritte der Technizität und Medialität von Erbgut und Zellen (Gewinnung, Auslese, Reinigung, Bevorratung, Kühlung u. a.) generell notwendig sind, ist erst durch die In vitro-Fertilisation zu breiterem Alltagswissen geworden. In diesem breiten Verständnis von „Same“, wie es sich schon bei Aristoteles im altgriechischen Wort *sperma* zeigt, ist der pflanzliche Same, der mit dem feuchten Boden zusammen keimfähig ist, die Ursprungsbedeutung der Metapher (die Samenbank als Spermatozoenbank ist der Saatgutbank nachgeordnet). Modern gesprochen handelt es sich beim pflanzlichen Samen mit fester Samenschale wie bei Linsen und Getreide um eine gut lagerungsfähige Form von Keimplasma, im Gegensatz zu Zwiebeln, Knollen oder einzelnen Geweben und Zellen (letzteres bei Mikroalgen und Bakterien). In all diesen Formen von Reproduktionseinheiten werden Gene im Medium ihrer potenziellen Manifestation („Keimplasma“; engl. *germplasm*) gespeichert. Der Same ist dabei mehr als seine DNA oder sein Genom. Er ist ein Embryo, der sich zweier Eltern verdankt und, wenn in die richtigen Medien gepflanzt, bereit, sein Genom auch phänomenal in Erscheinung zu bringen (vgl. ausführlich Karafyllis [24], dort auch mit weiterführender Literatur zu Samenbanken).

Gene sind Teile von Organismen und diese bestehen aus mindestens einer Zelle. Wer also mit Genen biotechnologisch arbeiten will, muss über sie verfügen können und das bedeutet, sie müssen in Biobanken in geeigneter Form langlebig vorgehalten werden. Dies ist sehr personal- und kostenaufwändig. Dabei leben die entstehenden Miniaturorganismen im Zustand der Latenz; bei gesammelten Pflanzensamen provoziert man künstlich durch teilweisen Wasserentzug und starke Kühlung die Samenruhe, eine Art Schlafzustand (Dormanz). In die Polarität von lebend/tot, die Epistemolog:inn:en als Kennzeichen der Molekularbiologie ansehen, wird ein Zwischenstadium eingeführt. Es ist kein Untoter oder Zombie, der nicht sterben darf, sondern ein Unlebender, der noch nicht leben darf. Samenbanken erleichtern und beschleunigen den Flow zwischen saatgutverarbeitenden und -erforschenden Betrieben („Züchtern“), Prüfbehörden (z. B. das Bundessortenamt) und Wissenschaftsinstitutionen. Gleichzeitig minimieren sie die Interaktion der Samen mit all denjenigen Lebewesen, die zu ihrer natürlichen oder künstlichen Formung und Verbreitung beigetragen haben, darunter auch Tiere. Anders ausgedrückt: Moderne Samenbanken dekontextualisieren den Samen von seinen Geschichten, verhelfen zur Vergabe von Eigentums- und Patentrechten und der Transformation in digitale Einheiten. Gleichzeitig sichern sie die genetischen Informationen bedrohter Sorten, Varietäten und Arten. Ein zukünftiges Aufwachsen können sie nicht garantieren, weder evolutionsbiologisch, noch ökologisch, noch politisch.

Das (sortierende) Sammeln verdankt sich seinerseits einer Metaphernübertragung aus dem Bereich des (Aus-)Lesens, wie die Wörter Sortenlese und Weinlese noch heute bezeugen. Hier wird der einsammelnde, aneignende und verwertbare Aspekt des Sammelns betont. Intentional handelt es sich um eine Verschiebung der sofortigen Triebbefriedigung des Aufessens bzw. -trinkens, weil die Lagerung für einen späteren Zeitpunkt – normalerweise die Aussaat in der nächsten Vegetationsperiode – vorgesehen ist. Das Lesen bedeutet also neben der eingangs festgestellten Fähigkeit zum Perspektivenwechsel eine Zähmung des Appetits. In dieser Hinsicht hat das Lesen als Sammeln in seiner Wechselwirkung mit dem Sammeln als Lesen (in Genombibliotheken, s. u.) eine besonders kreative Form der Unbestimmtheit erreicht (s. nachfolgendes Unterkapitel).

Eine der einfacheren Varianten ist die sog. *Genom-Bibliothek*, die das Genom eines Organismus in viele tausend Fragmente enzymatisch zerlegt und bestimmte Bakteriophagen sowohl als Speicher wie später auch als Vektor nutzt. Hans Blumenberg hob die entsprechende Dynamik der medialen Erzeugungen und Stabilisierungen im mikroskopischen Bereich hervor, der ähnlich wie der makroskopische sich ihm als ein Kampf um den besseren Wirt oder Nährboden darstellt: „auch Mikrobe und Virus haben das Recht auf ‚Befall' dessen, was für sie doch ‚Medium' ihres Lebens, der jeweils bessere Wirt ist, zu dem alles wandert, was wandern kann" (so Blumenberg [25], S. 95). Hat also schon das Virus eine infrastrukturelle Doppelfunktion, indem es Speichermittel und Transportmittel ist, so gilt dies umso mehr für seine Heimatinstitution, die Genombibliothek. Sie gehört zu den Biobanken, womit das Metaphernfeld der Bank und der Bibliothek interagieren. Beiden ist sowohl die Bestandserhaltung im Depot bzw. Magazin als auch die Mobilität der Objekte eigen. Dabei handelt es sich nur bei der Bibliothek (noch) um materielle Objekte (Bücher); in Banken wird immer weniger materielles Geld bewegt, sondern seine Wertzuschreibung auf Konten.

Das Sammeln von Samen ist die ältere Kulturtechnik. Dazu gehört das Anlegen lokaler Samenbanken in Dörfern und landwirtschaftlichen Stationen. So konnten sog. Landsorten bewahrt werden, die von Kleinbauern gezüchtet wurden; oft von Indigenen. Mit dem Aufkommen der Genetik entstanden um 1900 moderne nationale Saatgutbanken (zunächst die unter der Leitung von Nikolai Vavilov in St. Petersburg), die darauf abzielten, möglichst viele Sorten einer Kulturpflanze zu bevorraten. Sie sammelten ab und sie sammelten ein, von indigenen Völkern wie von Botanischen Gärten. Das Ziel war und ist die Züchtung von Elitesorten mit hochfunktionalen Merkmalen und dafür braucht es den Erhalt von Agrobiodiversität. Heute werden neben den Hochzuchtsorten und Landsorten auch Wildformen mitgesammelt (sog. *crop wild relatives*), um den Genpool einer Art möglichst komplett als Bestand vorliegen zu haben

(„core collection“).[9] Dahinter finden wir die Vorstellung einer Universalbibliothek, wie sie auch Leibniz vorschwebte (s. u.).

Sammlungsinstitutionen haben demnach etwas mit dem Lesen zu tun. Sie beherbergen Organismen als *Bestände* und halten sie für die Biotechnologie vor. Das bestandserhaltende Sammeln strebt Vollständigkeit an, weil züchterisch die Gesamtheit aller genetisch sich bereits verwirklichter Möglichkeiten (= der Genpool) interessant ist. Gegen diesen Hintergrund gelesen, ist die angeblich tote Metapher des Samensammelns für das Lesen möglicherweise doch sehr lebendig, weil sie produktive Unstimmigkeiten erzeugt.

2.6 Eine Lesbarkeit der biologischen Welt? (Eingedenk Hans Blumenberg)

Hans Blumenberg macht in seinem Klassiker *Die Lesbarkeit der Welt* (1981) auf zahlreiche Sinnbrüche in der jahrhundertelangen Metapherngeschichte der Lesbarkeit aufmerksam,[10] von denen hier nur wenige Berücksichtigung finden können und auch nur dann, wenn sie biotechnologisch relevant sind. Dazu gehören im Minimum folgende Unstimmigkeiten:

- Die Geschlossenheit des Buches (kanonischer Texte) versus die Offenheit der Welt.
- Das Buch, in dem schon alles geschrieben steht versus das Buch, in dem noch nichts geschrieben steht, also ein Buch mit leeren Seiten.
- Das Lesen als Wunsch des Lesers nach einer sinnstiftenden Intimität mit dem Autor.

Zum ersten Punkt. Die legitimatorische Geschlossenheit des Buches mit einem kanonischen Text wie der Bibel oder dem Quran steht in eigentümlichem Widerspruch zu einer offenen, evolvierenden Welt, wie sie ab etwa 1800 vorstellbar wurde. Mit Blick auf die Textmetapher des genetischen Codes hebt diese mit ihrem dogmatischen Anspruch aber letztlich „auf das alte Buch der Natur als den von Gott mit sakrosankter Endgültigkeit niedergeschriebenen Text der Schöpfung“ ab ([2], S. 398). Hier ergibt sich eine produktive Unstimmigkeit dahingehend, den genetischen Code nicht mehr eineindeutig zu denken, sondern als dynamisch mit dem Evolutionsgeschehen verwoben – die Umwelt gibt den Interpretationsrahmen vor, in dem sinnvoll gelesen wer-

9 Im Falle von Bakterien gestaltet sich die Situation anders, weil die meisten Bakterien ohnehin „wild“ vorkommen (von gezüchteten Hefestämmen, Lactobacillen u. a. abgesehen), wenn auch mit hohen, kaum zu beziffernden Biodiversitätsverlusten aufgrund der Umweltdegradation und -verschmutzung.

10 Weiterführend jüngst Waszynski [26].

den kann (EvoDevo). Darüber hinaus wäre in der Zukunft eine Brücke zur Quantenphysik zu schlagen.[11]

Zum zweiten Punkt: Das Buch, in dem alles schon geschrieben steht und in dem man nur noch nachlesen muss, was die Welt im Innersten zusammenhält, ist ein alter Traum. Er ist eng verbunden mit der Enzyklopädistenbewegung im 18. Jahrhundert und schon zuvor mit der Idee der Universalbibliothek bei G. W. Leibniz. Biobanken bilden zusammen mit Ganzheitsmetaphern wie der der universellen Lesbarkeit einen ideell und materiell vorstellbaren Zugriff auf das Ganze der Welt [24]. Dahinter kommt ein Naturideal der romantischen Naturphilosophie zum Tragen [27]. In der Ganzheit der Welt mit ihren einzelnen Bestandteilen, die immer wieder neu kombiniert werden können, sind auch die Potenziale in mathematischer Hinsicht endlich. Das Wissen um mögliche zukünftige Welten ist prinzipiell vorhanden, weil es durch eine mathematische Kombination an endlichen Möglichkeiten theoretisch gegeben ist im Sinne einer *mathesis universalis* (weiterführend [28]). Der Anspruch auf eine Vollständigkeit der Welt findet sich auch wieder als Vollzähligkeit, weil der Wunsch nach Anschaulichkeit nicht selten in Methoden der Prognostik und Berechenbarkeit überführt wird. Hier ergibt sich eine Unstimmigkeit zwischen der Lesbarkeits- und der Berechenbarkeitsmetaphorik. Weil Enzyklopädien nie abgeschlossen sind (denn sie können sich nicht selbst enthalten), wäre hier selbst bei theoretisch vollständiger Sequenzierung aller existierenden Genome auf diesem Planeten die Möglichkeit zur technischen Erweiterung und Neukombination immer noch gegeben. Die Metapher der Enzyklopädie ist technologieoffen, die des Buchs ist es nur eingeschränkt. Umgekehrt ist die Vorstellung, dass es ein Buch mit leeren Seiten gibt, nur schwer mit dem Schöpfungsgedanken und dem Buch der Natur zu verbinden.[12] Statt der Phylogenese käme hier die Ontogenese zum Zuge, die das Individuumsproblem in der Biologie adressiert. In der Bibliothek befänden sich dann immer auch Bücher mit leeren Seiten, die zum Teil selbst beschrieben werden müssen. Die Bibliothek würde so als Milieu bzw. Umwelt für Bücher verstanden [30]. Im Lesesaal jener Universalbibliothek sitzt ein Leser, der nicht nur durch seine Augen- und Handbewegungen liest, sondern der durch seine gesamte Physis atmend anwesend ist beim Lesen [31] als einem sinnstiftenden Akt des Lebens. Das Buch mit leeren Seiten kann gegen die Utopie der Synthetischen Biologie als einer *creatio ex nihilo* als mediale Schranke verstanden werden, so wie es die erste Zelle mit Keimplasma und Organellen ist, die zuhanden sein muss, bevor aus ihr ein technisch zugerichtetes, neues Lebewesen entstehen kann (vgl. [32], [33]). Blumenberg war der Ansicht, dass die „Metapher der Versprachli-

---

11 Blumenberg betont nicht umsonst im letzten Unterkapitel „Der genetische Code und seine Leser", wie wichtig die Grammatikunterstellung des Erbguts für den Physiker Erwin Schrödinger und nachfolgend auch für den Chemiker Erwin Chargaff war.

12 Eine besondere Rolle spielen für die Differenzierungsarbeit auch unter Machtgesichtspunkten die Benennungspraxen, wie Waszynski [29] hervorhebt.

chung" „ganz einem gegen das Ideal wissenschaftlicher Objektivierung gerichteten Konzept von ‚Sein'" dient ([2], S. 21).

Zum Dritten kommen wir auf die Appetitzügelung zurück, die beim Sammeln und Auslesen eine Hemmung der Begierde erfordert, um die Kontinuitätsbedingungen von Züchtung zu sichern. Blumenberg [2] sieht in dem altbekannten Verlangen nach der Lesbarkeit der Welt einen „Inbegriff des Sinnverlangens an die Realität". Sie soll das Wahrnehmbare und das exakt Prognostizierbare überbieten, d. h. an Sinn sogar mehr bieten als die „Robinson-Welt" der sinnlichen Erfahrung und die „Newton-Welt" der mathematischen Berechnung zusammen. Es geht um nicht weniger als deren willentliche Voraussetzung, dass die Welt prinzipiell sinnstiftend ist – eine Welt, die nicht erst technisch beherrscht werden muss, um verfügbar zu sein:

> Der Wunsch, die Welt möge sich in anderer Weise als der der bloßen Wahrnehmung und sogar der exakten Vorhersagbarkeit ihrer Erscheinungen zugänglich erweisen: im Aggregatzustand der ‚Lesbarkeit' als ein Ganzes von Natur, Leben und Geschichte sinnspendend sich erschließen, [...] [ist] Inbegriff des Sinnverlangens an die Realität, gerichtet auf ihre vollkommenste und nicht mehr gewaltsame Verfügbarkeit. Darin läßt er sich nur dem einen Wunsch nach unmittelbarer Intimität vergleichen, der Gott selbst möge sich als eßbar erweisen, so daß zugleich von ihm nichts bliebe und er doch ganz einverleibt würde: die Inkarnation als Ritual (so Blumenberg [2], S. 10).

Zuletzt bleibt die Frage, wie konservativ die Metapher der Lesbarkeit ist und dabei muss man nicht unbedingt an ein religiöses Sündenregister denken. Zumindest schwingt in der Metaphorik eine Nostalgie des Buches und der klassischen Bibliotheken mit, die ihrerseits durch die Digitalisierung im Umbruch begriffen sind. Das passt in die Zeit, denn zur Vermarktung der Buchkultur im digitalen Zeitalter wird ein „Retro-Charme" des Buches in Anschlag gebracht, indem der „uralte Ruhe- und Langsamkeitsdiskurs mit einem nicht minder alten Seelendiskurs verknüpft wird" ([34], S. 9). Die Lesbarkeit der Welt, so scheint es, findet trotz aller Unterstützungstechnologien gemütlich statt. Durch maschinelles Lernen wird der Leser sich wohl auch immer häufiger als Autor im Internet ‚wiederlesen' (Stichwort: Seelendiskurs), wenn auch ohne Entlohnung. Echte Bücher aber sind mehr als Texte. Sie können nicht nur inhaltlich beunruhigen, wie Sascha Michel feststellt (ebd.), oder gar süchtig machen; sondern sie können mit ihrem Papier, Klebstoff, Wachsbezug und vielem mehr als Medium und Habitat für Mikroben dienen [30]. Langfristig hilft dagegen kein Konservator. Die Ewigkeit der Schrift bleibt ein frommer Traum, aus dem sich die Digitalisierung speist. Die „Leseratte" und der „Bücherwurm" schaffen als Tierchen dasjenige, was der metaphorisch gemeinte Mensch gerne hätte: sich die Göttlichkeit der Schrift einzuverleiben und eine vordergründige Identität zwischen Natur und Geschichte herzustellen.

Literatur

[1] Kaminski A. Technik als Erwartung. Grundzüge einer allgemeinen Technikphilosophie. Bielefeld: transcript, 2010.
[2] Blumenberg H. Die Lesbarkeit der Welt. Frankfurt/M.: Suhrkamp 1981.
[3] Kay LE. Who wrote the Book of Life? A History of the Genetic Code. Berkeley, CA: Stanford University Press, 2000.
[4] Fox Keller E. The Century of the Gene. Cambridge, Mass.: Harvard University Press, 2000.
[5] Achtermeier D, Kosch L (Hg.). Mythen des Lesens. Über eine Kulturtechnik in Zeiten gesellschaftlichen Wandels. Bielefeld: transcript, 2024.
[6] Sontag S. AIDS und seine Metaphern. München, Wien, 1989.
[7] Otis L. Membranes. Metaphors of Invasion in nineteenth-century Literature, Science, and Politics. Baltimore: Johns Hopkins University Press, 2000.
[8] Pennisi E. ENCODE Project Writes Eulogy for Junk DNA. Science 2012,337,1159–61.
[9] McLeish T. A Meta-Metaphor for Science: The True and the Fictional within the Book of Nature. Interdisciplinary Science Reviews 2020,45(3),406–15.
[10] Benjamin W. Über das mimetische Vermögen [1933]. Gesammelte Schriften, Bd. II,1, Frankfurt/M.: Suhrkamp 1977, 210–13.
[11] Fox Keller E. Secrets of Life – Secrets of Death. Essays on Language, Gender and Science. London, New York: Routledge, 1992.
[12] Zuckerkandl E, Pauling L. Molecules as documents of evolutionary history. Journal of Theoretical Biology 1965,8(2),357–66.
[13] Sapp J. The new foundations of evolution: on the tree of life. Oxford, New York: Oxford University Press, 2009.
[14] Karafyllis NC. Mikroben als widerständige Objekte an und für sich. P Breil, A Kronberger (Hg.): Eigensinnige Objekte. Virtuelle Möglichkeitsräume zwischen Aufforderung und Entzug. Bielefeld: transcript 2025,309–29.
[15] Karafyllis NC. Wesentlich nicht-unnatürlich. Grundlagen biofaktischen Denkens. Kursbuch Nr. 218: Von Natur aus. Hg. von Armin Nassehi, Juni 2024,61–76.
[16] Gould SJ. Planet of the Bacteria. Washington Post Horizon, 1996,119(344),H1.
[17] Black M. Models and Metaphors: Studies in Language and Philosophy. Ithaca, NY: Cornell University Press, 1962.
[18] Zimmer J. Metapher. Bielefeld: transcript, 1999.
[19] Fox Keller E. Cognitive Functions of Metaphor in the Natural Sciences. Interdisciplinary Science Reviews 2020,45(3),249–67.
[20] Karafyllis NC. Biologisch, natürlich, nachhaltig. Philosophische Aspekte des Naturzugangs im 21. Jahrhundert. Tübingen: Francke, 2001.
[21] Karafyllis NC, Waszynski A. Das ganze Spektrum. Die Frühgeschichte der Deutschen Sammlung von Mikroorganismen (DSM). Acta Historica Leopoldina 2021,80,87–117.
[22] Karafyllis NC (Hg.). Biofakte. Versuch über den Menschen zwischen Artefakt und Lebewesen. Paderborn: mentis, 2003.
[23] Hauskeller M. Biotechnology and the Integrity of Life: Taking Public Fears Seriously. New York, 2016.
[24] Karafyllis NC. Die Samenbank als Paradigma einer Theorie der modernen Lebendsammlung. Dies. (Hg.): Theorien der Lebendsammlung. Pflanzen, Mikroben und Tiere als Biofakte in Genbanken, Freiburg: Karl Alber 2018,39–136.
[25] Blumenberg H. Der Untergang der Welt am Leben. In ders.: Die Vollzähligkeit der Sterne. Frankfurt a. M.: Suhrkamp, 2000,92–97.
[26] Waszynski A. Lesbarkeit nach Hans Blumenberg. Berlin, Boston: de Gruyter, 2021.

[27] Köchy K. Ganzheit und Wissenschaft. Das historische Fallbeispiel der romantischen Naturforschung. Würzburg: Königshausen & Neumann, 1997.
[28] Kirchhoff T, Karafyllis NC, Evers D et al. (Hg.): Naturphilosophie. Ein Lehr- und Studienbuch. Tübingen: Mohr-Siebeck, ^{2}2020.
[29] Waszynski A. Macht des Benennens. Mikroben als sprachliche Objekte in Sammlungskontexten. B Lindner-Bornemann, S Kürschner (Hg.): Die Sprache wissenschaftlicher Objekte. Interdisziplinäre Perspektiven auf die materielle Kultur in den Wissenschaften. Berlin, Boston: de Gruyter, 2024,205–36.
[30] Karafyllis NC, Waszynski A, Lammers U. Mikroben-Welten. NC Karafyllis, J Overmann, UJ Schneider (Hg.): Die kontaminierte Bibliothek. Mikroben in der Buchkultur. Leipzig: Leipziger Universitätsverlag, 2021,12–31.
[31] Schneider UJ. Atmen beim Lesen. Bibliotheken im Industriezeitalter. Wien: Turia+Kant, 2024.
[32] Köchy K. Lebensbegriffe in den Handlungskontexten der Synthetischen Biologie. Jahrbuch für Wissenschaft und Ethik 2014,18(1),133–72.
[33] Waszynski A, Karafyllis NC. Re-Collecting Microbes with Hans Blumenberg's Concept of Reoccupation (»Umbesetzung«): from Isolating/Cultivating towards Digitizing/Synthesizing. Zeitschrift für Medien- und Kulturforschung 2020,11(1),95–116.
[34] Michel S. Die Unruhe der Bücher. Vom Lesen und was es mit uns macht. Stuttgart: Reclam, 2020.

Hans G. Ulrich

3 Metaphern – Ein Kapitel zur Forschungsethik

Das Folgende ist – unter diesem Titel – ein Teilstück aus einer etwa zehnjährigen gemeinsamen Arbeit zwischen Walter Doerfler, einem Molekularbiologen und Virologen und mir, einem theologischen Ethiker. Es ist ein von mir für diese Konferenz ausgewählter Ausschnitt, der mir geeignet schien, weil er die Arbeit an Metaphern und mit Metaphern in der Molekularbiologie direkt verbindet mit der Arbeit an einer Metaphorologie, die ihrerseits in einen geistesgeschichtlichen Kontext gehört, der für beide, die Molekularbiologie und die Theologie von zentraler und brisanter Bedeutung ist. Enden werde ich freilich erst einmal nur mit einer Frage, die zu weiterer Arbeit einladen soll.

Der Bezug auf Metaphern hat sich im Laufe unseres Unternehmens, das zunächst experimentell auf ein noch zu findendes Ziel hin gestartet war, ergeben auf dem Hintergrund der damals (in den Jahren von 1980 bis 2000) akuten Diskussion um Gentechnik und um die ethischen Implikationen, die auch die Forschung betreffen mussten. Wenn wir etwas erforschen, dann tun wir etwas, das – weil es ein Tun ist – ethische Reflexion hinsichtlich vieler Fragen impliziert. Es schließt auch die Frage danach ein, ob diese oder jene Forschung dem – sagen wir – "gerecht" wird, was erforscht wird und zugleich dem, was uns Menschen als den Forschenden zukommt, sowohl hinsichtlich dessen, was wir als Forschungsergebnis gewinnen, als auch hinsichtlich der Folgen, die damit verbunden sind, dass es dieses Ergebnis gibt, also sozusagen nun „in der Welt“ ist oder in die Welt „gebracht“ worden ist.

Kurz gesagt: es geht bei diesem Unternehmen um Forschungsethik, und zwar so verstanden, dass wir – der Naturwissenschaftler und der Theologe – damit eine gemeinsame Erkenntnis- und Verstehensaufgabe haben. Wir waren damit auf einer gemeinsamen Linie, auch weil W.D. darauf insistierte, dass Forschung sich ohne Einschränkung, mit vollem Risiko und jeder Art von kritischer Offenheit, immer neu, ruhelos der Frage stellen muss, ob das, was sie findet – gemessen an den gegebenen Methoden, Theorie, Forschungstechniken etc. – zu halten ist, in diesem Sinne also "wahr" ist, und wo die markierbaren Grenzen sind. "Wahrheit" wird hier als methodisch gewonnene Wahrheit verstanden, so ist "Wahrheit und Methode" mitthematisiert und damit ist auch die Frage gestellt, welche Methoden zum Einsatz kommen – auch Methoden der Interpretation und des hermeneutischen Zugangs zu dem, was aufgefunden und irgendwie medial und sprachlich vermittelt wird. Es ist also angezeigt, dass in den Grenzen des methodisch Erfassbaren präsent wird, was wahr ist, aber doch zugleich jede Art von Aufmerksamkeit und Phantasie braucht, die über diese Grenzen beständig hinausgreift und doch – in Sprache – erfasst sein will, wenn es im „Kontext“ des Wissens eingefügt werden soll.

Durch das Präsenthalten des – und jetzt greife ich auf die Diskussion um die Metaphorologie zurück, wie sie durch Hans Blumenberg provoziert worden ist – also des

https://doi.org/10.1515/9783112215685-003

Präsenthaltens des „Unbegrifflichen“, also dessen, was nicht im Begriff erfasst ist oder (definitiv) nicht darin erfasst werden kann (das betrifft unterschiedliche Metaphern, auflösbare und nicht auflösbare, oder in Blumenbergs Unterscheidung einfache und absolute Metaphern – wie z.B. „Welt“, „Geschichte“ und „Leben“)[1],[2]].

Damit also sind wir im Feld der Metaphern – so jedenfalls kann die Disposition hinsichtlich der Wahrheitssuche mit Hans Blumenbergs Arbeit an der Metaphorologie angezeigt werden. Die Forschungsethik – theologische und philosophische – ist selbstverständlich an den darin implizierten erkenntnis- und wahrheitstheoretischen Fragen genuin beteiligt.

Ich schließe hier z.T. an Hans Blumenberg an, nicht um seine Arbeit an der Metaphorologie und seine Philosophie hier direkt zum Gegenstand werden zu lassen, sondern weil seine Arbeit an der Metaphorologie Schlüsselfragen abbilden lässt, die die geistesgeschichtliche Dramatik hervortreten lassen, in der wir uns auch in einem solchen Feld wie der Molekularbiologie bewegen – eine Dramatik, in die die Theologie jedenfalls tief verwickelt ist. Entscheidend ist an Blumenbergs Projekt – um das gleich anzuzeigen –, dass durch Metaphern, die das „Unbegriffliche“ präsenthalten, die technisch vermittelte Erschließung der „Welt“ in die Suche nach der wahren Wirklichkeit einbezogen wird.

„Technisch vermittelt“ – das heißt immer auch „sichtbar“ (wie mit der Metapher „Lesbarkeit“ der Welt verbunden). Das stellte sich in unserem Projekt für die Didaktik so dar, dass Walter Doerfler die mit Hilfe von Metaphern verbalisierten Vorgänge in biochemischer Formelsprache und anderen Zeichnungen an die Tafel skizzierte – so dass immer etwas auf seine Funktionalität hin Abgebildetes vor Augen war, das darauf hinwies, dass es hier (mikroskopisch) Sichtbares gibt, das es gilt zu „erkennen“ und zu „verstehen“.

3.1 Geistesgeschichtliche Disposition

Es geht dann im Besonderen auch um die Differenz und das Zusammenspiel von Erkenntnistheorie (Epistemologie) und Phänomenologie, einfach gesagt um die Frage, inwiefern die Wahrheit von etwas in der „Welt“ (eines Seienden) als “Erscheinung” seiner wahren “Wirklichkeit” (oder seines Wesens) zu fassen ist, und dies nur, wenn mit dem, was wissenschaftlich (methodisch – technisch) „erkannt“ werden kann, zugleich das präsent gehalten wird, das davon nicht „erfasst“ ist.

In dieser Spannung und Unterscheidung bewegen sich die verschiedenen Positionen und Projekte wie Blumenbergs Arbeit an der Metaphorologie, die – auch im Widerspruch gegen Heidegger (der der Wahrnehmung der Sprache als durchgehend metaphorisch folgt) – Wahrheit (diesseits der Metaphysik) nicht im „Erscheinen“ einer wahren Wirklichkeit (oder eines wahren Wesens) entgegen einer wie auch immer, auch mit technischen Mitteln, erfassten „Welt“, sucht, sondern in der Welt der Beschreibung, in der Welt des methodisch Erfassbaren verbleibt, aber zugleich das Unbegriffliche präsent-hält. Dabei sind freilich auch die Metaphern im Blick zu behalten, die hier für die Darlegung der gemeinsamen wissenschaftlichen „Arbeit" gebraucht werden. Jede Beschreibung von wissenschaftlicher Arbeit gebraucht signifikante Metaphern (wie die Metapher „Arbeit" selbst), die diese von verschiedenen Dramatiken – „Entdecken", „Freilegen,", „Erfassen", „Begreifen" etc. – bestimmt sein lassen. Wir bewegen uns so auf mehreren Ebenen, die wir nicht gleichzeitig diskutieren können, aber präsent halten müssen. Wir bewegen uns immer in mehreren metaphorisch artikulierten Feldern (oder „Systematiken" [3]), die freilich nicht gleichzeitig thematisiert werden können.

Wir bewegen uns – so Blumenberg –, um dies schon festzuhalten, immer schon im Horizont dessen, was er "absolute Metaphern" nennt, d.h. im Horizont solcher Metaphern, die präsent halten, was nicht oder niemals in Begriffen erfasst werden kann —wie "Welt" oder "Geschichte" – und so auch „Leben" oder „das Lebendige". Darin sich zu bewegen heißt, sich in einem Horizont zu bewegen, der nie überschritten (oder „weggewischt") werden kann, innerhalb dessen vielmehr Orientierung gewonnen wird – innerhalb dessen Verstehen gebraucht und möglich wird, das sich von Wissen unterscheidet, aber doch auch die Gewinnung von Wissen und die weitere Suche nach Wahrheit antreibt. Die Unterscheidung von „Wissen" und „Verstehen", die hier nicht zu entfalten ist, hat uns bei unserem Experiment immer geleitet – inklusive der biblisch-hebräischen Semantik bzw. Metaphorik, in der „Verstehen" verstanden werden kann als die Kunst des Unterscheidens.

Damit ist – freilich nur andeutungsweise – etwas von der geistesgeschichtlichen Disposition („Drama") angezeigt, in dem sich die Diskussion um die Metaphern bewegt, zumal – wie noch zu entfalten ist – signifikanter Weise oder auch paradigmatisch in der Molekularbiologie. Dies ist bei Blumenberg angezeigt in der Disposition, dass „Kosmos" (das ist die griechische Metapher für „Welt", eine absolute, also nicht auflösbare Metapher) und „Logos" korrelativ sind [4] – in dem Sinn, dass die niemals vollkommen erfasste kosmische Welt sukzessiv durch den „Logos" (auch den technisch vermittelten Logos) erschlossen werden kann – in einem verstehenden Erkennen, das sich je und je durch kosmologische Stimmigkeit als Verstehen ausweist. Die „kosmische Welt" kommt hier in dem Sinne also zur Sprache, als sie die gegebene Welt ist, in der wir uns aufhalten, und zugleich eine Welt ist, die uns als geordnete erscheint und schließlich auch der astronomisch erfasste Kosmos, der etwa durch seine „Strahlung" mit zu erfassen ist.

3.2 Metaphern in der Forschungspraxis

Die Genomforschung hat immenses Wissen über die durch das „Genom" (mit-)gesteuerten „biologischen" Vorgänge gewonnen, in denen sich das heraus"bildet" (alles metaphorisch gesagt), was uns „Menschen“ (so wie wir uns sehen) als Bio-Welt vor Augen kommt. Die Forschung hat damit Wissen über Vorgänge gewonnen, die zur Bildung dessen führen, was uns phänotypisch als „Mensch“ gilt und was – darauf kommen wir noch zu sprechen – zentral und entscheidend selbst zu dem gehört, was unsere Suche nach Erkenntnis und Verstehen ausmacht.

Das Erfassen des Vorgangs dieser “Genese” ist hinsichtlich der Dichte, Reichweite und Eigenart ihrer Komplexität und auch hinsichtlich der Schwierigkeit, Parameter für die Reduktion der Abbildung dieser Komplexität zu finden, nach Maßgabe dessen begrenzt, was die Heuristiken und (technisch vermittelten) Erschließungsmethoden (Datengewinnung und -verarbeitung) hergeben, die selbst in beständiger Weiterentwicklung sind.

„Metaphern“, wie sie hier im Gebrauch sind – wie die schon erwähnte Metapher „Steuerung“ von (biochemischen) Vorgängen – , halten präsent, was in welcher Richtung zu erschließen und was zugleich (noch) nicht erschlossen ist. Metaphern (darauf lenkt Blumenberg den Blick) verweisen (durchweg) auf „Funktionen“ – so „Genom“ auf die „Funktion“ einer strukturierten Generierung von „Genese“, und „Genese“ verweist auf die Funktion von „kontinuierlicher Abfolge“ auf ein „Produkt“, das wiederum auf seine „Funktion“ hin zu fassen ist. Eine „Funktion“ zu erfassen heißt, ein Woraufhin festzuhalten, an das Weiteres anschließen kann und wirklich auch anschließt.

Wenn wir von hier ausgehend diskutieren, welche Metapher wofür steht, mit welchen Implikationen und Folgen, so setzten wir damit voraus, dass zunächst durchaus offen scheint oder auch offen bleibt, welche Metapher wir einsetzen, weil zu prüfen ist, was mit dieser oder jener Metapher gewonnen wird für die weitere Erschließung, und was womöglich nicht, was wir aber erst wahrnehmen, wenn wir eine andere Metapher ausprobieren. Es macht einen weitreichenden Unterschied (so in einem Teil der Diskussion), ob etwa von einem gewissermaßen alles bestimmenden „Programm“ zu reden ist, das mit dem „Genom“ gegeben ist, oder – anders – im Blick auf den ganzen Vorgang der Genese – von einem „System“ des Zusammenwirkens oder einer „systemischen Kommunikation“ in Vorgängen, die nur als Ganzes dann den „Phänotyp“ herausbilden oder in der als Ganzes dieser Phänotyp herausgebildet wird. (Sprache, wie sie in der Diskussion aufzufinden ist.) „Kommunikation“ ist freilich eine sehr weiträumige Metapher, die aber dennoch kaum zu ersetzen ist, will man nicht Verengungen in Kauf nehmen, wie bei der Metapher „Programm“ oder auch beim Verzicht auf die Metapher „System“ [5].

So ist immer die Frage gegeben, wie gut, angemessen und nachvollziehbar die gebrauchten Metaphern, das, was sie in den Blick rücken sollen, wirklich präsent werden lassen, oder auch, ob das, was sie induzieren, diesem Präsentwerden dient oder davon wegführt. Anders gesagt: Die Metaphern haben eine je verschiedene heuristische Zielrichtung und Kraft, auch Suggestionskraft – und werden entsprechend daraufhin auch diskutiert (wie eben die Unterscheidung von genetischem „Programm“, „System“ der Genese, oder systemische „Kommunikation“). Ebenso ist das mit Metaphern angezeigte Erschließungsverfahren je different. Ein „Programm“ ist anders zu „lesen“ als ein „Text“, und ein „System“ zu beobachten ist etwas anderes als einer Kommunikation zu folgen. Auch die Metapher „Text“ (das Genom als „Text“ [6]) verweist auf eine Funktion. Anders als „Programm“, das auf Steuerung verweist, induziert „Text“ eher „Instruktion“ oder auch „Information“, die abgelesen wird. Und „Genom“ selbst verweist metaphorisch auf kontinuierliche „Genese“ und diese wiederum ist unterschieden von „Werden“, dessen Bedeutung völlig unbestimmt bleibt.

Diese Metaphern sind vielfach kritisch gesichtet worden – daraufhin, ob sie das anzeigen oder induzieren, was sich – technisch vermittelt, sichtbar – fassen lässt und erklärungskräftig bleibt, nicht nur heuristisch stimulierend. Dabei hat sich auch die Resistenz bestimmter Metaphern gezeigt, und zwar als wirklich bewährte Resistenz, wie vor allem die Metaphorik eines „skriptural“ verfassten systemisch kommunikativen Vorgangs. Dieser ist – so bestimmt – mit der Metapher „Text“ nicht zu erfassen, denn es geht um einen skripturalen Vorgang, in dem das Geschriebene selbst das ist, was schließlich in einem Produkt (wie ein 3D-Druck) realisiert wird.

Die kritische Arbeit an der Metaphorik ist etwa an der Leitmetapher „Buch des Lebens“ geleistet worden, durchaus, um sie in ihrer Brauchbarkeit oder ihrer bislang gegebenen Unersetzlichkeit zu bestätigen (Lily E. Kay [7]), so auch mit Blumenbergs Projekt und seiner Arbeit an der Metapher „Lesbarkeit der Welt“ [8]. Mit der Metapher der „Lesbarkeit“ ist eine Funktion angezeigt, mit der wir Menschen einen bestimmten, uns Menschen entsprechenden – auch technisch vermittelten – Zugang zu der „Welt“ gewinnen und sie in ihrer Ordnung erschließen und verstehen können. Wir bewegen uns damit (wie schon erwähnt) in der (womöglich doch gegebenen) Korrelation von Kosmos und Logos – also jener antiken Disposition der Wahrheitssuche.

Blumenberg hat – wie schon gesagt – von einigen Leitwörtern, die wir – wie die Metapher „Welt“ – beständig gebrauchen, als von „absoluten Metaphern“ gesprochen. Metaphern zeigen Funktionen an und bewähren sich darin, dass sie diese präsent halten. Die absoluten Metaphern halten präsent, was unbegrifflich ist, also nicht durch Begriffe eingeholt werden kann, aber doch mit-präsent gehalten werden muss, wenn nicht Erkenntnis, die darauf wartet, gewonnen zu werden, verloren gehen soll und mit ihr mögliches Verstehen. In dieser Hinsicht ist die Theologie nicht weniger gefordert, an der Metaphorologie zu arbeiten – zumal ihr Metaphern – im Vorgang der Überlieferung – ausdrücklich sozusagen aufgegeben sind – wie auch die Metapher „Welt“. Immer ist zu fragen, wie weit diese so ausdrücklich aufgegebenen Metaphern mit denen von der Philosophie erfassten, wie auch immer ausdrücklich gegeben, übereinstimmen. Wie ist es mit der Metapher „Leben“?

„Leben“ ist – wie „Welt“ und „Geschichte“ – eine absolute Metapher, die bei allem wissenschaftlichen (methodischen) Erfassen präsent hält, was in seiner ganzen unverkürzten möglicherweise Schritt für Schritt offenkundig werdenden Bedeutung zu erfassen und zu verstehen ist.

„Leben“ ist freilich bezogen auf den Menschen beides zugleich: das physische Leben und das von ihm gelebte Leben: bios und zoe.[9] So ist in der Bibel, im „Buch der Offenbarung des Johannes" vom „Buch des Lebens" (ἐν τῇ βίβλῳ τῆς ζωῆς) gesagt, dass darin die Namen derer geschrieben sind, die nach „ihren Werken gerichtet" werden. Das „Buch des Lebens" ist ein Geschichtsbuch, in dem Gott liest, kein Buch, das – wie es dann auch kritisch verhandelt wird (Lily E. Kay) – das Werden lebender Wesen in ihrer Spezifität beschreibt (durchaus auch in der Einheit von zoe und bios), das wir auf diese Weise gewärtigen können. Damit ist die Metapher in eine andere Dramatik versetzt, denn dieses Buch ist nicht uns zum Lesen gegeben. Aber sie provoziert die Wahrnehmung von uns Menschen, als solchen (paradigmatischen) Lebewesen, deren „Leben" aufgeschrieben ist.

Die Metapher wie sie in der Diskussion um die Molekularbiologie gebraucht worden ist, verweist nun auf uns Menschen (das meint die Funktion der „Sichtbarkeit" und der „Lesbarkeit"), die wir dieses „Buch" vor Augen bekommen oder auch zum Lesen aufgegeben bekommen. Die Frage ist damit gegeben, was uns damit wie mit welcher Beteiligung oder/und Funktion als Leser vor Augen kommt – das heißt – und zugleich – dass uns vor Augen kommt, wie in dem Buch die darin verzeichneten „Elemente" („Buchstaben" oder was immer) wodurch miteinander (in den Zellen) kommunizieren, und dies (bestimmten Rekonstruktionen entsprechend) bei gleichzeitigem Schreiben oder Fortschreiben.

Die Metapher eines skripturalen und (in sich) kommunikativen Ganzen (oder auch „Systems"), das den Vorgang der Genese eines spezifischen Lebewesens darstellt und zugleich (weil material vermittelt) vollzieht, legt sich offenbar dadurch wirklich nahe, dass durch das Sichtbarwerden der Struktur von „Elementen", die in ihrer Funktion als (gleichwohl sehr verschiedene Elemente) einer Kommunikation zu fassen sind, – etwa auch als „Information", die von Empfängern aufgenommen und verarbeitet wird, die dann weitere „Informationen" generieren und darin materialiter die zusammenhängenden Elemente entstehen lassen, und schließlich lebendige „Organismen" bilden.

Nun ist eine solche skizzenhaft verbalisierte Kennzeichnung voller weiterer Metaphern (wie „Information" oder auch „Instruktion"), die dann ihrerseits weitere Heuristiken in Gang setzen. Vieles spricht dafür, mehrere Metaphern zugleich zu gebrauchen, oder es ist auch unvermeidlich. Die sichtbare Struktur dessen, was „Gen" und dann auch das „Genom" genannt wird, bleibt jedenfalls ein (sichtbar) Gegebenes, das wir mit Metaphern in seiner Zugänglichkeit präsent halten. Sie drängen darauf – auch wenn dann etwa von Buchstaben-Sequenzen, von „Wörtern" oder „Patches" (Wort-Teilen) gesprochen wird –, dass wir uns in einer damit angezeigten Suchrichtung bewegen und von ihr geleitet weitere Entdeckungen machen. Das schließt die Bereitschaft ein, die Metaphern zu ändern, wenn sie in ihrer heuristischen Kraft erschöpft sind, und in ihrer Begrenzung zu kritisieren.

3.3 Das Endprodukt

Gehen wir von der Metapher „Kommunikation“ aus, in der die DNA mit ihrem – sagen wir – „Informationsbeitrag“ (statt „Programm“) beteiligt ist, kann unser menschliches Mitvollziehen (Lesen) darin bestehen, einzelne Teilvorgänge des kommunikativen Austausches sichtbaren Eigenschaften des Endprodukts zugeordnet zu beobachten, und damit zu realisieren, was sie in dem Gesamtvorgang „bedeuten“. So wird diese Kommunikation auf das Endprodukt hin in ihrer Funktionalität erfasst, das heißt hier daraufhin, was in ihr und durch sie jeweils auf das Endprodukt hin generiert wird. Wenn innerhalb dieser systemischen Kommunikation bestimmte Vorgänge als „Übersetzung“ oder „Transkription“ erfasst werden, so wird auch damit die Metapher „Kommunikation“ eingelöst und es können weitere Funktionen angezeigt werden. Wenn wir den Beschreibungen dieser inneren Kommunikation folgen – etwa mit Francois Jacob, „Logik des Lebenden“ [10] – dann begegnen uns dort eine Vielzahl von Metaphern, die je für sich zu verfolgen wären – auf das hin, was sie versprechen und was sie als schon erfasst zeigen, so z.B. die Metapher „Bauplan“ für Moleküle, mit der Implikation, dass Teile des Baus „ersetzt“ werden können. [10, 111] Wenn von systemischer Kommunikation zu reden ist, dann ist mitgegeben, dass es auch eine Kommunikation zwischen dem System und seiner Umwelt (Milieu) gibt – auch hier gibt es dichte Beschreibungen und neue Metaphern – das schließt dann auch das Kapitel der „Epigenetik“ ein, also die Beobachtung der Integration von Außeneinflüssen auf das Genom oder auf die innere Kommunikation des Ganzen.

Wir bleiben so innerhalb des durch die Metaphern angezeigten Erkenntnis- und Beobachtungsraumes. Was wir Menschen sehen und in seiner Funktionalität erfassen können, weil wir das jeweilige Produkt – das Endprodukt – sehen (identifizieren), entbirgt nichts Weiteres als eben dies in seiner verlässlichen Stetigkeit und Selbigkeit. Es wird als dieses identische Produkt fassbar. Wenn wir dann etwa vom Endprodukt eines „Organs“ sprechen, dann ist es freilich dieses „Organ“, weil wir auch das ganze Endprodukt, den ganzen Organismus, schon vor Augen haben – wie z.B. den, den wir „Mensch“ nennen. Wir bewegen uns somit auch immer schon rückwärts von dem ausgehend, was wir schon fertig sehen. Dies ist uns vor Augen, und damit ist dann, wenn es denn gelingt, auch seine Genese in der materiell vermittelten (technisch vermittelten) wahrnehmbaren Kommunikation in der ihr eigenen Sichtbarkeit vor Augen, wie dicht auch immer diese Kommunikation abgebildet werden kann.

Das, was da vor Augen kommt, die Kommunikation hat keinen anderen (substantiellen) „Inhalt“, keine andere Botschaft, aber doch dieses Ausgerichtet sein auf ein bestimmtes „Endprodukt“ in seiner Selbigkeit.

3.4 Vom Endprodukt aus

Von hier aus stellt sich (nach rückwärts) die Frage, ob das Ganze, das So-und-nicht-anders-Werden des Endprodukts mit der Metapher „Kommunikation“ (oder „systemische Kommunikation“) in seiner Genese metaphorisch als erfassbar versprochen werden kann, oder ob doch – wiederum metaphorisch – Weiteres präsent zu halten ist, damit wir auch das, was da generiert wird, das Endprodukt, „verstehen“ (und damit wohl auch erst seine Genese), das heißt – hätten wir eine geeignete Metapher – in seiner Funktion erfassen.

Das heißt: jede Kommunikation endet – zunächst – bei einem bestimmten Produkt – oder bei einer bestimmten Funktion, von wo sie dann weiterläuft. Hier kommt es dann auf lückenlose Kontinuität (oder „Integration“) an, so dass nicht etwa „Brücken“ fehlen, die zum nächsten Produkt oder zur nächsten Funktion führen.

Es ist – im vorbehaltlichen Vergleich gesagt – wie die Kommunikation von Ingenieuren, die schließlich eine bestimmte Maschine hervorbringen, indem sie diese Stück für Stück entwickeln, zusammensetzen etc., eine Maschine, die als Ganze eine bestimmte Funktion hat. Zur Ausführung dieser Funktion sind alle Einzelteile (Zwischenprodukte) und ihr Zusammenspiel entscheidend und insofern auch der ganze Vorgang ihrer Konstruktion – letztendlich um der gewollten Funktion der Maschine willen (wie z.B. ein Holzbrett in zwei Teile teilen, das heißt dann – wenn es die Maschine gibt – „zersägen“.) Diese Funktion gibt es nur mit dieser Maschine oder Abwandlungen davon. Diese Funktion kommt mit der Maschine in die zugängliche Welt.

3.5 Teleologie

Also: wir bräuchten eine Metapher für das Endprodukt des genetischen Vorgangs, den wir als Kommunikation (auf ein Endprodukt hin) erfassen – und den wir dann als letztlich koordiniert auf das Endprodukt hin in all seiner komplexen Gegebenheit verstehen, die seiner schließlich zu erwartenden Funktion oder den zu erwartenden Funktionen (vielleicht sind es sehr viele) entspricht.

Wir sind bei einer solchen Beschreibung bei dem, was – auch in der Genetik – als „teleologische“ Betrachtung verhandelt worden ist. Wir stehen ja vor der verwunderten Frage, wie die so zuverlässige Genese eines bestimmten Organismus in ihrer Kontinuität verstehend nachzuvollziehen ist. Die teleologische Fassung ist fundamental kritisiert worden, sofern mit ihr die Vorstellung verbunden wird, dass das „telos“ des Vorgangs (das „Sinn“, „Ziel“, „Zweck“, „vollkommene Erfüllung“ heißen kann) substantiell gefasst wird – und nicht funktional. Auf die Maschine übertragen hieße das, eine Maschine zu haben, die läuft, aber nicht sagen zu können, welche Aufgabe sie wirklich erfüllt, weil ihre Funktion möglicherweise gänzlich verschiedenen Aufgaben zugehören könnte, ohne dass von einer Zweckentfremdung zu reden wäre – so wenn man eine Motorsäge als Antrieb für etwas anderes benutzt.

Das heißt auf den Menschen übertragen: dieser Mensch, wie er erscheint, ist ein – irgendwie – gegebenes „Wesen“, das in einer bestimmten integrierten „Gestalt“ eben da ist, so wie der ganze Vorgang der Kommunikation auch einfach da ist. Das können wir feststellen, ohne die Funktion dieses Wesens ganz, vollkommen, „erkennen“ oder „verstehen“ zu können. Oder ist auch das nicht Fall? Dieser „Mensch“, der da generiert wird, gehört in dem Modell Kosmos-Logos zum „Kosmos“, wenn diese Metapher so gebraucht wird, dass sie alles umfasst, was uns – lesbar – vor Augen kommt. Der Mensch gehört dazu – wie auch immer diese Zugehörigkeit – etwa mit der Frage nach dem „Menschen im Kosmos“ – bestimmt werden kann. Kurz gesagt: Die Genetik und die Metaphern helfen uns nicht, den Menschen (als Endprodukt) in seiner Funktion oder Bedeutung (für uns) zu erfassen, sondern nur in seiner Genese als dieser Organismus, dessen weitere Bestimmung offen bleibt. Oder ist das nicht der Fall? Müssen wir nicht (wie bei der Maschine) eben diese (teleologische) Bestimmung mit-präsent haben (metaphorisch), um die Genese in ihrer Zielgerichtetheit und Bestimmtheit wirklich zu erfassen – also die Genese genau dieses dann so genannten „Menschen“? Oder kann dies offenbleiben und insofern auch die Genese (von uns) verändert werden?

3.6 Nietzsches Frage

Hier sind wir mit der wohl allzu direkten Frage konfrontiert, die Nietzsche in seiner „Genealogie der Moral – Dritte Abhandlung „Was bedeuten asketische Ideale“ – ausgesprochen hat: „Wozu Mensch überhaupt“? Gemeint ist der Mensch, der sich selbst nicht in der Welt verorten kann, weil er die „Welt“ als „wahre Wirklichkeit“ (die Welt in ihrer Wahrheit) nicht erfasst, nicht erfassen kann, sondern – siehe „Wahrheit und Lüge“ – nur in einer „Welt“ lebt, die er sich durch Metaphern zurechtgelegt hat. [1][1]

Wir nähern uns damit der geistesgeschichtlichen Dramatik, in die wir mit der Frage nach den Metaphern in der Molekularbiologie geraten, und zwar so, dass sie genuin dahinführt und nicht irgendwie herangetragen ist. Oder ist das nicht der Fall?

Wozu Mensch überhaupt? Hier fehlt die Funktion (anders als bei allen auffindbaren Elementen im Vorgang seiner Genese, die eine bestimmte begrenzte Funktion haben), wenn „Mensch“ einfach da ist, und „Mensch“ eine (absolute) Metapher ist, die Unbegriffliches – wiederum in einem bestimmten kommunikativen Zusammenhang – präsent hält und eine Funktion anzeigt, die uns wie die „Lesbarkeit der Welt“ – so befragt – vor Augen kommt.

---

1 Siehe zu diesem Zusammenhang von Metaphorologie und Weltorientierung bei Nietzsche [1].

Es müsste – um in der Metaphorik „Kommunikation“ zu bleiben – mit dem Endprodukt „Mensch“ eine weitere Kommunikation wie auch immer anschließen. Dann wäre es auch möglich von der Funktion zu sprechen, die mit dem „Menschen“ gegeben ist. Was aber schließt an das zunächst „finale“ Endprodukt an?

Sollen wir mit Francois Jacob zunächst jedenfalls hier aufhören und – im Sinn der „Logik des Lebenden“ – sagen:

> In den Laboratorien von heute wird nicht mehr das Leben befragt. Man versucht nicht mehr, seine Umrisse zu erfassen. Man bemüht sich lediglich Struktur, Funktion und Geschichte der lebenden Systeme zu analysieren. Kommt aber den lebenden Systemen eine Finalität zu, so ist keine Biologie mehr möglich, ohne sich unaufhörlich auf das Projekt der Organismen zu beziehen, auf den »Sinn«, den allein schon die Tatsache ihrer Existenz ihren Strukturen und Funktionen gibt.
>
> Der Unterschied zwischen dieser Einstellung und dem lange Zeit vorherrschenden Reduktionismus ist offensichtlich. Um wissenschaftlich zu sein, mußte sich bisher die Analyse vorerst jeder Überlegung enthalten, die über das zu erforschende System und seine funktionelle Rolle hinausging. Die von jeder Beschreibung geforderte Genauigkeit verlangte die Beseitigung jenes Elements von Finalität, das der Biologe in seiner Analyse nicht zulassen wollte.
>
> Heute ist [dagegen] die Struktur nicht mehr von ihrer Bedeutung zu trennen; das gilt nicht nur für den Organismus, sondern auch für jene Folge von Ereignissen, in deren Verlauf sich der Organismus entwickelt hat. Jedes lebende System entsteht aus einem bestimmten Gleichgewicht zwischen den Elementen einer Organisation. [10,318–19]

Also – bedarf es doch der Bedeutung des Endprodukts, die dann nach rückwärts verfolgt werden kann und auch auf weitere Erkenntnisse drängt. So sind wir bei der Frage nach der Bedeutung von „Mensch“, der ein Anschluss folgt. Wozu Mensch überhaupt? Was schließt hier an? Nachdem die Frage des Übergangs zum Menschen (als Übergang vom Organischen zum Lebenden) weitgehend bearbeitet ist (Jacob) geht es jetzt wieder um einen Übergang.

Lily E. Kay und andere haben diese Frage nicht direkt bearbeitet, aber doch auf eine mit der Tatsache der gegebenen „systemischen, material (skriptural) vermittelten Kommunikation gegebene „Verschmelzung von Schöpfung und Offenbarung und deren ontologische Bedeutung verwiesen“. Also: mit dem Erscheinen des Menschen in der für ihn gegebenen Genese wird „etwas“ offenbar. Was in der genetischen Kommunikation generiert wird, offenbart zugleich, dass im Ganzen dessen, was es gibt (Metaphern „Welt“, „Kosmos“) „Mensch“ in eben der (teleiotes) Bestimmtheit und Vollkommenheit, in der er stetig und selbig erscheint, gegeben ist. Dieser Mensch wird uns präsent (offenbar), indem er generiert wird und indem wir diese Genese in ihrer Selbigkeit beobachten und erfassen. Es wird uns Menschen präsent, dass mit uns ein Wesen erscheint, das seine eigene Genese selbst beobachtet – und so an der Kommunikation seiner Genese mitgewirkt hat – das kann dieser Mensch nun auch „von außen“ fortsetzen.

Ist das alles? Mit Nietzsche tritt hier (wenn wir nicht zuerst noch auf Kants Grundfragen eingehen sollen, die in die Frage einmünden „Was ist der Mensch?“) der

Philosoph auf den Plan, der die Grundfrage der Philosophie und ihrer Wahrheitssuche – die Frage „warum ist etwas und nicht vielmehr nichts" – mit der Frage „wozu Mensch?" vermittelt gesehen hat. Martin Heidegger hat den Menschen als „Da-Sein" gedacht, das dadurch ausgezeichnet ist, dass es nach dem „Sein" des Seienden fragt – hinter alle Funktionalitäten zurück, bis auf den letzten Grund zurück, über das hinaus, was er mit seiner Erkenntnis für sich gewinnt und worin er sich behauptet (Blumenberg). Das ist er denn, der Mensch, dass durch ihn, das, was ist, in seinem wahren Wesen erscheint. Das ist mitnichten damit schon erschienen, dass er seine Genese erfasst – im Gegenteil, das sagt ihm nichts über das, was er in Wahrheit ist. Eben dagegen steht das Projekt der Metaphorologie von Blumenberg. Der Logos, der dem Menschen zugänglich ist, enthält nichts, was nicht (im „Kosmos") uns zugänglich, technisch vermittelbar eingeschrieben ist – und seine, des Menschen, Wahrheitsfindung ist es, die den Logos präsent werden lässt, nichts aber, was über oder hinter dem Kosmos (im Sein des Seienden) zu finden wäre.

Die Kritik der Metaphysik folgt für Blumenberg keiner Kehre, die in eine „Seinsgeschichte" hineinführt, in der sich „das Sein" entbirgt. In dieser „Seinsgeschichte" freilich nimmt der Mensch einen entscheidenden Ort ein. Nicht dass sich die Seinsgeschichte um ihn dreht, aber durch ihn wird diese als solche präsent, es wird präsent, dass es etwas geben muss, das so und nicht anders (abgekürzt gesagt) zu „denken" ist. Im Unterschied dazu die Geschichte des Logos in seiner Korrelation zum Kosmos, den wir durch den Logos, – inklusive – unserer Technik, erfassen. Metaphern wie die „Lesbarkeit der Welt" versprechen, dass der Kosmos im Logos – in Wahrheit – durchaus erschlossen wird.

In seiner Beschreibung des Projekts der „Metaphorologie" Blumenbergs hält Haverkamp fest, dass es als „Variationsmuster der funktionalen Korrelation von Kosmos und Logos" „klar begrenzt ist": „Es umfasst die Tradition von Aristoteles bis Nietzsche. Kein schicksalhafter Verfall ist in ihr zu befürchten, wie er bei Heidegger und Nietzsche nach Sokrates einsetzt und in Aristoteles' Bearbeitung der platonischen Philosophie greifbar wäre, aber es ist ein ‚Mut zur Vermutung' aufzubringen, der auf neue Gestalten drängt." [2,55]

Wir befinden uns damit in einer geistesgeschichtlichen Dramatik, die, so wie sie Nietzsche intoniert hat, direkt mit der Metaphorologie verbunden ist, und zwar direkt mit der in der Genetik entstandenen Metaphernbildung – weil diese auf die Frage „wozu Mensch?" hindrängt, – wenn sie wirklich vollständigen Erkenntniswert haben soll, etwa schon wegen des Wunders der gegebenen Stetigkeit der Genese dieses Menschen, so dass nicht etwa eine zweite Gattung „Mensch" entstanden wäre.

Das sind die Sachverhalte, die wir, Walter Doerfler und ich, in unserem Experiment ausgiebig diskutiert haben. Bei der Feststellung „ecce homo!" kann die Wahrheitssuche nicht enden, sowohl nach rückwärts als auch von diesem Menschen aus weiter. Sie drängt auf die Frage „wozu dieser Mensch?", sie drängt auf die Frage nach seiner „Bedeutung", sie drängt auf die Frage, was ist dieser Mensch mit seiner Suche nach Wahrheit, die doch nicht stehen bleiben kann dabei, dass der Mensch sich seiner Genese vergewissert und darin sich behauptet.

Nietzsche schreibt in seiner Schrift „Über Wahrheit und Lüge im außermoralischen Sinn" zu Beginn:

> In irgend einem abgelegenen Winkel des in zahllosen Sonnensystemen flimmernd ausgegossenen Weltalls gab es einmal ein Gestirn, auf dem kluge Tiere das Erkennen erfanden. Es war die hochmütigste und verlogenste Minute der ‚Weltgeschichte': aber doch nur eine Minute. Nach wenigen Atemzügen der Natur erstarrte das Gestirn, und die klugen Tiere mußten sterben. – So könnte jemand eine Fabel erfinden und würde doch nicht genügend illustriert haben, wie kläglich, wie schattenhaft und flüchtig, wie zwecklos und beliebig sich der menschliche Intellekt innerhalb der Natur ausnimmt; es gab Ewigkeiten, in denen er nicht war; wenn es wieder mit ihm vorbei ist, wird sich nichts begeben haben. [11,369]

Der abgründige Mangel des menschlichen Intellekts (es ist nicht nur eine Schwäche) wird durch die Metaphernbildung kompensiert oder verdeckt (auch – so Nietzsche – durch die Begriffsbildung). Metaphern machen das Gegebene, wie auch immer technisch vermittelt fassbar, auf den Menschen hin, auf das „Subjekt" Mensch hin zurecht, lassen es also in ihren Funktionen ihm zugänglich erscheinen. So wird seine Wahrheitssuche befriedigt, in der er gefangen ist, weil er in der Metaphorik gefangen bleibt. Es dreht sich alles um den Menschen, der Mensch dreht sich wie ein Falter um „die Flamme Eitelkeit" (370) – sei es mit der Phantasie der Metaphern oder dem mathematischen Kalkül. So behauptet sich der Mensch in der Unwahrheit – anders als die Selbstbehauptung des Menschen bei Blumenberg, der gegen Nietzsche (und Heidegger) diesem Menschen – auch mit Hilfe der Technik – das Ganze der Wahrheit einzuholen versprochen sieht.[2] Nietzsche dagegen beschreibt den Menschen als den, der – wegen seines abgründigen Mangels – immer neue Täuschungen (auch als Schutzmauer gegen die Mächte, die gegen ihn einstürmen) generiert und so immer neue Metaphern (oder auch Mythen) hervorbringt.

Nietzsche widerspricht der Korrelation von Kosmos und Logos, der Mensch verschwindet mit seinem Intellekt, wie auch immer er einen Logos erfassen sollte, im Kosmos. Ausdrücklich: die Wahrheit erscheint nicht in empirischen Dingen. (Anders auch Paul Ricoeur, der gleichermaßen gegen Heidegger und Blumenberg spricht.)

Nietzsche sieht beide, den metaphorisierenden Menschen und den Menschen des Kalküls (und der Begriffe) hinsichtlich ihrer Möglichkeit, die wahre Wirklichkeit zu fassen, gleichauf.

> Beide begehren über das Leben zu herrschen: dieser, indem er durch Vorsorge, Klugheit, Regelmäßigkeit den hauptsächlichsten Nöten zu begegnen weiß, jener, indem er als ein ‚überfroher Held' jene Nöte nicht sieht und nur das zum Schein und zur Schönheit verstellte Leben als real nimmt. [11,383]

2 Siehe zu Blumenbergs Metaphorologie: [12].

Also: es gilt für den Menschen mit seiner Wahrheitssuche, die nicht anders kann, sich eine Welt zurechtzumachen und so über das Leben zu herrschen, um sich zu behaupten. Die entscheidende Angriffsfläche, sich die Welt zurecht zu machen, ist das „Leben", dessen Nöten der Mensch zu begegnen sucht – kein anderes oder vielleicht „höheres" Ziel? Insofern sind wir mit den Biowissenschaften im Zentrum dieser Weltbeherrschung. So braucht es kein „Wozu?", der Mensch genügt sich selbst, er selbst ist das „Wozu". Warum solle es um eine andere „Wahrheit" oder wahre Wirklichkeit gehen, der er zugehörte, zu der er vordringen könnte, oder die mit ihm zur Erscheinung käme? Was sollen solche „asketischen Ideale", die von dieser Welt und der Behauptung darin wegführen? So bleibt der Mensch bei sich selbst, kreist um seine Selbst-Erhaltung und vergewissert sich deshalb seiner Genese, da sollte alles immer gut gehen.

Damit sind jene Fragen und Probleme der Metaphorologie angezeigt, die zumeist ohne diese Hintergrunds-Dramatik verhandelt werden, die in der Frage angezeigt ist, was Menschen hinsichtlich der Erforschung des Lebens zukommt, was vielleicht menschlicher Hybris entspringt, was so viel heißt wie „Gott" spielen, oder eben den „Übermenschen" zu realisieren. Solche Fragen verdanken sich der angezeigten Dramatik, sie bewegen sich innerhalb dieser Dramatik, sind ihr verhaftet, in ihr gefangen, und insofern in Auseinandersetzung mit der darin enthaltenen Wahrheitsfrage zu bearbeiten.

So ist schließlich auch die Frage gegeben, ob wir dieser Dramatik (schicksalhaft?) ausgeliefert sind, auf welcher Seite wir auch immer uns finden, auf der Verfallsseite, sofern Metaphern uns nur täuschen, oder auf der Seite der zu steigernden Selbstbehauptung, auf der Metaphern uns Erkenntnis versprechen.

Noch einmal zum letzteren: Es liegt durchaus nahe zu fragen, ob nicht die Tatsache, dass wir Menschen mit uns verfügbaren, auch technischen Mitteln unsere Genese erfassen können, darauf hinweist, dass diese Konstellation eben so eingerichtet ist. Im Kontext der Metaphorik von der „Lesbarkeit der Welt", hieße das, dass der hier zu lesende Text (was immer er an innerer Kommunikation enthält) an uns als seine potentiellen Leser gerichtet ist, damit sie ihn lesen und sich darin selbst „erfasst" finden als die, die so und nicht anders, so in verlässlicher Stetigkeit und Identität in Erscheinung treten werden. Das sollte an „wozu" genügen. Der Mensch ist einer, der sich seiner Erscheinung in der Welt selbst vergewissern kann. Diese Sicherheit, diese „Herrschaft" ist seine Wahrheit. Oder – in der Metaphorik der systemischen Kommunikation beschrieben – kommt es uns Menschen zu, an dieser Kommunikation teilzunehmen, derer wir uns vergewissern können. Diese – so kommt doch ein Sollen ins Spiel? – sollten wir so festhalten. Was, wer würde uns autorisieren, in den Text einzugreifen? Kann die Metapher „Text lesen" je bedeuten, den „Text" verändern, statt ihn versuchen zu verstehen?

Wenn wir der positiven Funktion von Metaphern folgen, induzieren Metaphern einen bestimmten Umgang mit dem metaphorisch gefassten Gegebenen. Es liegt offensichtlich auf der Hand, dass ein Text darauf wartet, korrigiert, verändert oder wie auch immer als solcher bearbeitet zu werden – wenn er nicht wie die 10 Gebote auf steinerne Tafeln geschrieben erscheint (und auf diese Weise, so festgehalten, als dieser so verschriftete Text weitergegeben und tradiert werden kann. In der Metaphorik systemischer Kommunikation geht es überdies darum, dass beständig Veränderungen geschehen – freilich innerhalb der (wie zu erfassenden) Zielgerichtetheit auf das bestimmte gleichbleibende finale, in der systemischen Kommunikation beschlossene vollkommene, identische Endprodukt. Jede wie auch immer herbeigeführte Veränderung kann nicht anders, als in diesem System zu bleiben, und das heißt innerhalb der Selbst-Erfassung des Menschen hinsichtlich seiner teleologisch erfüllten (leiblichen) Verfasstheit, denn diese ist nicht als allgemeine Erkenntnis festzuhalten, sondern gilt es, als so gegeben und überliefert, weiter zu überliefern.

Eine spezifische Grenze ist – in dieser Logik – dort markiert, wo der Eingriff in das Genom vorgeburtlich vorgenommen wird und so ein „Individuum" geboren wird, das von anderen Menschen in seiner Genese mitbestimmt worden ist und sich daher in einer spezifischen Hinsicht abhängig oder fremdbestimmt wissen muss, anders als alles, was ihm („von Natur" „schicksalhaft") mitgegeben, vererbt wird. Hier greifen verschiedene Felder von Metaphern ineinander. Es kommt hier die Differenz von „schicksalhaft-kontingent" (innerhalb der Geschichte der menschlichen Genese) auf der einen Seite und „historisch ursächlich fremdbestimmt" hinzu.

Das Problem also bleibt, ob das – in der für jeden Menschen gleichen Genese – erfasste Endprodukt „Mensch", so wie er es selbst von Metaphern geleitet erfasst, schon erfüllt sein kann, und damit auch das Verstehen seiner Genese. Anders, wenn sein Verstehen darüber hinausgreifen müsste, um des Phänomens „Mensch" uneingeschränkt gewärtig zu werden.

Das verspricht die Metapher vom „Übermenschen", die etwa im Sinne eine Verschmelzung von Technik ("cybernetic organism") und menschlicher Natur eine „transhumane" Existenz meint. So ist auch Nietzsches „Übermensch" verstanden worden. Das „Trans" in „Transhumanismus" ist freilich mehrdeutig, es kann zum einen unbegrenzte Steigerung anzeigen – ein beständiges Transzendieren, oder es kann einen Sprung in eine andere Existenz, in eine „neue Gestalt" bedeuten. Es kann auch (Blumenberg) das Neue als ein immer Neues, das immer den Vorrang hat vor dem Gegebenen, so verstanden werden, dass dieses immer Neue, das immer mögliche Neue für die „wahre Wirklichkeit" einsteht, die in ihrer Wahrheit nicht anders „erscheinen" kann als in diesem Vorgang des beständigen Hinzukommens (wie auch immer dieser Vorgang zu beschreiben ist) des Neuen. Dies kann die Differenz von „renovatio" und „revolutio" einschließen, wiederum ein Metaphernpaar, das eine eigene Dramatik enthält.

Die metaphorisch versprochene Wahrheitsfindung richtet sich gegen jene Disposition (von Heidegger), in der Wahrheit (wahre Wirklichkeit) anders als in der Korrelation von Kosmos und Logos präsent wird, und so auch eine andere Wahrheit ist, die – gleichwohl nicht metaphysisch gedacht – in einer anderen „Geschichte" erscheint, in der Geschichte des wahren und wirklichen Seins. Gegen diese Fortführung der Metaphysikkritik wehrt sich Blumenberg.

Die schon angezeigte Frage, was in dem Geschehen der Erschließung der „wahren Wirklichkeit“ dem Menschen zukommt, inwiefern überhaupt durch ihn diese Erschließung stattfindet, inwiefern dies sein „Wozu?“ ist, dass der Mensch derjenige ist, der sich seines So-Da-Seins vergewissern kann (weil Kosmos und Logos korrelieren), hat hier ihren geistesgeschichtlichen Kontext. Mit dem Menschen und durch den Menschen wird „offenbar“ (offenkundig), worum (um mit Nietzsche zu reden) sich alles dreht, nämlich um ihn selbst – dass er sich als dieser Mensch behaupten kann, dass er sich vergewissern kann, dass seine Erscheinung, so wie sie sich tradiert, eingelöst ist. Alle Metaphern verbleiben in diesem Horizont einer so eingelösten menschlichen Existenz. Nun legt aber die Beschreibung der Genetik durchaus ein bestimmtes Weiterfragen nahe – nämlich danach, was an dieses Endprodukt „Mensch“ anschließt, wenn es nicht dabei bleiben soll, dass dieser Mensch – in welcher Dynamik der Veränderung auch immer – „identisch“ reproduziert wird und sich dessen vergewissert, dass er so – wie er im Genom „verschriftet“ ist – tradiert wird, statt ihn weiter zu entwickeln, jedenfalls auch zu verändern oder gar in einen anderen zu verwandeln. Das hieße hier „Mensch bleiben“.

3.7 Zum Schluss: Der verbleibende Horizont

In der gemeinsamen Arbeit an Beschreibungs-Aufgaben in der Molekularbiologie hat die Wahrnehmung der dabei gebrauchten Metaphern und ihrer Diskussion dazu verholfen, ein Forschungsfeld auszumachen, auf dem Theologie, Philosophie und Biowissenschaft – am Beispiel der Molekularbiologie – gleichermaßen tätig sind, und zwar untrennbar, wenn der das Forschungsfeld bestimmende Horizont nicht eingeschränkt werden soll. Darüber hinaus aber hat sich bestätigt, dass die Frage nach dem Gebrauch von Metaphern in der Molekularbiologie direkt mit der grundlegenden Frage „wozu überhaupt Metaphern?“ verbunden ist, weil dort der Gebrauch der Metaphern mit der Arbeit am Selbst-Verständnis des „Menschen“ verbunden ist, wenn denn das Selbst-Verständnis des Menschen auch seine leibliche Verfassung, wie sie in der Genetik zu erfassen ist, genuin einschließt und wenn diese leibliche Verfassung dem Menschen so vor Augen kommt, dass er gefragt ist, wie, was er damit – auch von sich selbst – durch das „Lesen“ zu „verstehen“ hat. Wäre nicht jedenfalls eine grundlegende Aufgabe des Verstehens damit gegeben, dass das stetig Bleibende der Genese und die Modalitäten ihrer Veränderung in ihrer Disproportion gesehen würden – und so der „Text“ ein lesender bleibt – in einem nicht beschränkten Horizont?

Literatur

[1] Blumenberg H. Theorie der Unbegrifflichkeit. Hrsg. v. A. Haverkamp, Frankfurt am Main, Suhrkamp, 2007.

[2] Haverkamp A, Mende D. (Hrsg.) Metaphorologie: Zur Praxis von Theorie. Technische Universität Dresden. Originalausgabe, erste Auflage, Frankfurt am Main, Suhrkamp, 2009.

[3] Lakoff G, Johnson, M. Leben in Metaphern. Konstruktion und Gebrauch von Sprachbildern. Zehnte Auflage, Heidelberg, Carl-Auer Verlag, Heidelberg, 2021.

[4] Blumenberg, H. Metaphorisierte Kosmologie, in: Paradigmen zu einer Metaphorologie. In: Archiv für Begriffsgeschichte (6–142) 106–122, Hamburg, Meiner Verlag, 1960.

[5] Villányi D, Lübcke, T Soziologische Systemtheorie und Metaphorik – Zur Epistemologie der Metapher des Systems. In: Junge M (Hg.): Metaphern und Gesellschaft, Wiesbaden, VS Verlag für Sozialwissenschaften, 2011, S. 31–48.

[6] Bock von Wülfingen B. Genom als Text: Die Schriftmetapher revisited. In: metaphorik.de 2016 (26). Online verfügbar unter https://www.metaphorik.de/sites/www.metaphorik.de/files/journal-pdf /met26-bvwuelf.pdf.

[7] Kay L E. Das Buch des Lebens. Wer schrieb den genetischen Code?, München, Hanser, 2000.

[8] Blumenberg H. Die Lesbarkeit der Welt, Frankfurt am Main, Suhrkamp, 1981.

[9] Weiß M G (Hg.). Bios und Zoë. Die menschliche Natur im Zeitalter ihrer technischen Reproduzierbarkeit, Frankfurt am Main, Suhrkamp, 2009.

[10] Jacob, F. Logik des Lebenden. Von der Urzeugung zum genetischen Code, Frankfurt am Main, Fischer, 1972.

[11] Nietzsche F. Über Wahrheit und Lüge im außermoralischen Sinne (1873). In: Nietzsche F, Colli G, Montinari M (Hrsg.). Kritische Gesamtausgabe, III,2. Nachgelassene Schriften 1870–1873, Berlin, De Gruyter,1988, S. 369–384.

[12] Mende D. Metapher – zwischen Metaphysik und Archäologie. Schelling, Heidegger, Derrida, Blumenberg, München, Paderborn, Fink, 2013.

Domenico Schneider

4 Eine wissenschafts- und verkörperungsphilosophische Betrachtung der Metapher in wissenschaftlicher Praxis

4.1 Einleitung

Die nachstehenden Überlegungen zu einer Betrachtung der Metapher in wissenschaftlichen Praxen sind zweifach motiviert. Zum einen soll im Rückgang auf die lebendige Leiblichkeit an die verkörperte und intermodale Zugangsweise von Metaphern erinnert werden, um sie nicht nur für die alltäglichen Belange der Sprachverwendung kenntlich zu machen, sondern sie ebenfalls für die theoretisierende und wissenschaftliche Praxis hervorzuheben. Dieser Gesichtspunkt meines Artikels wird durch Erläuterungen zu George Lakoffs und Mark Johnsons [1-4] Metapherntheorie bewerkstelligt. Zum anderen soll im Ausgang einer Eigenschaftsliste zu Metaphern von Max Black [5, S. 75–76] die *Entstehungsdynamik* von Metaphern näher angeschaut werden. Black hat in seinem Text *Die Metapher* eine recht offen gelassene Entstehungsvielfalt der Metapher im fünften Punkt dieser Liste formuliert. Daher stelle ich die These auf, dass die Metaphern in unserer heutigen technisierten Welt gerade im Hinblick auf ihr Entstehen durch Technik und Instrumentarien geprägt sind. Letzteres soll mit Ian Hackings [6] Ansatz einer instrumentellen Intervention vertieft werden. Um überhaupt eine moderne, naturwissenschaftliche Praxis zu entwickeln, bedarf es Instrumente und letztlich ein *damit* zusammenhängendes, mediales Denken in Modellen und Theorien, welches eine zentrale Rolle in der Entstehung von wissenschaftlichen Metaphern spielt.

Der Artikel gestaltet sich im Weiteren wie folgt: in einem ersten Abschnitt wird die sprachanalytische Debatte zwischen Max Black und Donald Davidson einführend aufgerollt, um vor allem den Punkt der Notwendigkeit einer Entstehungsdynamik für Metaphern zu erfragen. Dabei wird insbesondere die fehlende Leiblichkeit herausgestellt, die dann in einem zweiten Abschnitt schlaglichtartig ergänzt wird. Beides wird in einem Abschnitt zur *Ergonomie* des wissenschaftlichen Instrumentariums für eine Verlängerung der Metaphorik von bildgebenden Verfahren näher beleuchtet. Abschließend wird im Rückgang auf Hacking die These formuliert, dass die Entstehungsdynamik von wissenschaftlichen Metaphern zumindest zum Teil durch die wissenschaftliche Umwelt-Mensch-Relation bestimmt ist, welche im Wesentlichen technisch vorstrukturiert ist. Diese führt letztlich für Wissenschaftler und Wissenschaftlerinnen zu einer spezifischen *Technoimagination* [7, S. 177], die eine andere Beziehung von Mensch und Welt mit sich bringt, die im öffentlichen Diskurs notwendigerweise zu Schwierigkeiten führen muss.

https://doi.org/10.1515/9783112215685-004

4.2 Klassische Metapherntheorie und Naturwissenschaften

Die klassischen Metapherntheorien, die im deutschsprachigen Raum am besten sicherlich durch Anselm Haverkamp [8, 9] zusammengetragen worden sind, befassen sich überwiegend mit sprachinternen Gesichtspunkten der Metapher. Referenz, Bedeutung, Übertragung, Analogie, Etymologie, lokutionäre, illokutionäre und perlokutionäre Aspekte, Narration, Prädikation, Übersetzung, Schema, Rhetorik usw. beziehen sich als Bestandstücke einer Metapherntheorie auf die sprachinterne Gebundenheit. Sicherlich werden in all den verschiedenen Theorien, die Haverkamp heranzieht, ebenso über die sprachinternen Mechanismen hinausgehende Gesichtspunkte erwähnt. Dies geschieht spätestens dann, wenn einzelne Metaphern näher erläutert werden müssen und die Gegenständlichkeiten, die durch die Metapher benannt werden, zum Vorschein treten. Beispielsweise analysiert Paul Henle in seinem Text *Die Metapher* den folgenden in Englisch geschriebenen und in Deutsch übersetzten Text, der auf John Keats zurückgeht:

„When by my solitary hearth I sit
And hateful thoughts enwarp my soul in gloom
[Wenn ich einsam in meinem Haus sitze
Und haßerfüllte Gedanken meine Seele in Trübsinn hüllen]“ [10, S. 84].

Bei einer Analyse der Metapher – und Henle bewerkstelligt dies auch so [10, S. 84–85] – kann man das *Umhüllen* erklären, in dem man als Beispiel auf eine Decke eingeht, die den menschlichen Körper zum Wärmen umhüllt, um die Metapher aus diesem Gedicht zu bestimmen. Man verlässt bei dieser Erklärung offensichtlich den rein sprachinternen Bereich und geht auf die Gegenstandsbezüge zurück. Abgesehen aber von solchen notwendigen Analyseakten, die auf lebensweltliche Grundlagen eingehen, beschäftigt sich eine Vielzahl der Metapherntheorien, die Haverkamp heranzieht, letztlich mit Fragen zur Sprache, was sicherlich seine Berechtigung hat, sofern es um die hermeneutischen Bereiche von geisteswissenschaftlichen Denkweisen oder eben Literatur selbst geht. In diesen Bereichen – Geisteswissenschaft und Literatur – kann das, was gängig unter Metapher verstanden wird, am deutlichsten hervortreten. Landläufig wird unter einer Metapher ein sprachliches Stilmittel oder ein sprachlicher Ausdruck verstanden, der von einem bekannten Bedeutungszusammenhang in einen neuen Zusammenhang überträgt [5, S. 56–58; 10, S. 80–81; 11, S. 42] und sich dabei eines *Vergleichs* oder einer *Analogie* bedient. Dass diese Definition nicht hinreichend erscheint, lässt sich an den umfangreichen Ansätzen erkennen, die gerade bspw. die Vergleichstheorie kontrovers diskutieren [5, S. 65–68; 12, S. 29–31]. Wichtig scheint aber auf dem ersten Blick der Umstand zu sein, dass es im Rahmen von Geisteswissenschaft und Literatur zunächst um *sprachinterne* Fragestellungen geht.

All dies ändert sich jedoch eklatant, sobald man naturwissenschaftliche Praktiken näher betrachtet. Hier werden abgesehen vom alltäglichen Sprechen – worin es bereits zuhauf tote und lebendige Metaphern gibt – die gesamten wissenschaftlichen Praktiken in Form von Modellieren, Theoretisieren, und Experimentieren virulent. Die naturwissenschaftliche Verschriftlichung scheint bereits voller Vergleiche, Modelle und Übertragungen zu sein, wodurch sie also insgesamt schon metaphorisch angereicht ist. In dem von Andrew Ortony [13] herausgegebenen Sammelband *Metapher and Thoughts* gibt es eine eigene ausgewiesene Sektion über den Zusammenhang von Metaphern und Naturwissenschaften. Dedre Gentner und Michael Jeziorski [14] machen hierin deutlich, dass die westliche Wissenschaftlichkeit einen eindeutigen Wechsel von der Metapher zur Analogie durchlaufen hat. Diesem Paradigmenwechsel liegt sicherlich der Wunsch zugrunde, dass man jeher in den Naturwissenschaften das metaphorische Sprechen als eine abträgliche Eigenschaft im Diskurs verstanden hat. Die Wissenschaft müsse frei sein von metaphorischen Beschreibungen und in ihren Bezügen auf den wissenschaftlichen Gegenstand zurückkommen. Gentner und Jeziorski arbeiten sich hierbei in ihren Beispielen an der Modellbildung ab [14, S. 447–448, 456–462]. Das Rutherfordsche Atommodell als Analogie zum Planetenmodell wird erwähnt und Robert Boyles Ansatz eines Kügelchenmodells, um chemische Prozesse zu verstehen, werden näher mit Carnots Überlegungen zu diesen Naturerscheinungen verglichen. Vereinfacht gesagt, erscheint das Prinzip der Analogiebildung im Sinne Gentner durch eine lebensweltliche Verbindung gegeben zu sein, die Anknüpfungspunkte im Meskosmos aufgreift und damit der menschlichen einfachen und unverstärkten Sinnlichkeit nahe kommt.

Der Wissenschaftstheoretiker Richard Boyd problematisiert in seinem Text *Metaphor and theory change: What is "metaphor" a metaphor for?* die Sonderstellungen der metaphorischen Verwendung in den Wissenschaften. Wohingegen in der Literatur die Metapher durchaus ein Substitutionsmittel sein kann, was sicherlich nicht für alle metaphorischen Verwendungsweisen gilt, kann das, was in den Naturwissenschaften durch die Metapher geleistet wird, nur durch ein ostensives, also zeigendes Verständnis entstehen [15, S. 483, 504]. Durch das Hinweisen auf die Gegenständlichkeiten werden wissenschaftlich tradierte Begrifflichkeiten zumeist für mehrere Wissenschaftsgenerationen fixiert [15, S. 483]. Dieses führt für Boyd zu einer Konzeption von *theoriekonstitutiven Metaphern*, die eine Reihe von untypischen Eigenschaften mit sich bringt. Am prominentesten erscheint mir für den Anspruch dieses Artikels die schlechte Anschlussfähigkeit an die Öffentlichkeit: „In important respects, however, these theory-constitutive metaphors are highly atypical. In the first place, they undergo a sort of public articulation and development that is uncharacteristic of literary metaphors" [15, S. 487]. Es fehlt letztlich eine Art geordnete und nicht trivialisierende Eintrittsmöglichkeit einer theoriekonstitutiven Metapher in den *sensus communis*. Diesen Sachverhalt differenziert Boyd nochmals über die Gegenüberstellung von *literarischen Interaktionsmetaphern*, die gerade dem sprachliebenden und literaturbegeisterten Menschen zugänglich sind, gegenüber den *theoriekonstitutiven Metaphern* der naturwissenschaftlichen Betriebsamkeit. Die literarischen Interaktionsmetaphern besitzen gerade eine konzeptionell offene Endlichkeit (conceptual open-endedness), wohingegen theoriekonstitutive Metaphern recht eng gebunden an einem programmatischen Forschungsparadigma kleben bleiben und hierdurch eben hermetisch sich verschließen [15, S. 488–489]. Letztere werden gerade explizit geschaffen und kreiert, um wirkliche Aufgaben in den Naturwissenschaften zu erledigen und Ergebnisse dauerhaft für die Zukunft zu sichern. Wie Boyd später in seinem Artikel festhält, scheint aber gerade so etwas wie Referenz – Bezug im Weitesten Sinne – eine dynamisch sich verändernde Angelegenheit zu sein [15 S. 504–505]. Zumindest zielt die Schaffung von theoriekonstitutiven Metaphern in den gängigen Fällen auf Analogien und Vergleiche ab, die einerseits verkümmerte Metaphern sind, aber andererseits durch oftmals technisierte Anhängsel dem nicht-wissenschaftlichen Sprachgebrauch enthoben werden. Die Zeichenkette H_2O als ein Formelzeichen für Wasser kann hier als ein solches Beispiel genannt werden, auch wenn hier aus guten Gründen schwerlich von einer Metapher im literarischen Sinne die Rede sein kann.

Eine andere Schwierigkeit, die im Übrigen auch durch das Computermetaphernbeispiel bei Boyd angerissen wird [15, S. 486–487], besteht darin, welche Auswirkung technische Werkzeuge in der Metaphernbildung etablieren. Beispielsweise wird die Computermetapher, wie Boyd ebenfalls erwähnt, herangezogen, um das phänomenale Bewusstsein auf Basis von neuronaler Vernetzung im Gehirn zu erklären. Ein klassisch gewordener Ausspruch von Daniel Dennett aus seinem Buch *Consciousness Explained* zum Gehirn soll exemplarisch diese metaphorische Beschreibung erläutern: „Now we are ready to turn this standard idea upside-down. Just as you can simulate a parallel brain on a serial von Neumann machine, you can also, in principle, simulate (something like) a von Neumann machine on parallel hardware, and that is just what I am suggesting: Conscious human minds are more-or-less serial virtual machines implemented – inefficiently – on the parallel hardware that evolution has provided for us“ [16, S. 218]. Das Gehirn wird mittels einer virtuellen Maschine selbst konzipiert. Es gäbe zu dieser kontrovers diskutierten Position inhaltlich viel zu sagen, was jedoch von der Thematik der Metapher wegführt. Wichtig für das in diesem Artikel besprochene Thema – naturwissenschaftliche Praktiken und Metaphern – scheinen aber die folgenden zwei Gesichtspunkte im Hinblick auf das Verwenden von instrumentellen Vorrichtungen bzw. weitergedacht überhaupt Medien zu sein: Erstens, werden innerhalb der naturwissenschaftlichen Praxis wissenschaftliche Instrumente benutzt, um die Objekte und Forschungsgegenständlichkeiten überhaupt verständlich zu machen. Dies führt dann zu dem, was Ian Hacking eben *Intervernieren mittels Instrumenten* nennt, um die Realität der Gegenständlichkeiten zu erklären [6, S. 249–453]. Mit diesem Intervenieren auf Basis von Instrumenten entwickelt sich jedoch eine spezifische wissenschaftliche Sprechweise, die nur und ausschließlich Sinn im Hinblick auf das Instrumentarium hat, aber trotzdem in den Praxen der Wissenschaftler und Wissenschaftlerinnen eine eigenständige, wie Boyd es nennen würde, *theoretisierende Metaphorik* mit sich bringt. Zweitens, können solche so geschaffenen Metaphern eben aus ihren originären wissenschaftlichen Praxen heraustreten und sich in andere Bereiche, etwa in philosophischen Debatten zum Gehirn, einnisten und dort den Diskurs zumindest zeitweise bestimmen. Nichts anders scheint mir letztlich am Beispiel der Beschreibung durch *eine virtuelle Maschine* im Hinblick des *Gehirns* geschehen zu sein. Ein anderes gängiges Beispiel stellt der Vergleich mittels der Phrase des „Quantensprungs" dar, was darauf hindeutet, dass ein außerordentlicher Fortschritt geschehen ist: „Seine Schulleistungen kamen einen Quantensprung seines Verstehens gleich, nachdem er Nachhilfe genommen hat." Auf diesen Gesichtspunkt der Erweiterung von Metaphern mit Rückgang auf ein technisches Instrumentarium wird im Laufe des Artikels zurückzukommen sein.

Die genannten Autoren – Gentner, Jeziorski, Boyd – gehen zu Beginn ihrer Ausführungen auf Max Blacks Text *Die Metapher* ein, um die grundlegenden Eigenschaften zu Metaphern zu erläutern. Dies macht insofern Sinn, als die möglichen Kandidaten, Substitutionstheorie und Vergleichstheorie, ebenfalls für naturwissenschaftliche Metaphorik herangezogen werden können: Die Übertragung des Planetenmodells (zentraler kugelförmige Stern (Sonne) wird von Trabanten (Planeten) auf Kreisbahnen oder Ellipsen umkreist) auf das Atommodell (mit einem Kern als zentralen Körper und diesen umkreisenden Elektronen) hat sich als erfolgreich herausgestellt und kann als eine Übertragung in Form eines *Vergleich* – hier sogar eine Analogie – gewertet werden. Ferner diskutiert Black neben der Vergleichstheorie auch die Substitutionstheorie, die formal als eine Art hermeneutisches Entschlüsseln für die Metaphern verstanden werden kann. Eine wörtliche Bedeutung L wird durch einen metaphorischen Ausdruck M ersetzt. Demnach müsse man als Anwender, Leser oder Rezipient lediglich im funktionalen Sinne eine Art Umkehrung vollziehen, d. h. es ergibt sich eine Metaphorizierung als $f: L \rightarrow M$, wobei L als *literarischer Bedeutungszusammenhang* und M als metaphorischer Bedeutungszusammenhang verstanden werden kann. Das Verstehen des Rezipienten wäre demnach eine Suche nach einer Umkehrfunktion f^{-1}, die eine Art Rückübersetzungen garantiert: „Diese [die „figurative" Sprache] geht davon aus, daß jede Sprachfigur, die semantischen Wechsel mit sich bringt [...], aus einer Umwandlung der *wörtlichen* Bedeutung besteht. Der Autor liefert nicht die von ihm beabsichtigte Bedeutung, m, sondern eine Funktion von ihr, $f(m)$; Aufgabe des Lesers ist die Anwendung der inversen Funktion, f^{-1}, um so zu $f^{-1}f(m)$ zu gelangen, d. h. zu der ursprünglichen Bedeutung, m" [5, S. 65]. Diese hölzern wirkende Idee, wie Metaphorizierung und ihr Verstehen ablaufen könnte, lässt sich sicherlich nicht beim Verstehen wiederfinden, obgleich im Rahmen von semantic web und überhaupt semantischen Suchmaschinen derartige Ansätze überlegt worden sind. Zumeist scheitern solche Ansätze wie das des Semantic webs vor allem an der Überkomplexität und der zeitlich immer kürzer werdenden Dynamik wie neue Metaphern in einer digital-datafizierten Netzkultur sich ergeben. Ted Cohen hat in seinem Artikel *Figurative Rede und figurative Akte* bereits vor der Entwicklung des Massenmediums Computer festgestellt, dass eine Algorithmisierung der Metapher nicht möglich ist [12, S. 29–31]. Metaphern entstehen nach Cohen mit einer gewissen Unvorhersagbarkeit.

Von diesen offensichtlichen Problematiken der Substitutionstheorie abgesehen, weist Black der Subsitutionstheorie, damit diese, wie oben beschrieben, funktionieren kann, eine zugrundeliegende Analogie oder Ähnlichkeit zwischen M und L zu, damit diese in Beziehung treten können [5, S. 66]. Bei den genannten Suchmaschinen geschieht dies zumeist durch Merkmalslisten, die zusätzlich in einer Baumstruktur geordnet werden und somit ein semantisches Netz durch so genannte Marker (Identifier) eindeutig zuordnen können. Mit solchen Beziehungsmarkern wäre dann ein Vergleich möglich, was dann zur Vergleichstheorie führt [5, S. 66]. Black kritisiert jedoch diese Art von Vergleichstheorie berechtigterweise, da letztlich unklar bleibt, ob mit einer derart starren Fixierung die natürliche Sprache in ihrer Überkomplexität nicht doch letzten Endes vage bliebe. Black bemerkt hierzu zusammenfassend: „Der Haupteinwand gegen eine Vergleichstheorie besteht darin, daß sie an einer vagen Unbestimmtheit leidet, die an Leere grenzt" [5, S. 67]. Bekanntlich bietet Black seine *Interaktionstheorie* als Alternative, um den Menschen als den Benutzer von Metaphern ins Spiel zu bringen. Dabei verbessert Black die Vergleichstheorie indem er den dynamischen Charakter der Metapherentstehung bereits mittels eines Ähnlichkeitsansatzes anspricht: „Es wäre in einigen [...] Fällen aufschlußreicher zu sagen, die Metapher schafft Ähnlichkeiten [similarity], statt zu sagen, sie formuliert eine bereits vorher existierende Ähnlichkeit" [5, S. 68]. Der Ähnlichkeitsbegriff bleibt fragwürdig, da er selbst philosophisch unklar erscheint: Entsteht die Ähnlichkeit auf einer figurativ-sinnlichen Ebene (bspw. Tischbein und die Länglichkeit eines tatsächlichen menschlichen Beins), einer bereits abstrakten Zuschreibung oder durch eine andere kontingente Zuordnung (historisch, narrativ, u. a.)? Von dieser Problematik abgesehen, werden die Ähnlichkeiten eben *geschaffen* und liegen nicht bereits in irgendeiner Weise vor. Die Interaktionstheorie bezieht sich dann auf die Metapher als Interaktion zweier zusammenwirkender Vorstellungen, welche ein *„System miteinander assoziierter Gemeinplätze [system of associated comonplace]"* verbindet [5, S. 71].

Donald Davidson [17] hat das Prinzip der Ähnlichkeit in gewisser Hinsicht ebenfalls aufgegriffen. In seinem Text *Was Metaphern bedeuten* zeigt er, dass die Metaphern uns auf Gleichheiten aufmerksam machen, betont jedoch dabei, dass dies kein hinreichendes Kriterium darstellt, um das Wesen der Metapher vollumfänglich zu bestimmen [17, S. 52–54]. Mit seinem Text lehnt Davidson insgesamt die Vorstellung ab, dass Metaphern einen zusätzlichen kognitiven Gehalt beim Verstehen von Metaphern hätten; d. h. die Metapher hat neben ihrer buchstäblichen Bedeutung keine weitere. Man müsse die Wörter letztlich in ihrem Verwendungsbereich untersuche, um die Funktionsweise von Metaphern zu extrapolieren [17, S. 50–51]. Sofern man berücksichtigt, dass Black mit seinen Gemeinplätzen den Kontext mit berücksichtigt sehen möchte, erscheinen Black und Davidson sich in dieser Hinsicht einig zu sein. Dabei bezieht sich Davidson auf Gottlob Frege und erklärt, dass die Metapher in den jeweiligen speziellen Bedeutungen den Bezug zu gewöhnlichen Kontexten auf identische Weise festlegt, wie es andere Wörter tun. Demnach kann das Verstehen von Metaphern genauso wie bei gewöhnlichen Wörtern, bei den beispielsweise nur ein Gegenstandsbezug vorliegt (bspw. ist die Zeichenkette *Auto* eben durch einen Bezug zu einem vierrädrigen motorisierten Fahrzeug bestimmt), durch den *Gebrauch* als einen Prozesse des Lernens etabliert werden. Für Davidson lässt sich das Verstehen der Metapher daher über den Umgang mit Sprache selbst erklären und steht damit den nicht-metaphorischen Wörtern in nichts nach. Insgesamt lässt sich die Metapher nicht mittels ihrer Bedeutung oder metaphorischen

Wahrheit hinreichend verständlich machen, vielmehr scheint ihr Gebrauch in dem dazugehörigen Kontext entscheidend zu sein: „Was die Metapher auszeichnet, ist nicht die Bedeutung, sondern ihr Gebrauch – in dieser Hinsicht verhält sie sich wie das Behaupten, Anspielen, Lügen, Versprechen oder Bemängeln." [17, S. 68]. Die Metaphern erscheinen in Davidsons Ansatz kontextsensitiv. Wörter haben jeher eine ausgefranste Bedeutung und dies gilt umso mehr für die Metaphern, deren Bedeutung deutlicher durch den Kontext fixiert wird. Dabei geben uns die Metaphern einen speziellen Blick auf die Dinge der uns umgebenden Welt (objektive und soziale Welt gleichermaßen gedacht), wie Davidson mit Bezug auf Black formuliert [17, S. 71]. Wichtig für Davidson erscheint, dass man aber die *Wirkung* der Metaphern – und hier meint Davidson sicherlich den Prozess des Verstehens von Metaphern – nicht mit einer spezifischen kognitiven Bedeutung verwechseln sollte: „Der Irrtum [...] besteht darin, daß sie [Autoren, die den Metaphern einen spezifischen kognitiven Gehalt zuschreiben] sich an die Inhalte der Gedanken klammern, die durch die Metapher ausgelöst werden, und diese Inhalte in die Metapher selbst hineinlesen" [17, S. 71]. Sofern man auf der Ebene einer Sprache bleibt, die in schriftlichen Zeichenketten vorliegt, hat Davidson sicherlich eine zutreffende Kritik formuliert. Nichtsdestoweniger scheinen mir beide Ansätze, also ebenso Blacks Ansatz, die Dimension der verkörperten Sprache nicht zu berücksichtigen. Im Wesentlichen verhandeln beide geschriebene Sprache, die der Rezipient eben nur lesend erfasst und dabei zumindest potentiell ein Wörterbuch zur Hand hätte, um sich bei problematischen und unklaren Metaphern über die wörtliche Bedeutung zu verständig. Diese Art der Sprachauffassung und ihre an der Verschriftlichung orientierten Durchdringung scheint einerseits auf den ersten Blick ideal zu einer naturwissenschaftlichen Verwendung von Metaphern zu passen, denn der naturwissenschaftliche Unternehmungsgeist findet neben der umfangreichen Arbeit in Laboren, in der Feldforschung und an experimentellen Untersuchungen überwiegend in verschriftlichter Form statt. Historisch gesehen sah und sieht sich die gesamte sprachanalytische Philosophie in einem ähnlichen Fahrwasser verortet. Andererseits verbleibt der Mensch in der naturwissenschaftlichen Betriebsamkeit eben auch Mensch, der nicht ausschließlich naturwissenschaftlich denkt, sondern durch eine individuelle Entwicklung an der Sprachgemeinschaft teilhat, die nicht naturwissenschaftlichen Ursprungs ist. Dieser Teil der alltäglichen und lebensweltlich orientierten Sprache ist bekanntlich selbst durchzogen von Metaphern und metaphorischen Konzepten, die nicht ohne einen Rückgang auf den lebendigen menschlichen Körper verständlich werden. Ferner scheint dieser Rückgang aus dem Umstand gerechtfertigt, dass die meisten räumlichen Metaphern in der naturwissenschaftlichen Sprache selbst nur durch Konzepte verständlich werden, die auf einen leiblich interagierenden Körper zurückgehen. Dieser Punkt soll im nächsten Abschnitt aufgegriffen und erläutert werden.

Bevor auf die verkörperte Seite des metaphorischen Verstehens eingegangen wird, soll abschließend in diesem Abschnitt eine Grundidee des Artikels mit Hilfe von Blacks sieben Punkteprogramm überlegt werden [5, S. 75–76]. Verkürzt stellt Black folgende sieben Punkte zusammen, von denen der fünfte hier explizit zitiert wird: 1. metaphorische Aussagen besitzen einen Hauptgegenstand und einen untergeordneten Gegenstand, 2. Gegenstände aus (1.) sollten eher als „Systeme von Dingen“ und weniger als Dinge selbst verstanden werden. 3. der Hauptgegenstand wird durch ein System von assoziierten Implikationen bzgl. des untergeordneten Gegenstandes durchstrukturiert, 4. diese Implikationen sind gegeben durch (a) *Gemeinplätze* über den untergeordneten Gegenstand und (b) abweichender Implikationen, „die vom Autor *ad hoc* entworfen sind.“, 5. „Die Metapher selegiert, betont, unterdrückt und organisiert charakteristische Züge des Hauptgegenstands, indem sie Aussagen über ihn einbezieht, die normalerweise zum untergeordneten Gegenstand gehören.“ 6. es findet ein metaphorischer Transfer statt, der in einer Bedeutungsverschiebung bei Wörtern besteht, die zur selben Familie oder zum selben System wie der metaphorische Ausdruck gehören, 7. es gibt keine einfache Ursache („ground“) für das Gelingen und Versagen von Metaphern. Alle genannten Punkte bedürften genauerer Überlegungen und kommen sowohl beim Erstellen (Produzentenseite) als auch beim Verstehen bzw. Wirken (Rezipientenseite) mit unterschiedlicher Gewichtung zum Zuge, was ergänzend, hier aber nicht weiter ausgeführt, nochmals die lokutionären, illokutionären und perlokutionären Gesichtspunkte, kurz die sprechakttheoretischen Aspekte, von Metaphern mit einbeziehen müsste [12, S. 32–48]. Der fünfte Punkt sowie der vierte Punkt mit (b) erscheinen insofern zentral zu sein, als hier die Entstehungsdynamik von Metaphern angedacht wird. Zum einen können mit 4 (b) – inwieweit dieses *können* in ein *müssen* übergeht, scheint unklar zu sein – Metaphern eine Autorschaft ab dem Moment des Hervorbringens aufweisen. Wie dies bei toten Metaphern („Tischbein“) geschehen sein kann, bleibt sicherlich ein dunkler und nicht mehr aufweisbarer Prozess der Sprachentstehung. In der naturwissenschaftlichen Praxis erzeugen die Wissenschaftler und Wissenschaftlerinnen die Metaphern entlang ihrer Forschungsgegenständlichkeiten, die in den meisten Fällen mit spezifischen Forschungsinstrumenten hervorgebracht werden. Mit dem fünften Punkt tritt zum anderen durch das, was dann in den einzelnen Metaphern der Hauptgegenstand und der untergeordnete Gegenstand darstellt, etwas an der Entstehungsdynamik von Metaphern hervor, was nicht ausschließlich der Autorschaft des Produzenten anheimfällt, sondern vielmehr durch eine eigene *Spannung der Bezugsverflechtungen der Begriffe* strukturiert wird. In den Naturwissenschaften handelt es sich um theoriebeladene und technisch-instrumentelle Begriffe. Wenn die Metaphern in der naturwissenschaftlichen Arbeitstätigkeit nur *vermittels* des technischen Instrumentariums verstanden werden kann, werden diese eine nicht unerhebliche Rolle in der Entstehungsdynamik von naturwissenschaftlichen Konzepten an dieser Stelle ihrer Spannungsentladung und Bezugsverdeckung spielen. Dieser Aspekt wird im letzten Abschnitt mit Hackings wissenschaftstheoretischem Ansatz eines *Eingreifens* mittels *Technik* aufgegriffen.

4.3 Verkörperte und technisch-mediale Metaphorik

4.3.1 Verkörperungstheoretische Grundlagen von Metaphern

Die Sprache ohne den lebendigen Körper zu denken, entspricht einer philosophischen und geisteswissenschaftlichen Auffassung des Menschen, die eindrücklich durch den Cartesianischen Dualismus beschrieben ist: Der menschliche Geist – und für Descartes ging es hierbei auch um die menschliche Seele – muss radikal von allen physischen, d. h. ausgedehnten Dingen, also insbesondere dem lebendige Körper, d. i. vor allem der menschliche Leib, unterschieden werden [18, S. 176–213]. Die Sprache als ein rein geistiges Phänomen käme daher völlig ohne den menschlichen, lebendigen Leib aus. Nach diesem Paradigma müssen alle deskriptiven, sprachwissenschaftlichen Zugänge zum Phänomen der Sprache nur durch sprachinterne Konstituenten der Sprache, wie Referenz und Bedeutung, genügen, um Sprache zu erschließen. Vom cartesianischen Dualismus aus gesehen, lässt sich in der abendländischen Philosophie eine philosophisch-historische Entwicklung nachzeichnen, die diesem Paradigma im Wesentlichen folgt und bis in die Bereiche der modernen Philosophie reicht. Ausschnittsweise sollen hier a) auf die Anfänge und weiteren Fortführungen der sprachanalytischen Philosophie hingewiesen werden, worin Wittgenstein [19, 20] mit seinem *Tractatus* und den *Philosophische Untersuchungen*, Carnap [21] mit seinem Text *Scheinprobleme in der Philosophie: Das Fremdpsychische und der Realismusstreit* und einigen zentralen Artikeln und Quine [22] mit *Wort und Gegenstand* je eigene Schwerpunkte dieses sprachanalytischen Zugangs setzten. Die hier in a) erwähnten Werke und Denker müssen als Ausgangspunkt für die gesamte sprachanalytische Strömung gesehen werden, welche aber insgesamt einen völlig vom menschlichen Körper entkoppelten Weg der Sprachanalyse und der mit der Sprache verbundenen Inhalte wählt. Weiterhin wird b) auf das computationalistisches und neurofunktionelles Verständnis des Geistes bzw. des Gehirns verwiesen, wie man es etwa bei Daniel Dennett oder Thomas Metzinger finden kann. Auch in dieser philosophischen Strömung reicht ein wie auch immer *verdrahtetes neuronales Netz* ohne einen lebendigen Körper völlig aus, um Modelle des Geistes und der Sprache zu entwickeln. Schließlich führt dies zu c) spezifischen Formen des Transhumanismus und der Philosophie der künstlichen Intelligenz, bei denen grundsätzlich ein *rechnerisches Bild des Geistes* vorherrscht und kein lebendiger Körper benötigt wird. Der philosophische Verkörperungsansatz – Embodiment – bricht mit dieser vorherrschenden Vorstellung des Menschen und insbesondere eines Konzeptes von Sprache, welches unabhängig vom menschlichen, interagierenden Körper wäre [2, 23–26]. Damit wird die zentrale These vertreten, dass kognitive, mentale und perzeptive Fähigkeiten inklusive der Sprache auf den lebendigen Leib unter Berücksichtigung der sensomotorischen Kapazitäten des menschlichen Körpers zurückzuführen sind.

Die mit dem Verkörperungsansatz vertretenen Thesen besitzen sicherlich ihre Grenzen darin, dass beispielsweise die Sprache nach einer *hinlänglichen* Verfestigung, Vergemeinschaftung und Beherrschung, ebene eine vom Körper losgelöste symbolische Form darstellt. Sie erscheint uns in diesem Sinne ebenso vom konkret Leiblichen losgelöst erlebbar zu sein, womit ein Reduktionismus auf bloße Leiblichkeit auszuschließen ist, d. h. es muss bei allen Zugeständnissen des Verkörperungsansatzes gesehen werden, dass es Facetten der Spracherscheinung und des Spracherwerbs gibt, die eben nicht völlig verleiblicht sind. Die Sprache ermöglicht als enaktive, symbolische Form eine *Distanz* zu den weltlichen Dingen. Hiervon abgesehen, erfahren wir als Menschen seit unserer Geburt *Widerständigkeiten* und *Erlebnisse* die wiederkehrend sind und damit bestimmte Strukturen im Verstehen festlegen: Gravitation, Hindernisse, Kräfte, die mit der Hand ergriffenen Gegenstände und die damit verbundenen taktilen und funktionellen Objekteigenschaften werden beständig erlebt und schreiben mit dieser Erfahrung ein dazugehöriges Verstehen fort. Die Widerständigkeiten und Erlebnisse werden primär durch den lebendigen Körper erfahren, wodurch ein Verstehen auf Basis der sensomotorischen Gegebenheiten etabliert wird. Das von Johnson entwickelte Konzept im Hinblick auf diese wiederkehrenden Strukturen nennt er *image schema* und seit Michael Krois' Text *Tastbilder – Zur Verkörperungstheorie ikonischer Formen* [27] wird der deutsche Begriff *Bildschema* oder *bildschematische Strukturen* verwendet. Das bekannteste Bildschema ist das *Behälterschema* (container schema), [1, S. 23]. Beständig erfahren wir seit unserer Geburt das Behälterschema, welches darin besteht, dass es ein Innen und ein Außen geben muss, welches zumindest partiell durch eine Begrenzung abgetrennt ist. Der eigene Körper, welcher Nahrung zu sich führt und Atemluft einatmet, fungiert als Behälter. Trinkgefäße, Eimer, Schüsseln, die Spielzeugkiste usw. dienen uns als Behälter für Flüssigkeiten, Schüttgut und andere Gegenstände, die in diesen Behältern aufbewahrt werden. Johnson macht an diesem Beispiel zentrale Eigenschaften dieser kognitiven Verstehensweise des Behälters fest und motiviert damit das Konzept des *Bildschemas*: „In sum, image schemata operate at a level of mental organization that falls between abstract propositional structures, on the one side, and particular concrete images, on the other" [1, S. 29]. Man hat es daher weder mit konkreten Bildern noch mit verbalisierbaren Propositionen zu tun. Die bildschematischen Strukturen emergieren als Verstehensstrukturen aus der leiblichen Interaktion und setzen sich in andere Bereiche fort. Johnson selbst fasst die zentrale Idee zu den bildschematischen Strukturen wie folgt zusammen:

> [...] in order for us to have meaningful, connected experiences that we can comprehend and reason about, there must be pattern and order to our actions, perceptions, and conceptions. A schema is a recurrent pattern, shape, and regularity in, or of, these ongoing ordering activities. These patterns emerge as meaningful structures for us chiefly at the level of our bodily movements through space, our manipulation of objects, and our perceptual interactions. It is important to recognize the dynamic character of image schemata [1, S. 29].

Neben dem Behälterschema stellen die Autoren Lakoff und Johnson weitere Schemata vor: *Pfadschema, Kraftschema, Balance-* bzw. *Gleichgewichtsschema, Hindernisschema,* usw. Das Entscheidende bei diesen Schemata besteht darin, dass sie intermodal und gekreuztmodale Verstehensstrukturen erzeugen: Sie werden (a) primär durch den sensomotorisch agierenden Körper festgelegt, im Laufe der Zeit stabilisiert und erneut in vergleichbaren Kontexten aufgerufen. Sie können (b) sich in Form von wahrnehmungsmäßigen Situationen neu gestalten und befestigen. Das *Gleichgewicht* kann beispielsweise bei einem schief hängenden Gemälde erkannt werden. Ähnliche visuelle, ferner auditive, taktile u. a. sensorische Modalitäten können teilweise durch diese bildschematischen Strukturen mit bestimmt sein. Die Bildschemata können (c) bei kognitiven Prozessen im Mentalen, d. h. hier dem Denken als Prozess, beteiligt sein. Ein klassisch gewordenes Beispiel besteht in der Fähigkeit des mentalen Rotierens. Schließlich finden sich (d) die Bildschemata als *metaphorische Erweiterungen* in der Sprache wieder. Diese Konzepte bilden ein Skelett in Form von räumlichen Metaphern innerhalb jeder Sprache, die ohne einen leiblich agierenden Körper schwerlich verständlich werden können. Für das *Behälterschema* wird in einigen europäischen Sprachen die Präposition *in* verwendet: Peter geht *in* das Haus; Luft ist *im* Schlauch; Wut hat sich *im* Bauch angesammelt; Florian ist *in* Sieglinde verliebt; usw. In anderen Sprachen kann dies durch eine andere grammatikalische Struktur, etwa durch Prä- oder Suffixe an verbalen oder nominalen Wörtern, gegeben sein. Andere Beispielsätze für andere Bildschemata lassen sich bei Lakoff und Johnson finden [2–4, 28]. Es muss betont werden, dass die *metaphorischen Erweiterungen* auf Basis von bildschematischen Strukturen lediglich ein Skelett bzw. ein Gerüst für die Metaphorik einer Sprache bilden, womit ein Reduktionismus der gesamten Metaphorik auf derartige räumliche Bildmetaphorik ausgeschlossen ist. Wegen der komplexen Bildungsmöglichkeiten von Metaphern und der Vielzahl von andersartigen Metaphern, die sich nicht auf eine derartige Raummetaphorik zurückführen lassen, können nicht alle metaphorischen Erscheinungen durch bildschematische Strukturen gebildet werden.

Nichtsdestoweniger bilden bildschematische Struktur aufgrund ihrer modalübergreifenden Verstehensmöglichkeiten eine Basis für *fortführende* Metaphern, die komplexerer Natur sind. Im Laufe des Artikels werde ich hierauf nochmals zurückkommen. Eine für die *Entstehungsdynamik* von Metaphern wichtiger Zusammenhang besteht in der von Johnson ursprünglich stammenden Motivation für eine Heraushebung von verkörperten Verstehensstrukturen, die in der Betonung der *Imaginationsfähigkeit* besteht: „My use of the term [schema] derives from its original use as it was first elaborated by Immanuel Kant. He understood schemata as a nonpropositional structures of imagination“ [1, S. 19]. Die wissenschaftliche Arbeitsweise ist durchzogen von einer Reihe von technischen *bildgebenden* Verfahren, die in einer intrinsischen Art unsere Imagination aufrufen, um uns ein modellhaftes Bild der Welt zu erzeugen. Im Anschluss an Flusser kann man von einer medial erzeugten Technoimagination [7, S. 171–222] sprechen, d. h. der wissenschaftlich arbeitende Mensch imaginiert nicht primär über den zu erforschenden Gegenstandsbereich sein Forschen sondern vielmehr über die medial vermittelten Instrumentarien. Es scheint naheliegend zu sein, dass die technischen Metaphern sich im Wechselspiel von technischen Instrumentarium und modellierter Gegenständlichkeit aufhalten. Gerade hier wird dieses Wechselspiel ebenfalls durch eine ganze Reihe von bildschematischen Strukturen verstärkt, was in der Natur der *Raummetaphorik* der bildschematischen Strukturen selbst liegt und was zugleich dem Umstand geschuldet ist, dass die naturwissenschaftlichen Gegenstandsbereiche mit *materiellen Dingen* zu tun haben. In solch einem Zusammentreten werden gerade die basalen bildschematischen Strukturen wie Behälter-, Balance-, Kräfte-, Hindernis- und Pfadschema virulent: Biologische Zellen oder Organe können durch Membranen bzw. Zellwände als *Behälter* aufgefasst werden, Potentiale und Felder werde in *Gleichgewicht* oder *Ungleichgewicht* gedacht, auf Teilchen und Moleküle wirken *Kräfte*, diese beschreiben ferner *Wege* und werden durch *Hindernis* an ihrer Fortbewegung gestört, usw. Die Liste kann beliebig fortgesetzt werden und im Weiteren kann nur selektiv auf einige Beispiele eingegangen werden, um diese auffallende Verschränkung zu betonen. Um dies zu bewerkstelligen, werden die zentralen Eigenschaften bildschematischer Strukturen nochmals zusammengefasst: a) bildschematische Strukturen stellen basale Strukturen des Verstehens dar, die von physisch-räumlichen Interaktionen als Erfahrungsstrukturen herstammen, b) bildschematische Strukturen wirken präreflexiv und sind von propositionalen Überzeugungen verschieden, d. h. sie sind nicht-propositional, c) bildschematische Strukturen kommen in verschiedenen Erscheinungsweisen vor, womit sie sich in unterschiedlichen Verstehensstrukturen *überkreuzen* (cross-modal structures of understanding), namentlich lassen sich vier Bereiche nennen: leibliche Interaktion (leibliches Verstehen), Kognition (mentales Verstehen), Wahrnehmung (perzeptives Verstehen), metaphorische Erweiterung mittels Raummetaphern (sprachliches Verstehen).

4.3.2 Intuitives Design und technische Werkzeuge – Metaphern der Instrumente

Im folgenden Abschnitt werden einige Beispiele herangezogen, um die *Entstehungsdynamik* von naturwissenschaftlicher Metaphorik zumindest partiell näher zu bestimmen. Dabei werden die Ergebnisse aus den vorigen Abschnitten zusammengetragen, um einen Ausblick auf die Vielschichtigkeit dieser Entstehungsdynamik naturwissenschaftlicher Metaphorik zu verdeutlichen. Mit dem Konzept einer *Entstehungsdynamik* wird auf den oben diskutieren fünften Punkt in Blacks Liste Bezug genommen. Die Metaphern entstehen zumeist in stark kontextsensitiven Zusammenhängen, womit man auf die *Umgebung* und die *lebensweltlichen* Bedingungen naturwissenschaftlicher Praxis zurückgeworfen wird. Mit lebensweltlichen Bedingungen sind hier die *vertrauten* und *nicht hinterfragten, technisch-medialen Bedingungen* naturwissenschaftlicher Umgebungspraxis gemeint. In einer ersten Sichtung dieser Umgebungspraxis lassen sich nach Jörn Hurtienne [29–31] eine ganze Reihe von bildschematischen Strukturen in den medialen Interaktionsschnittstellen wieder erkennen, womit das *Design* der Mensch-Maschine-Interaktion oder spezieller Mensch-Computer-Interaktion angesprochen wird. Im Bereich der Ergonomie spielen Bildschemata eine explizite Rolle in der Verbesserung dieser Schnittstellen zwischen Mensch und Instrument. Tastaturen, Regler, Knöpfe, Bildschirme und andere bildgebende Verfahren, aber auch Werkzeuge und Instrumente der Naturwissenschaftler können hierunter verstanden werden. Diese habe zumeist eine eigene Geschichte, die im Hinblick auf ihre Schnittstellen und Bedienbarkeit neben den *eigentlichen* zugrundeliegenden Modellen und Methoden unentbehrlich für das naturwissenschaftliche Forschen sind. Einfache Beispiele wie etwa die Schieberegel, die als Potentiometer für die zu verstärkenden Signale, Felder, Lautstärke usw. dienen, gehen nach dem bildschematischen Prinzip vor: *oben ist mehr, unten ist wenig*. Andere Regler und Armaturen für flüssige Medien im ingenieurwissenschaftlichen und medizintechnischen Bereichen rufen ähnliche bildschematische Strukturen bei der Steuerung von Stoffströmen hervor: Hindernis-, Blockade- und Wegschema werden mit diesen Reglern explizit angesprochen. Durch die Digitalisierung und Computerisierung geraten die ursprünglichen Anzeiger (bspw. Zeiger von Zeigermessgeräten) in die zweidimensionalen Anzeiger (Displays) der Forschersoftware auf einem Computer, womit nochmals auf eine andere Art und Weise im Sinne der Ergonomie bildschematische Strukturen im Design der Software selbst eingebettet sind. Neben zweidimensionalen piktoralen Repräsentationen (Buttons, scrollbare Regler, u. a.) kann die Software direkte *numerische Voreinstellungen* (d. h. explizite Zahlenwerte) auf Basis der in die technischen Instrumente gegossenen Modelle abverlangen.

All dies führt im Alltag des naturwissenschaftlichen Arbeitens zu einer eigenen Metaphorik, die technisch-medialer Natur ist, womit die durch Boyd formulierte theoriebasierende Metaphern durch eben diese technisch-medialen Metaphern ergänzt werden müssen. Diese Metaphorik betrifft sowohl das Kommunizieren der Wissenschaftler und Wissenschaftlerinnen untereinander, als auch die bereits verschriftlichte Form der Artikel und Veröffentlichungen, in denen ein nicht unerheblicher Teil auch die Methoden und Instrumente darstellen und reflektieren muss. Die technisch-wissenschaftlichen Instrumente spiegeln einen Forschungsstil bzw. ein Forschungsparadigma ihrer jeweiligen Forschergeneration wider [32]. Sie führen zu typischen bildgebenden, technischen und naturwissenschaftlichen Verfahren, die selbst eine eigenständige Metaphorik etablieren. Im *technischen Bild* liegen neben theoriebeladenen Erkenntnissen ferner mannigfaltige Probleme, die oben bereits durch einen fehlenden sinnvollen Eintritt in den *sensus communis* erklärt worden sind. Als Beispiel möchte ich hier zum einen die bildgebenden Verfahren der Neurowissenschaften und die Geschichte des Mikroskop schlaglichtartig diskutieren, um die Art und Weise des theoretisierenden und technisch-medialen Metaphorisieren zu durchleuchten.

Das bildgebende Verfahren des fMRT basiert auf dem BOLD-Signal, welches eine *indirekte* Methode ist und auf die magnetische Eigenschaft des Hämoglobins zurückzugreift, wobei hier der Oxygenierungsgrad des Hämoglobins eine Rolle spielt. Auf einer tieferliegenden Ebene nutzt man den Eigendrehimpuls (Spin) und das damit verbundene magnetische Dipolmoment von Atomkernen, welches gerade die Grundlage für die Kernspinresonanz bildet. Diese technischen Details, die an dieser Stelle nur genannt werden und nicht in ihren mathematisch-ingenieurwissenschaftlichen Grundlagen dargestellt werden kann, bleiben zumeist unbekannt im Hintergrund der wissenschaftlichen Erforschung der Neurowissenschaft, die sich im Rahmen eines Aufgaben-neuronale-Aktivitäts-Paradigmas mit bestimmten Atlanten von Gehirnregionen[1] und ihrer Aktivität im Zuge von expliziten Aufgaben gegenüber den Probanden beschäftigen. Am Bildschirm selbst verbleiben bereits *interpretierende* Thermobilder (Farbskalen von Blau über Grün und Gelb bis Rot), die in Anbetracht der Tatsache, dass die Voxel-Muster-Analyse recht grob im Verhältnis zur eigentlichen Größe von Neuronen ist, nur eine geringe Auflösung zur Verfügung stellen: Sofern bei Experimenten von „neuronaler Aktivität" die Rede ist, werden all diese Ebenen der indirekten Bilderstellung im besten Fall metaphorisch mitgedacht oder schlichtweg ignoriert. Diese vielschichtigen Probleme der Neurowissenschaften werden nur bedingt von der Neurophilosophie reflektiert, wohingegen wissenschaftstheoretische Überlegungen in Form einer *kritischen Neurowissenschaft* [33, 34] die metaphorischen Abhängigkeiten des Sprechens über Gehirnfunktionen von ihren zugrundeliegenden bildgebenden Verfahren mit herausstellen. Anstatt weiterhin an dem Paradigma von *positiven Aufgaben* für Probanden festzuhalten, geht man beim *Resting state fMRI* von einem *negativen-Aufgabesituation* (task-negative state) aus, um die Methode der funktionellen Magnetresonanztomographie angepasst an den eigenfunktionalen Aktivität des Gehirns zu begegnen. Es wird vielfach diskutiert, ob dieser Paradigmenwechsel sinnvoll und gerechtfertigt ist. Hiervon abgesehen, scheint aber mit dieser Forschungsänderung ein metaphorischer Wechsel einher zugehen, der von einer *task-positiv state* zu einem *task-negative state* übergeht.

Eine ähnliche Herangehensweise lässt sich durch Hackings Überlegungen zu einer wissenschaftlichen Praxis erkennen, die von einem *gelungenen* und *vorstrukturierten Eingreifen* ausgeht, anstatt bloß das Theoretisieren und Beobachten als wissenschaftliche Praxis zu deklarieren. Dieses vorstrukturierte Eingreifen hängt im hohen Maße von den bildgebenden Verfahren ab, die als Grundlage für die Modellbildung und die Theoretisierung der beobachteten Gegenstandsbereiche dienen. In seiner Aufarbeitung einer Geschichte der Mikroskopie [6, S. 319–323], wird zum einen gezeigt, dass das Sprechen über das, was mit dem Mikroskop gesehen wird, vom Stand der Instrumentarien abhängt. Vom Leeuwenhoek-Mikroskop über das Auflichtmikroskop nach Robert Hooke bis hin zu den modernen Zeiss-Mikroskopen und schließlich neueren Transmissionselektronenmikroskopen gelangt man zu unterschiedlichen Auffassungen und Modellen, von dem was gesehen wird. Nach Hacking war man in dieser Geschichte der Mikroskopie erst im 19. Jhdt. gesichert davon ausgegangen, dass man mit dem Mikroskop tatsächlich ein *Abbild der Realität* wahrnimmt. Aber selbst an die-

1 Funktionelle Gehirnatlanten haben selbst eine eigene Historie, worin etwa das Wernicke-Areal, Broca-Areal oder die bekannten Körperprojektionen nach W. G. Penfield lediglich den Beginn einer Verortung von funktionellen Zentren des Gehirns darstellen.

ser Stelle bedarf es einer klareren Sprechweise, denn es macht gerade bei modernen bildgebenden Verfahren eher Sinn von einer *Wechselwirklichkeit* auf Basis eines spezifischen Instrumentariums zu sprechen als von einem Abbild der Realität: Beim Elektronenmikroskop handelt es sich um „Abbildungen von Wechselwirkungen zwischen dem Objekt und der das Bild auslösenden Strahlung" [6, S. 345]. Diese Wechselwirkungen und Wechselwirklichkeiten bedürfen nach Hacking auch expliziter weiterer Ergänzungen durch andere wissenschaftliche Methoden, wie es Hacking anhand der Theoriebildung der Blutkörperchen in der Biochemie verdeutlicht: „Die Mikroskopie wird von sich aus niemals vollständig Auskunft geben über diese Körperchen [Blutkörperchen] [...]. Die Biochemie muß zu Hilfe gerufen werden" [6, S. 335]. Hacking macht deutlich, dass andere wissenschaftliche Methoden neben der Elektronenmikroskopie, in diesem Fall mit Hilfe von spektroskopische Analysegeräte herangezogen werden müssen, um ein vollständigeres Bild der Objektbereiche, hier eben Blutkörperchen, zu erhalten. All diese Schritte eines gelingenden Eingreifens in die Objektbereiche ist im Alltag durch spezifische Metaphern, des *Messens*, des *Kalibrierens*, des *Modellierens*, des *Kalkulierens*, des *Experimentierens* und des *Erstellens von hypothetisch-deduktiven Schemata* [6, S. 348–363] vielschichtig metaphorisch besetzt. Die Metaphorik, die dann im *Spezifischen* zu finden wäre, ist an dieser Stelle unüberschaubar, denn die wissenschaftliche Verzweigung ist derart fortgeschritten, dass jede Forschergruppe und Forschergeneration entlang ihrer Objektbereiche und eben gewählten Instrumentarien *spezifische Sondermetaphern* einführt. Zumeist führen diese Sondermetaphern neben mathematisierten Formeln zu diagrammatischen und piktoralen Darstellungen (Kurven, Diagramme usw.) auf Basis der jeweiligen Modelle, die immer mit den Messgeräten bzw. Instrumenten und daher schließlich medial gedacht werden müssen.

4.4 Zusammenfassung und Ausblick

Die *Entstehungsdynamik* von naturwissenschaftlichen Metaphern steht im Vordergrund dieses Artikels. Dabei wurden zwei Aspekte deutlich hervorgehoben. Zum einen muss im Rahmen des alltäglichen naturwissenschaftlichen Agierens die verkörperte Seite der Metaphorik berücksichtigt werden. Dies trifft sowohl auf die theoretisierende Modellierung der Objektbereiche als auch auf die medial-technischen Instrumentarien zu. Hierbei wurde auf die von Lakoff und Johnson entwickelte Metapherntheorie zurückgegriffen. Zum anderen scheinen die Objektbereiche des naturwissenschaftlichen Arbeitens nicht ausschließlich durch das Theoretisieren, Modellieren und Beobachten gegeben zu sein. Vielmehr legen die technischen Instrumente selbst die Forschungsparadigmen und eine dazugehörige Metaphorik fest. Die naturwissenschaftlichen Metaphern besitzen neben einer allgemeinen Sprechweise (Kalibrieren, Kalkulieren usw.) eine forscherspezifische Sprache, der weiter nachgegangen werden muss. Schließlich bleibt offen, wie neben den theoretisierenden ferner die technisch-medialen Metaphern sinnvoll in einen *sensus communis*, d. h. in die breite Öffentlichkeit geraten kann. Dies scheint eine zentrale Aufgabe der *Wissenschaftskommunikation* zu sein und wie mein Artikel versucht hat zu zeigen, muss auf die technisch-mediale Umgebungspraxis von Wissenschaftlerinnen und Wissenschaftler eingegangen werden. Nur so kann ein vollständiges Bild wissenschaftlicher Praxis und die Art der metaphorischen Sprechweisen verständlich werden und zugleich eine Hypostasierung von Wunsch- und Falschvorstellung wissenschaftlicher Ergebnisse vermieden werden. Ein Punkt, der an dieser Stelle ergänzt werden müsste, besteht in dem unausgesprochenen Umstand, dass viele wissenschaftliche Tatsachenergebnisse in der zeitgenössischen Wissenschaft vielmehr in Formen von *statistisch gestützten Forschungsergebnissen* bestehen. Sicherlich gilt dies nicht für alle naturwissenschaftlichen Aufbereitungen, aber hier liegt nochmals eine tieferliegende Metaphorik, der Hacking in seinem Buch *The Taming of Chance* [35] ansatzweise nachgegangen ist.

Literatur

[1] Johnson, M.: The body in the mind: The bodily basis of meaning, imagination, and reason. University of Chicago press, Chicago, 1986.
[2] Lakoff G., Johnson M.: Philosophy in the Flesh. Basic Books, New York, 1999.
[3] Lakoff G., Johnson M.: Metaphors we live by. University of Chicago press, Chicago, 2008.
[4] Lakoff G., Johnson M.: Philosophy in the Flesh: The Embodied Mind and Its Challenge to Western Thought. University of Chicago press, Chicago, 2013.
[5] Black M.: Die Metapher. In: Haverkamp, A. (Hrsg.): Theorie der Metapher. Wissenschaftliche Buchgesellschaft, Darmstadt, 1996 [1954].
[6] Hacking, I.: Einführung in die Philosophie der Naturwissenschaften. Reclam, Stuttgart, 1996.
[7] Flusser, V.: Kommunikolgie. Bollmann Verlag, Mannheim, 1996.
[8] Haverkamp, A. (Hrsg.): Theorie der Metapher. Wissenschaftliche Buchgesellschaft, Darmstadt, 1996.
[9] Haverkamp, A. (Hrsg.): Die paradoxe Metapher. Suhrkamp, Frankfurt am Main, 1998.
[10] Henle P.: Die Metapher. In: Haverkamp, A. (Hrsg.): Theorie der Metapher. Wissenschaftliche Buchgesellschaft, Darmstadt, 1996 [1958].
[11] Richards I. A.: Die Metapher. In: Haverkamp, A. (Hrsg.): Theorie der Metapher. Wissenschaftliche Buchgesellschaft, Darmstadt, 1996 [1936].
[12] Cohen, T.: Figurative Rede und figurative Akte. In: Haverkamp, A. (Hrsg.): Die paradoxe Metapher. Suhrkamp, Frankfurt am Main, 1998 [1975].
[13] Ortony A. (Hrsg.): Metaphor and Thought. Cambridge University Press, Cambridge, 1993 [1979].
[14] Gentner, D., Jeziorski M.: The shift from metaphor to analogy in Western science. In: Ortony A. (Hrsg.): Metaphor and Thought. Cambridge University Press, Cambridge, 1993.
[15] Boyd R.: Metaphor and theory change: What is "metaphor" a metaphor for? In: Ortony A. (Hrsg.): Metaphor and Thought. Cambridge University Press, Cambridge, 1993.
[16] Dennett D.: Consciousness Explained. Little, Brown, Boston, 1991.
[17] Davidson D.: Was Metaphern bedeuten. In: Haverkamp, A. (Hrsg.): Die paradoxe Metapher. Suhrkamp, Frankfurt am Main, 1998 [1978].
[18] Descartes R.: Medidationes de Prima Philosophia – Mediationen über die Erste Philosphie. Reclam Verlag, Stuttgart, 1986.

[19] Wittgenstein L.: Tractatus logico-philosophicus Logisch-philosophische Abhandlung. Suhrkamp Verlag, Frankfurt am Main, 2003.
[20] Wittgenstein L.: Philosophische Untersuchungen. Suhrkamp Verlag, 9. Auflage, Frankfurt am Main, 2003.
[21] Carnap R.: Scheinprobleme in der Philosophie: Das Fremdpsychische und der Realismusstreit. Suhrkamp, Frankfurt am Main, 1966.
[22] Quine W.v.O.: Wort und Gegenstand. Reclam Verlag, Stuttgart, 1980.
[23] Merleau-Ponty M.: Phänomenologie der Wahrnehmung. De Gruyter, Berlin, 1966.
[24] Varela F., Thompson E., Rosch E.: The Embodied Mind. Cognitive Science and Human Experience. MIT Press, Cambridge, 1991.
[25] Gallagher, S.: How the Body Shapes the Mind. Oxford University Press, New York, 2005.
[26] Wild M., Hufendiek R., Fingerhut J. (Hrsg.): Philosophie der Verkörperung: Grundlagentexte zu einer aktuellen Debatte. Suhrkamp Verlag, Berlin, 2013.
[27] Krois J.M.: Tastbilder – Zur Verkörperungstheorie ikonischer Formen. In: Bredekamp H., Lauschke, M.: Bildkörper und Körperschema. Akademie Verlag Actus et Imago, Berlin, 2013.
[28] Schneider D.: Dynamik des Verstehens – Eine phänomenologische Untersuchung der Dynamik bildschematischer Strukturen. Logos Verlag, Berlin, 2017.
[29] Hurtienne, J.: How Cognitive Linguistics inspires HCI: Image schemas and image-schematic metaphors. International Journal of Human-Computer Interaction, 33 (1): 1–20, 2017.
[30] Hurtienne J, Huber S, Baur C: Supporting user interface design with image schemas: The ISCAT database as a research tool. In: Hedblom M. M., Kutz O. (Hrsg.): Proceedings of the Sixth Image Schema Day. CEUR Workshop Proceedings, Vol 3140, 2022.
[31] Baur C, Wienrich C, Hurtienne J: Form follows mental models: Finding instantiations of image schemas using a design eesearch approach. In: Mueller F, Greuter S, Khot RA, Sweetser P, Obrsit M (Hrsg.) DIS'22: Designing Interactive Systems Conference: 586–598, 2022.
[32] Bredekamp H., Schneider B., Dünkel V. (Hrsg.): Das Technische Bild – Kompendium zu einer Stilgeschichte wissenschaftlicher Bilder. De Gruyter, Berlin, 2008.
[33] Choudhury S. (Hrsg.), Slaby J. (Hrsg.): Critical Neuroscience: A Handbook of the Social and Cultural Contexts of Neuroscience. Wiley-VCH, Weinheim, 2012.
[34] Craver, C.F.: Explaining the Brain: Mechanisms and the Mosaic Unity of Neuroscience. Clarendon Press, Oxford, 2007.
[35] Hacking, I.: The Taming of Chance. Cambridge University Press, Cambridge, 1990.

Joachim Boldt

5 Maschinenmetaphern und Ethik in der Synthetischen Biologie

Abstract: Das Ausmaß, in dem Maschinenmetaphern in der synthetischen Biologie verwendet werden, ist auffällig. Diese Metaphern beinhalten eine spezifische Sichtweise auf Organismen sowie auf den wissenschaftlichen und technologischen Fortschritt. Ausdrücke wie „genetically engineered machine“, „genetic circuit“ und „platform organism“, die aus den Bereichen Elektronik, Automobilbau und Informationstechnologie stammen, heben bestimmte Aspekte der Funktionsweise von Lebewesen hervor, während sie gleichzeitig andere Aspekte wie evolutionäre Veränderungen und Interdependenzen in Ökosystemen ausblenden. Da letztere Aspekte z. B. für die Risikobewertung von unkontrollierten Verwendungen synthetischer Organismen relevant sind, ist es ethisch geboten, sich diese Implikationen der Maschinenmetaphern bewusst zu machen. Darüber hinaus wird aus der Perspektive der Maschinenmetapher die Betrachtung eines Lebewesens als „moral agent“ bzw. „moral patient“ zweifelhaft. Wenn man Lebewesen, einschließlich Menschen, als Maschinen ansieht, wird es schwierig, die Zuschreibung eines moralischen Status zu rechtfertigen. Schließlich verstärkt die Maschinenmetapher den Glauben an das Potenzial der synthetischen Biologie, eine alleinige entscheidende Rolle bei der Lösung gesellschaftlicher Probleme zu spielen, und verdeckt die Rolle alternativer und begleitender technologischer, sozialer und politischer Maßnahmen.[1]

5.1 Einführung

Ein wichtiger Teil der moralischen Herausforderungen der Gentechnik rührt von Missverständnissen her, die durch die Verwendung von Metaphern gefördert werden, so der Philosoph Peter Janich [1]. Was Janich in Bezug auf die Metapher der genetischen Information schreibt, gilt auch für die Maschinenmetapher der synthetischen Biologie. Die Maschinenmetapher steht für ein spezifisches Verständnis der synthetischen Biologie. Sie kann sowohl als Ausdruck dieses Verständnisses von Synthetischer Biologie gelesen werden als auch daraufhin befragt werden, welchen Einfluss sie auf die resultierende Forschung hat [2, 3].

1 Dieser Text ist zuerst erschienen als: Boldt, J. Machine metaphors and ethics in synthetic biology. *Life Sci Soc Policy* 14, 12 (2018). https://doi.org/10.1186/s40504-018-0077-y. Übersetzung ins Deutsche vom Autor.

https://doi.org/10.1515/9783112215685-005

Zum einen beinhalten Metaphern Denkweisen über die Ontologie des eigenen Forschungsobjekts und über die Natur der eigenen Forschungstätigkeit selbst. In Bezug auf die synthetische Biologie ist beispielsweise immer wieder umstritten, ob die von der Maschinenmetapher vorgeschlagenen ontologischen Merkmale angemessen erfassen, was ein Organismus tatsächlich ist und wie er beschrieben und erklärt werden kann [4–6]. Zum anderen können solche ontologischen Annahmen ethische Implikationen haben für z. B. die Wahrnehmung von Fragen der Sicherheit, für das, was man als gerechtfertigte Handlungs- und Reaktionsweisen gegenüber dem Objekt ansieht, und für das, was man einer Technologie als Werkzeug zur Lösung spezifischer Probleme zutraut. Im Folgenden sollen einige der ontologischen Annahmen der Maschinenmetapher herausgearbeitet und analysiert werden. Dabei wird nicht im Mittelpunkt stehen, ob diese Annahmen das, was ein Organismus ist, als solches adäquat erfassen. Stattdessen wird sich die Argumentation darauf konzentrieren zu beschreiben, welche ethisch problematischen Implikationen ein von der Maschinenmetapher inspiriertes Verständnis der synthetischen Biologie und ihrer Forschungsobjekte haben kann. Damit wird hier nicht argumentiert, dass die Maschinenmetapher von vornherein und in jeder Hinsicht als sachlich nicht adäquat abgelehnt werden sollte. Die Maschinenmetapher kann beispielsweise dabei helfen, kontrollierbare Ursachen für molekulare intrazelluläre Prozesse zu suchen und zu identifizieren, und der gezielte Eingriff in diese Regelmäßigkeiten kann dazu beitragen, z. B. einzellige Organismen mit wertvollen neuen Eigenschaften zu entwickeln. Es wird jedoch argumentiert, dass man sich vor Augen halten sollte, dass die Maschinenmetapher eine Metapher ist und als solche bestenfalls Teile der Eigenschaften von Organismen adäquat erfasst. Man sollte sich darüber im Klaren sein, dass diese Diskrepanz die Erwartungen an Organismen und die Art und Weise, wie man sich ihnen gegenüber verhält, auf ethisch relevante Weise beeinflussen kann.

5.2 Die Maschinenmetapher und ihre Implikationen

In der synthetischen Biologie werden, um nur einige Beispiele zu nennen, einzellige Organismen als "genetically engineered machines" [7], intrazelluläre molekulare Prozesse als "genetic circuits" [8] und gentechnisch veränderte Organismen als "platform organisms" bezeichnet [9]. Offensichtlich nutzt die synthetische Biologie die Metapher der Maschine und ihre Varianten, insbesondere ihr informationstechnisches Äquivalent, den Computer, als zentrales konzeptionelles Mittel zur Beschreibung, Erklärung und darauf aufbauenden Veränderung molekularer intra- und interzellulärer Prozesse.

Die Verwendung von Maschinenmetaphern zur Beschreibung und zum Verständnis natürlicher Objekte und Prozesse ist kein neues Phänomen. Im siebzehnten Jahrhundert wurde zu diesem Zweck die mechanische Uhr verwendet, im achtzehnten Jahrhundert war die Waage eine einflussreiche Metapher, im neunzehnten Jahrhundert übernahm die Dampfmaschine diese Rolle, und im zwanzigsten Jahrhundert und bis heute hat der Computer, die informationsverarbeitende Maschine, diese älteren Maschinenmetaphern ersetzt [10, 11]. Alle diese Maschinen sind von Menschen entworfene und hergestellte Artefakte, deren strukturelle und materielle Beschaffenheit als Mittel zur Erreichung eines vordefinierten Zustands dient und somit einen bestimmten Zweck für den Menschen erfüllt. In Anbetracht der Tatsache, dass Lebewesen nicht von Menschen entworfen wurden und ihre Beschaffenheit evolutionstheoretisch nicht mit einem bestimmten vorausgesetzten Zweck erklärt werden kann, den sie erfüllen sollen, mag die weit verbreitete Verwendung von Maschinenmetaphern in der modernen Wissenschaft überraschen. Da es jedoch möglich ist, Organismen oder Teile von Organismen so zu erklären, als ob sie dafür entworfen wären, einen bestimmten Zweck zu erfüllen, lassen sich auch entsprechende kausale Beziehungen in Organismen identifizieren, die ihre zweckmäßige Neugestaltung und ihr Re-Engineering ermöglichen. In diesem Sinne fügen sich Maschinenmetaphern nahtlos in ein Konzept der Naturwissenschaften ein, demzufolge man, wenn man ein Objekt versteht, prinzipiell in der Lage sein sollte, es zu bauen, und demzufolge der erfolgreiche Bau eines Objekts als ein Experiment gilt, das die theoretischen Hypothesen stützt, die zu seinem Entwurf geführt haben [12].

Vor diesem Hintergrund kann die weit verbreitete Verwendung von Maschinenmetaphern in der synthetischen Biologie als Ausdruck des Elans gesehen werden, mit dem die synthetische Biologie rationale Design- und Bauideale in die Biologie einführt. Diese ingenieurwissenschaftliche Methodik ist ein wichtiger Bestandteil der multidisziplinären Forschungsansätze der synthetischen Biologie. Biologie, Chemie, Physik, Informatik und Ingenieurwissenschaften sind Teil dieses Hintergrunds, wobei ingenieurwissenschaftliche Ansätze im Mittelpunkt stehen [13, 14]. Ingenieurwissenschaftliche Prinzipien und Ansätze wie Design, Modularisierung und Standardisierung legen es nahe, die Maschinenmetapher für die Objekte der Analyse und der Eingriffe zu verwenden.

Darüber hinaus fügt sich die Maschinenmetapher nahtlos in ein größeres Narrativ darüber ein, was die synthetische Biologie ist und worauf sie abzielt. Diesem Narrativ folgend ist die synthetische Biologie der jüngste Schritt in der Entwicklung wissenschaftlicher Bottom-up-Erklärungen von Makroobjekten und ihrem Verhalten, der Analyse, und der darauf folgenden Ermöglichung des Nach- und Neubaus, der Synthese [15]. Auf der untersten Ebene analysiert die Physik die Bewegung und Struktur von Atomen, indem sie subatomare Strukturen und Teile identifiziert und analysiert. Auf der nächsten Ebene analysiert die Chemie komplexe Moleküle, indem sie die einfacheren Moleküle und Atome, aus denen komplexe Strukturen bestehen, unter die Lupe nimmt. Auf einer weiteren Ebene werden lebende Moleküle, d. h. Organismen, zum Gegenstand der Analyse. Dies ist der Bereich der "analytischen" molekularbiologischen Forschung, die das Verhalten von Organismen auf ihre inneren molekularen genetischen Strukturen zurückführt. Auf jeder Ebene erlaubt es das analytische Wissen, technologisch einzugreifen, die fraglichen Objekte zu verändern und neue Objekte zu entwickeln. Dies ist die "synthetische" Seite der einzelnen analytischen Wissenschaften. In der Chemie zum Beispiel können natürlich vorkommende Verbindungen wie Zucker oder Vitamine synthetisch hergestellt werden, und darüber hinaus können auch Verbindungen synthetisiert werden, die in der Natur nicht vorkommen, wie zum Beispiel Kunststoffe. Es wird erwartet, dass die synthetische Biologie zu ähnlichen Entwicklungen in Bezug auf Organismen führen wird. Synthetische Biologie wird in der Lage sein, natürlich vorkommende Organismen nachzubauen und mittels DNA-Synthese neuartige Organismen zu schaffen [16].

Diese einfache Darstellung einer Linie wissenschaftlichen Fortschritts und des Stellenwerts der synthetischen Biologie darin ist eng mit einer ontologischen Annahme verbunden. Wenn die Erklärung komplexer Moleküle darauf hinausläuft, dass man die einfachen Moleküle kennt, die in der komplexen Struktur enthalten sind, und wenn die Erklärung der Funktion eines Organismus gleichbedeutend ist mit der Identifizierung und Analyse der genetischen Struktur dieses Organismus, dann geht man offensichtlich davon aus, dass die Funktionsweise eines komplexen Objekts das Ergebnis der Gesetze und Regelmäßigkeiten ist, die das Verhalten der Teile dieses Objekts bestimmen. Wenn man also die Teile eines Objekts und ihre Funktionen kennt, kann man das Gesamtverhalten des betreffenden Objekts zuverlässig vorhersagen. Diese ontologische Annahme ist das Bindeglied zur Maschinenmetapher. In Bezug auf übliche Maschinen gelten dieselben Prinzipien der Teil-Ganzes-Beziehung und der Vorhersagbarkeit in umgekehrter Reihenfolge. Wenn man eine Maschine entwirft und zusammenbaut, geht es darum, Teile mit zuverlässigen und vorhersehbaren Funktionen zu kombinieren, um ein komplexes Ergebnis zu erzielen, das seinerseits aufgrund der Zuverlässigkeit seiner Teile bestimmte Funktionen und Zwecke auf zuverlässige und vorhersehbare Weise erfüllt. Wenn das, was man in der synthetischen Biologie tut, von der obigen Darstellung korrekt erfasst wird, muss man folglich davon ausgehen, dass die Objekte der eigenen Forschung wichtige ontologische Aspekte mit jenen Entitäten teilen, die man "Maschinen" nennt. Überträgt man die relevanten Merkmale des Maschinenparadigmas auf den Bereich der synthetischen Biologie und der einzelligen Organismen, so ergibt sich die folgende Liste: Erstens ist das Verhalten eines einzelligen Organismus anhand seiner molekularen, genetischen Bestandteile zu erklären. Einzellige Organismen können also entworfen und Teil für Teil aufgebaut werden. Zweitens wird durch den Entwurf und den Bau eines Organismus eine bestimmte Funktion im Organismus verankert. Diese Funktion erfüllt aus der Sicht des Designers einen bestimmten Zweck. Drittens kann das Verhalten des entstehenden Organismus bei ausreichender Kenntnis seiner Teile zuverlässig vorhergesagt werden [17].

5.3 Antizipation möglicher Folgen für Umwelt und Ökosysteme

Wenn man beabsichtigt, ein zuverlässiges Objekt mit bestimmten Funktionen zu bauen, und wenn man davon ausgeht, dass die Zuverlässigkeit und Vorhersagbarkeit des Objekts ein Ergebnis der Zuverlässigkeit und Vorhersagbarkeit des Verhaltens seiner Teile sind, ist ein natürlicher Ausgangspunkt die Analyse dieser Teile. Sobald man davon ausgehen kann, dass man ausreichende Kenntnisse über die Teile hat, muss die Bestimmung des Verhaltens des Objekts im Prinzip eine Frage der Berechnung sein. Verhält sich das Objekt wiederum auf unvorhergesehene Weise, was möglicherweise zu unbeabsichtigten Nebeneffekten führt, muss die Ursache des Fehlers im inneren Aufbau des Objekts vermutet werden. Stellt man sich nun vor, dass es sich bei diesem Objekt um ein elektronisches Gerät handelt, so deckt diese Perspektive die Anforderungen an den Bau sicherer Maschinen und den Umgang mit Nebenwirkungen hinreichend ab, so kann man annehmen. Stellt man sich das Objekt hingegen als Organismus vor, gibt es gute Gründe, an der Angemessenheit dieser Sichtweise zu zweifeln.

Zum einen entwickeln sich die Organismen weiter. Evolution ist ein Prozess, der zufällige Mutationen innerhalb eines Genoms beinhaltet. Zufällige Mutationen sind per Definition ein unvorhersehbarer Prozess. Dies steht jedem Versuch entgegen, einen stabilen, zuverlässigen Organismus zu entwerfen, der seine Designfunktion von Generation zu Generation beibehält. Evolutionäre Veränderungen sind daher ein Haupthindernis für die Entwicklung von Organismen, deren Verhalten über lange Zeiträume hinweg vorhergesagt werden kann. Um diesem Problem zu begegnen, wurde beispielsweise vorgeschlagen, in gentechnisch veränderte Organismen genetische Schaltkreise einzufügen, die Toxine produzieren. Unter normalen Bedingungen sind die genetischen Schaltkreise unterdrückt und exprimieren das Toxin nicht. Stellt man fest, dass sich der Organismus in unbeabsichtigter Weise vermehrt oder die ihm zugewiesene Umgebung verlässt, kann man den Genschaltkreis aktivieren, indem man z. B. einen Metaboliten hinzufügt. Dann wird das Toxin produziert und die Organismen sterben ab. Wie die Erfahrung zeigt, neigen aber auch diese "suicide genes" dazu, im Laufe der Zeit zu mutieren, wodurch ihre Funktionalität beeinträchtigt wird [18].

Zum anderen interagieren Organismen in vielfältiger Weise miteinander und mit ihrer Umwelt. In mikrobiellen Multispezies-Gemeinschaften beeinflussen sich die Bakterien gegenseitig durch direkten physischen Kontakt, metabolische Abhängigkeiten und koordinierte Signalsysteme und halten so das Gleichgewicht des Ökosystems aufrecht [19]. In Bezug auf mikrobielle Gemeinschaften erfordert die Modellierung solcher Zusammenhänge eine enge und kontinuierliche Zusammenarbeit zwischen theoretischen und experimentellen Disziplinen [10]. Die Modellierung eines Multispezies-Ökosystems, das nicht auf Mikroben beschränkt ist, wäre offensichtlich eine noch größere Herausforderung. Einerseits ist dies für die molekularbiologische Forschungspraxis keine große Überraschung. Andererseits erscheinen solche Mehrebenen-Interaktionen überraschend, wenn man sich auf das Maschinenparadigma beschränkt. Um eine zuverlässige Maschine zu bauen, würde man die Zahl der externen Faktoren, die die Funktionsweise der Maschine beeinflussen können, auf diejenigen beschränken, die notwendig sind, damit die Maschine ihren Konstruktionszweck erfüllt. Wenn man Organismen als Maschinen betrachtet, würde man also nicht erwarten, dass sie auf diese vielfältige Weise mit der Umwelt interagieren. Dies kann dazu führen, dass mögliche negative Auswirkungen von gentechnisch veränderten Organismen in der Umwelt unterschätzt werden, da sie einerseits Produkte der synthetischen Biologie sind und als Maschinen bezeichnet werden, andererseits aber immer noch natürliche Lebewesen sind.

Zusätzlich zu zufälliger Mutation und Wechselwirkungen in Ökosystemen stellen auch Reproduktion und Wachstum die Ideale der Maschinenperspektive in Frage. Maschinen sollen Entitäten sein, deren Verhalten nicht nur vorhersagbar und zuverlässig ist, sondern sie sollen ihre Funktionen auch effizient erfüllen. Bis zu einem gewissen Grad sind Wachstum und Vermehrung von Mikroorganismen eine Voraussetzung dafür, dass sie beispielsweise einen bestimmten wertvollen Stoffwechselstoff in größeren Mengen produzieren können. Oberhalb dieser Grenze jedoch verbrauchen Wachstum und Vermehrung Energie, die sonst im Stoffwechselprozess zur Herstellung größerer Mengen des benötigten Stoffes verwendet werden könnte. Die Tendenz des Lebens, sich sowohl in Bezug auf Individuen als auch in Bezug auf Generationen zu erhalten, konterkariert also ab einem bestimmten Punkt den Versuch, Organismen als effiziente Produktionsanlagen zu nutzen. Die Optimierung von Organismen in dieser Hinsicht wäre daher gleichbedeutend mit der Entwicklung von nicht-lebenden biologischen molekularen Netzwerken, wie z. B. genetischen zellfreien Produktionssystemen.

Zu den sicherheitsrelevanten Merkmalen natürlicher Organismen, die sich nur schwer in das Maschinenparadigma einfügen lassen, ist anzumerken, dass evolutionäre genetische Veränderungen kleine, schrittweise Veränderungen sind. Mutagenese ist eine selektive Veränderung des Genoms und baut auf dem Design auf, wie es sich bis zu diesem Zeitpunkt entwickelt hat, unabhängig davon, ob ein neues Design besser in eine ökologische Nische passt als bestehende Organismen. Auf den ersten Blick scheint die Maschinenmetapher nicht dazu aufzufordern, radikal genetisch veränderte Organismen zu entwickeln, anstatt sich enger an bekannte Organismen zu halten. Wenn sich natürliche Organismen durch die Funktionsweise einer Maschine erklären lassen, könnte der Bau einer Maschine genauso gut darin bestehen, eine leicht veränderte natürliche Vorlage nachzubauen. Wenn man jedoch den Inhalt der Maschinenmetapher in Bezug auf die Beziehungen zwischen Teilen und Ganzem und die Konzepte des wissenschaftlichen Fortschritts berücksichtigt, muss die Beschränkung auf die Neugestaltung natürlicher Organismen als eine unnötige Einschränkung der eigenen wissenschaftlichen und technologischen Fähigkeiten erscheinen. Der Nachbau natürlicher Organismen kann ein erster Schritt sein, um die Behauptung zu untermauern, dass man die Funktionsweise von Organismen genau analysiert und erklärt hat. Der ultimative Beweis für diese Behauptung ist jedoch die Entwicklung und Konstruktion von Organismen, die in der Natur nicht vorkommen. Der Verzicht auf die Erforschung potenzieller Vorteile, die nur neuartige Organismen haben können, wäre eine unkluge Beschränkung auf die ausgetretenen Pfade der Natur, eine Beschränkung, die aus wissenschaftlicher oder technologischer Sicht nicht mehr zu rechtfertigen ist, sobald genügend Wissen über genetische Teile vorhanden ist. Das Streben nach Neuem wird also in diesem Paradigma aus erkenntnistheoretischen Gründen und aus Gründen der Erkundung des Neulands der organismischen Funktionen und ihres möglichen Nutzens vorangetrieben. Überlegungen zur Sicherheit sind kein fester Bestandteil dieser Perspektive, sondern müssen sozusagen von außen hinzugefügt werden. Auf die Spitze getrieben könnte die Entwicklung neuartiger genetischer Organismen auch Organismen mit DNA aus alternativen Aminosäuresystemen umfassen. Da diese xenobiologischen Organismen weniger in der Lage sind, mit natürlichen Organismen zu interagieren, könnten sie in einigen Fällen sogar Sicherheitsvorteile bieten [20]. Generell gilt jedoch: Je radikaler sich ein Organismus genetisch von natürlichen Organismen unterscheidet, desto weniger kann man seine Auswirkungen auf die Umwelt vorhersagen, einschließlich der negativen Folgen. Wie das Beispiel invasiver Arten zeigt, bestehen solche diese Risiken durchaus.

Zusammenfassend lässt sich sagen, dass zufällige Mutationen und evolutionäre Veränderungen sowie Wechselwirkungen zwischen Organismus und Umwelt Merkmale von Organismen sind, die den Versuch, ihr Verhalten zuverlässig vorherzusagen, in Frage stellen. Mutationen verändern die interne genetische Struktur eines Organismus, was zu veränderten Funktionen führen kann, und sie treten, da es sich um Zufallsmutationen handelt, auf unvorhersehbare Weise auf. Die Wechselwirkungen zwischen Organismus und Umwelt umfassen eine große Anzahl von Variablen und Bezugsgrößen, was den Versuch, die Entwicklung von Ökosystemen mit mehreren Arten über größere Zeiträume hinweg zu modellieren, schwierig macht. Aus Maschinenmetaphern- Sicht sind Merkmale von Organismen wie Mutagenese und vielschichtige Umweltinteraktionen unerwartet und unerwünscht. Um eine zuverlässige Maschine zu bauen, möchte man zufällige Änderungen an der Konstruktion vermeiden, die sich auf die Funktion der Maschine auswirken, und man möchte die Zahl der externen Faktoren, die die Funktionsweise der Maschine beeinflussen können, auf diejenigen beschränken, die notwendig sind, damit die Maschine ihren Zweck erfüllt. Wenn man sich also ganz auf die Perspektive des Maschinenparadigmas beschränkt, kann man potenzielle Risiken und Nebenwirkungen übersehen, wenn ein genetisch veränderter Organismus für eine Anwendung in der Umwelt konstruiert wird. In der Logik dieses Paradigmas werden nur wenige Sicherheitsrisiken für Umwelt und Ökosysteme antizipiert und die ontologischen Annahmen des Paradigmas erklären gleichzeitig das Herstellen umfassend gentechnisch veränderter und in diesem Sinne neuartiger Organismen zum ultimativen Erfolgsbeweis für das Paradigma selbst.

Die Behauptung, dass im Maschinenparadigma Eigenschaften wie evolutionäre Veränderungen und Interaktionen innerhalb von Ökosystemen eher ausgeblendet werden, bedeutet nicht, dass die Maschinenmetapher für Organismen gänzlich untauglich ist oder generell als unzweckmäßig gelten muss. Das Maschinenparadigma kann in vielerlei Hinsicht hilfreich sein, wenn man genetische Strukturen analysiert und neuartige genetische Netzwerke entwickelt. Es bedeutet jedoch, dass bei Anwendungen in der Umwelt zusätzliches Fachwissen erforderlich ist, um die Risiken für die Umwelt zu bewerten. Dieses Fachwissen muss sich auf evolutionären Wandel und Wechselwirkungen in Ökosystemen konzentrieren, d. h. es muss Fachwissen aus den Bereichen Ökosystembiologie, Evolutionsbiologie und Entwicklungsbiologie umfassen. Dies ist natürlich keine Neuigkeit für die bestehenden Sicherheitsbewertungen von zur Freisetzung vorgesehenen gentechnisch veränderten Organismen. Diese und andere multidisziplinäre Sicherheitsbewertungsverfahren gibt es bereits. Das Wissen um die möglichen Auswirkungen der Maschinenmetapher auf die Wahrnehmung entsprechender Risiken unterstützt die Bedeutung dieser Verfahren.

Ein weiterer Punkt ist hier noch zu erwähnen. Mutagenese und Neuheit unterscheiden sich in Bezug auf die Herausforderungen der Sicherheitsbewertung. Zunächst einmal erschwert die Mutagenese die Sicherheitsbewertung eines jeden veränderten Organismus. Bei Organismen, die leicht veränderte Versionen einer natürlichen Vorlage sind, kann sich die Risikobewertung jedoch auf die Erfahrungen mit dieser Vorlage stützen. Im Gegensatz dazu wird man bei der Bewertung der Freisetzung eines neuartigen synthetischen Organismus vor größere Herausforderungen gestellt, da schon die Auswirkungen dieses Organismus in seiner jetzigen Form, d. h. vor der möglicherweise in Zukunft auftretenden evolutionären Weiterentwicklung, auf bestehende Ökosysteme schwer zu beurteilen sind. Schließlich gibt es in diesem Fall keine natürliche Vorlage, die als Grundlage für eine Risikobewertung dienen könnte. Diese Herausforderung kann letztlich im Fall radikal veränderter Organismen auch die Forderung plausibel machen, auf die Freisetzung ganz zu verzichten. Abgemildert werden könnte diese Herausforderung, wenn man neuartige Organismen nicht schlagartig, sondern schrittweise, ausgehend von einer nicht radikalen Version des synthetischen Organismus über immer weiter sich vom Vorbild entfernende Varianten, einführt und dieses Verfahren genügend Zeit lässt, um jede Version des Organismus und ihre Auswirkungen auf die Umwelt kennen zu lernen.

5.4 Maschinen und „Moral Agents"

Solange sich die synthetische Biologie auf die gentechnische Veränderung von Einzellern beschränkt, mag die Diskussion über den moralischen Status der veränderten Entitäten abwegig erscheinen. Auch Szenarien zukünftiger Modifikationen von komplexeren Organismen wie Säugetiere und Menschen, wie beispielsweise die Rekonstruktion des Mammuts durch die Veränderung von Elefantenkeimzellen oder die gentechnische Veränderung der menschlichen Keimbahn zur Verbesserung des

Immunsystems [15], scheinen solche Fragen eher nicht aufzuwerfen, da bei derartigen Modifikationen alle wesentlichen Fähigkeiten von Tieren und Menschen erhalten bleiben und es kaum Grund gäbe zu der Annahme, dass sich der moralische Status des Mammuts oder des genetisch veränderten Menschen vom moralischen Status des Elefanten oder des nicht gentechnisch veränderten Menschen unterscheiden sollten. Was sich jedoch ändern würde, wenn sich die synthetische Biologie mehrzelligen Organismen, Säugetieren und Menschen zuwendet, ist, dass der Maschinenmetapher folgend ein Verständnis von Leben und moralischem Status importiert wird, das in Spannung steht zu der Art und Weise, wie wir die Zuschreibung von moralischem Status üblicherweise vornehmen und begründen.

Viele ethische Theorien, darunter der Utilitarismus und die Deontologie, stimmen darin überein, dass eine notwendige Bedingung für moralisches Handeln die Fähigkeit ist, sich von den eigenen Interessen zu distanzieren und über diese Interessen von einem bewertenden Standpunkt aus nachzudenken, der das Wohlbefinden und die Interessen oder die Rechte anderer berücksichtigt. Im Utilitarismus beispielsweise ermöglicht diese reflektierende Distanzierung eine Bewertung möglicher Handlungen im Hinblick auf die Auswirkungen der Folgen dieser Handlungen auf die Interessen anderer, die von den Handlungen betroffen sind. In der kantischen Deontologie besteht die Distanzierung darin, zu bewerten, ob die Maxime der eigenen geplanten Handlung (d. h. die Aussage, dass man in einer bestimmten Situation eine Handlung eines bestimmten Typs ausführen will, um einen bestimmten Zweck zu erreichen) in einer hypothetischen Welt, in der alle moralisch Handelnden dieser Maxime folgen würden, aufrechterhalten werden könnte.

Die Fähigkeit, sich von den eigenen Interessen zu distanzieren, die einen sonst zu einem bestimmten Verhalten veranlassen würden, ist mit dem Maschinenparadigma nicht leicht zu vereinbaren. Zunächst einmal scheint diese Distanzierung die Fähigkeit zu beinhalten, jede Vorhersage über das eigene zukünftige Verhalten zu widerlegen, indem man einfach anders handelt. Wird man mit einer Vorhersage seines Verhaltens konfrontiert oder hat man den Verdacht, dass jemand eine bestimmte Regelmäßigkeit seines Verhaltens in der Vergangenheit ausnutzen will, von der er annimmt, dass sie sich in der Zukunft fortsetzen wird, kann man sein Verhalten ändern und entgegen diesen Erwartungen handeln, wenn man ein Interesse daran hat, nicht vorhersehbar zu sein. Die Aussetzung des eigenen Handelns und die Reflexion darüber scheinen zudem am besten als interpretative Tätigkeit zu verstehen zu sein. Bei der Bestimmung von Interessen oder Maximen geht es um die Bestimmung von Handlungen, zu denen jemand, der seinen Interessen bzw. Maximen folgt, neigt. Es ist oft und überzeugend argumentiert worden, dass Handlungen keine Entitäten sind, die unmittelbar als das wahrgenommen werden können, was sie sind. Ihre Identität hängt von den Zielen ab, denen sie dienen sollen. Diese Ziele können vielfältig sein und sind mit größeren Erzählungen darüber verknüpft, wer die oder der Handelnde ist und welche Art von Leben sie oder er führt. Ob ich zum Beispiel den Rasen mähe, Sport treibe, meiner Frau einen Gefallen tue oder meinen Nachbarn ärgere, lässt sich nicht allein anhand meiner Bewegungen erkennen. Mein Handeln zu verstehen, setzt Wissen über mich, meine Beziehungen, meine Gewohnheiten und meine Pläne voraus [21]. Dieses Wissen wiederum setzt Wissen darüber voraus, wie es ist, Emotionen zu erleben, in Beziehung zu anderen zu stehen und möglicherweise Sinn im Leben als Ganzes zu finden und zu verstehen. Wenn man versucht zu erkennen, was eine Handlung ist, muss man also die fraglichen Ereignisse im Hinblick auf verschiedene Erzählungen interpretieren, die ihnen einen Sinn geben, und diejenige auswählen, die am besten zu dieser spezifischen und anderen meiner Handlungen zu passen scheint. Wenn man auf vergangene Handlungen zurückblickt, helfen diese Erzählungen zu verstehen, was man tatsächlich getan hat und warum. Gleichzeitig bestimmen diese Erzählungen, wie man in Zukunft handeln wird, wenn man nach vorne blickt. Sie lassen bestimmte Optionen sinnvoller erscheinen als andere und veranlassen einen daher zu bestimmten Handlungen.

Nehmen wir an, man baut einen Roboter, der mit einer künstlichen Intelligenz ausgestattet ist, die es ihm ermöglicht, erstens sein Verhalten zu ändern, wenn er mit Vorhersagen dazu konfrontiert wird. Zweitens: Der Roboter denkt über Erzählungen nach, die seinen Handlungen einen Sinn geben, und wendet diese Erzählungen an, um sein künftiges Verhalten zu gestalten. Drittens basieren diese Erzählungen auf dem Wissen darüber, wie es ist, Emotionen zu erleben, mit anderen in Beziehung zu stehen und dem Leben als Ganzem einen Sinn zu geben. Wie es scheint, gäbe es in diesem Fall keinen Grund, dem Roboter nicht den Status eines „moral agent“ zuzuschreiben, es sei denn, es stellt sich heraus, dass der Roboter diese Eigenschaften nicht wirklich besitzt, sondern sie vortäuscht [22].

Aber gäbe es gleichzeitig einen guten Grund, diesen Roboter als Maschine zu bezeichnen, d. h. als ein Objekt, dessen Verhalten sich durch Teile erklären lässt, die effektiv angeordnet sind, um bestimmte Verhaltensziele zu erreichen? In Anbetracht der Tatsache, dass dieser Roboter aufhören kann, das zu tun, wofür er konstruiert wurde, wenn er über seine Konstruktionsziele informiert wird, und in Anbetracht der Tatsache, dass er seine Ziele und seine Zukunft ständig formt und umgestaltet, indem er seine Handlungen im Hinblick auf größere Erzählungen darüber interpretiert, was wichtig ist und seinem Leben einen Sinn verleiht, erscheint dies wenig plausibel. Während dieser Roboter auf der Mikroebene der Bitverarbeitung und der elektronischen Steuerung der Gliedmaßen durchaus als Maschine beschrieben werden kann, würde diese Beschreibung auf der Makroebene nicht mehr passen.

In ähnlicher Weise mögen isolierte Prozesse auf der Ebene molekularer Interaktionen im menschlichen Körper in sinnvoller Weise mit Maschinen vergleichbar sein, aber der Mensch als handelnder und reflektierender Gesamtorganismus, der zu moralischem Handeln fähig ist, ist es kaum. Die Anwendung der Maschinenmetapher auf den Menschen würde darauf hinauslaufen, die Realität der Fähigkeit in Frage zu stellen, sich von seinen Interessen zu distanzieren, falsche Vorhersagen über sein Verhalten zu widerlegen und seine Zukunft gemäß größerer menschlicher Lebenserzählungen zu gestalten. Da dies die Voraussetzungen für moralisches Handeln sind, würde die Anwendung der Maschinenmetapher auf den Menschen darauf hinauslaufen, die Realität der menschlichen Fähigkeit zu moralischem Handeln in Frage zu stellen.

Man kann diesen Gedankengang mit der Annahme des genetischen Determinismus vergleichen. Nach dieser Annahme ist die DNA ein Bauplan, der die phänotypischen Merkmale und das Verhalten determiniert. Da die phänotypischen menschlichen Eigenschaften und das Verhalten durch das Erbgut bestimmt werden, sei der Genotyp die eigentliche Ursache für das menschliche Verhalten, so dass der Glaube an die moralische Handlungsfähigkeit des Menschen eine Illusion sei [23]. Die Maschinenmetapher eignet sich gut für ähnliche Behauptungen, da ihr Erklärungsschema, wonach Teile zuverlässig Verhaltenseffekte der Einheit als Ganzes verursachen, keinen Raum für jene Erklärungsschemata lässt, die Zuschreibungen moralischen Handelns unterstützen.

5.5 Maschinen und „Moral Patients"

Die umfassende Modifikation des menschlichen Genoms mit den Mitteln der synthetischen Biologie ist Science-Fiction, auch wenn Ansätze zur Veränderung genetischer Schaltkreise in Säugetierzellen zur Verhinderung von Krankheiten bereits erforscht werden [24]. Die Modifikation des Genoms von mehrzelligen Organismen, einschließlich Insekten, ist jedoch bedeutend näher an der Realität [25]. Diese Organismen besitzen nach geläufigen Alltagsüberzeugungen und in üblichen lebensweltlichen Praktiken nicht den Status von „moral agents", entsprechend kann die Anwendung der Maschinenmetapher auf diese Organismen ihren moralischen Status in dieser Hinsicht nicht untergraben. Sowohl üblichen Alltagsüberzeugungen zufolge, als auch nach Maßgabe vieler ethischer Theorien haben einige Tiere jedoch einen moralischen Status in dem Sinne, dass der Schutz ihres Wohlergehens eine moralische Verpflichtung darstellt. Diesen Tieren Schaden zuzufügen, stellt prima facie ein moralisches Unrecht dar, das durch andere, übergeordnete moralische Verpflichtungen gerechtfertigt werden muss, um akzeptabel zu sein. Man kann also sagen, dass einige Tiere den Status von „moralischen patients" haben. Es stellt sich dann die Frage, ob die Anwendung der Maschinenmetapher auf diese Tiere die Praxis untergraben kann, ihnen den Status von „moral patients" zuzuschreiben und sie entsprechend zu behandeln.

In der Tierethik werden verschiedene Eigenschaften als Voraussetzungen benannt, die ein Organismus erfüllen muss, um als „moral patient" zu gelten. Die Fähigkeit, Leiden und Freude zu empfinden, ist zum Beispiel ein intuitiv naheliegender erster und grundlegender Kandidat. Erfahrungen von Leid und Freude sind keine neutralen Wahrnehmungen, sondern beinhalten ein Element der Bewertung. Das Erleben von Schmerz und Freude ist mit Bedürfnissen, Wünschen, Interessen oder, als übergreifender Begriff, Einstellungen („attitudes") verbunden [26]. All diese Begriffe legen die Vorstellung nahe, dass tierisches Verhalten der relevanten Art als ein Spannungsverhältnis zwischen einem wahrgenommenen Ist-Zustand und einem antizipierten Soll-Zustand verstanden werden muss. Metaphorisch gesprochen legen Beschreibungen im Sinne von Wünschen, Interessen und Einstellungen im Gegensatz zu Kausalbeschreibungen nahe, dass Verhaltensketten nicht durch Ausgangsbedingungen nach Gesetzen des tierischen Verhaltens vorangetrieben werden, sondern auf Zugkräfte zurückzuführen sind, nämlich auf die Attraktivität oder Unattraktivität verschiedener möglicher zukünftiger Zustände. Die Abwägung dieser Handlungsmöglichkeiten nach den für das Tier wichtigen Aspekten führt ein Element menschenähnlicher Handlungsfähigkeit ein, das im Konzept, ein "subject of a life" sein zu können, zum Ausdruck kommt [27]. Wenn dies ein korrektes Verständnis der Bedingung dafür ist ein „moral patient" zu sein, können der Status von „moral patient" und „moral agent" als Zuschreibungen an Organismen entlang einer Linie der zunehmenden Fähigkeit, zu den eigenen Motivationszuständen Stellung zu beziehen, interpretiert werden. Die Vermeidung von Schmerz, die Suche nach Vergnügen, das Vorhandensein von Bedürfnissen, das Vorhandensein von Wünschen, das Verfolgen von Interessen und die Gestaltung des eigenen Lebens gemäß Erzählungen können als Schritte entlang dieser Linie einer zunehmenden Fähigkeit verstanden werden, unmittelbare Handlungsimpulse zu suspendieren und die eigene Zukunft in Übereinstimmung mit evaluativer Reflexion zu gestalten [28].

Auch hier steht diese Fähigkeit, Subjekt eines Lebens zu sein, in Spannung zur Annahme des Maschinenparadigmas, dass das Verhalten eines Objekts durch interne Teile zu erklären ist, die dieses Verhalten effektiv, zuverlässig und vorhersehbar verursachen. Die Anwendung der Maschinenmetapher auf Tiere, die den Status eines „moral patient" haben, schwächt diese moralischen Statuszuschreibungen, da sie die Annahme in Frage stellt, dass das Verhalten eines Tieres eine grundlegende Form der Handlungsfähigkeit eines Wesens sein kann, das ein Subjekt seines Lebens ist.

Es bleibt unbenommen, dass die Anwendung der Maschinenmetapher auf genetische Prozesse und Netzwerke in höher entwickelten Organismen dazu beitragen kann, technologisch und auch medizinisch nützliches Wissen über diese Prozesse zu sammeln. Wendet man diese Metapher aber auf Tiere und Menschen als ganze Organismen an, werden Merkmale des Verhaltens dieser komplexen Organismen und darauf aufbauende Zuschreibungen von moralischem Status unverständlich.

5.6 Speerspitze von Wissenschaft und Technologie

Die Maschinenmetapher fußt auf einer ontologischen Vorstellung, der zu Folge das Verhalten eines jeden komplexen Objekts durch Bezugnahme auf seine Teile erklärt werden kann. Eine vollständige Erklärung der Wirklichkeit als Ganzer beginnt demnach bei den einfachsten Teilen, geht über die Zwischenstufen zunehmender molekularer Größe und Komplexität und endet mit der Erklärung hochentwickelter Organismen und Menschen. Im Prinzip sollten die Erklärungen des Verhaltens der komplexen Organismen so die Erklärungen des Verhaltens der Teile auf jeder Zwischenstufe enthalten, da diese als Teilmenge der Erklärungen auf höchster Ebene betrachtet werden können. Hält man sich strikt an dieses Paradigma, so sind Erklärungen, die z. B. auf teleologischen Konzepten, „folk psychology" oder narrativen Darstellungen historischer Ereignisse beruhen, nur dann gültig, wenn nachgewiesen werden kann, dass sie auf physiologische, chemische und physikalische Erklärungen zurückgeführt werden können. Die letztgenannten Erklärungen erscheinen dann als "echtere" Erklärungen, während die erstgenannten bestenfalls Abkürzungen für diese echten Erklärungen sind.

Aus der Sicht des Maschinenparadigmas ist die Bevorzugung von Erklärungen auf der Ebene von Teilen eine Bevorzugung von Erklärungen, die sich auf kausale Gesetze oder gesetzesähnliche Regelmäßigkeiten beziehen, da diese Regelmäßigkeiten Grundlage für zuverlässige Vorhersagen und zuverlässige Vorhersagen wiederum Voraussetzung für das Herstellen stabil funktionierender Maschinen ist. Teleologische und narrative Erklärungen von Ereignissen sind dagegen von Mehrdeutigkeit und Unsicherheit begleitet. Die Absicht einer Person lässt sich beispielsweise nicht, wie erwähnt, direkt aus ihrer Handlung als physischem, beobachtbarem Ereignis ableiten, sondern hängt vom größeren Rahmen der langfristigen Pläne, beruflichen Ziele, privaten Bestrebungen, situativen Neigungen und vielen anderen Einstellungen, Charaktereigenschaften und Zielen der Person ab. Jedes dieser Merkmale kann eine Rolle dabei spielen, zu verstehen, warum die Person auf eine bestimmte Weise gehandelt hat, und somit ihre Absicht zu erfassen. Selbst wenn die Person selbst ein mögliches Ziel auswählt und erklärt, dass es ihre Absicht war, dieses und nicht ein anderes Ziel zu erreichen, bleiben notwendigerweise Zweifel, ob sie letztlich richtig liegt, und es können andere überzeugende Geschichten angeboten werden, die ein neues Licht auf ihr Verhalten werfen. Akademische Disziplinen wie die Geschichts-, Sozial- und Politikwissenschaft müssen zwangsläufig mit diesen Unklarheiten und Unsicherheiten zurechtkommen. Nach ihren eigenen Maßstäben wird dadurch der Anspruch auf Wissen und Angemessenheit von Erklärungen nicht untergraben. Vom Standpunkt der Maschinenmetapher aus gesehen müssen diese Wissensansprüche jedoch zweifelhaft erscheinen.

Auch unter den Naturwissenschaften kann die synthetische Biologie in Aufnahme der Implikationen der Maschinenmetapher eine besondere Rolle beanspruchen. Während die Physik bereits eine analytische Genauigkeit erreicht hat, die unter anderem die Herstellung neuartiger synthetischer Elemente ermöglicht, und die Chemie chemische Reaktionen bereits so weit analysiert hat, dass die Synthese neuartiger Verbindungen wie z. B. Kunststoffen möglich wird, ist die Biologie nun genau an der Schwelle angelangt, an der das gezielte Entwerfen, Anordnen und Umordnen genetischer Teile in einem solchen Maße möglich wird, dass die daraus resultierenden gentechnisch veränderten Organismen als "neuartig" angesehen werden können. Folgt man diesem Erklärungsschema, dann muss die synthetische Biologie als derzeitige Speerspitze des wissenschaftlichen und technologischen Fortschritts gelten. Aus der

Perspektive der Maschinenmetapher ist sie eine Disziplin, die im Begriff ist, das bisher genaueste Wissen über Organismen zu generieren und dieses Wissen in zuverlässige technologische Mittel zur Veränderung und Kontrolle von Verhalten umzusetzen [29].

Viele der aktuellen großen gesellschaftlichen und globalen Herausforderungen betreffen Leben und unseren Umgang mit Leben. Eine wachsende Bevölkerung muss mit Nahrungsmitteln versorgt werden. In weiten Teilen der Erde können aufgrund von Trockenheit keine Nutzpflanzen mehr wachsen. Ölverschmutzungen bedrohen marine Ökosysteme. All diese Probleme sind bekannt, und es ist offensichtlich, dass der Einsatz der verfügbaren technologischen Mittel bisher nicht zu dauerhaften Lösungen geführt hat, und dass auch soziale und politische Maßnahmen zur Lösung keine entscheidende Wirkung gezeigt haben.

Stellt man sich ganz auf den Boden des Maschinenparadigmas, dann wird man, wenn man nach neuen Lösungen sucht, in erster Linie auf Technik setzen und nicht auf soziale und politische Maßnahmen, da letztere ex hypothesi nicht von wirklich zuverlässigem Wissen informiert und geleitet würden. Im Bereich der Technologie wiederum liegt es aus dieser Perspektive nah, sich den neuesten, vermeintlich vielversprechendsten Entwicklungen zuzuwenden. Vor dem Hintergrund des Maschinenparadigmas kann die synthetische Biologie damit nicht nur als einer unter anderen, sondern vielmehr als der wichtigste Kandidat für die Lösung gesellschaftlicher und ökologischer Probleme angesehen werden.

Kritiker dessen, was als "technological fixes" für gesellschaftliche Probleme bekannt geworden ist, argumentieren seit langem, dass diese Ansätze unter einer Reihe von Nachteilen leiden [30]. Wenn beispielsweise gewinnorientierte Unternehmen in reichen Teilen der Welt Technologien entwickeln und in Niedriglohnländern einsetzen und vermarkten, kann dies zu globaler Ungleichheit beitragen und wirtschaftliche Abhängigkeiten verfestigen. Darüber hinaus bieten Hightech-Anwendungen keine nachhaltigen, langfristigen Lösungen, wenn die lokalen Kenntnisse und Ressourcen nicht ausreichen, um die Anwendung zu reparieren und funktionsfähig zu halten. Folglich kann die Entscheidung für Low-Tech-Lösungen oder Alternativen zu technischen Lösungen oder die Änderung gesellschaftlicher Rahmenbedingungen, z. B. in Bezug auf Bildung und Ausbildung, oft bessere Ergebnisse versprechen als (isolierte) technologische Lösungen. Die Maschinenmetapher kann dazu verführen, diese vielfältigen Verflechtungen von Technologie in gesellschaftliche, soziale und ökonomische Zusammenhänge zu unterschätzen.

Auch dies ist kein Argument dafür, die Maschinenmetapher aufzugeben, und es ist auch kein Argument dafür, auf die Entwicklung von Anwendungen der synthetischen Biologie und die Bewertung ihres potenziellen Nutzens zu verzichten. Es ist vielmehr ein Argument dafür, bei den Hoffnungen und Versprechungen, die sich mit der synthetischen Biologie verbinden, realistisch zu bleiben, das gesamte Feld möglicher technologischer und sozialer Lösungen für gesellschaftliche Probleme im Auge zu behalten und die Anwendungen der synthetischen Biologie in einen gesellschaftlichen Kontext einzubetten, der eine langfristig sichere und gerechte Nutzung ermöglicht.

5.7 Schluss

Die Maschinenmetapher in der synthetischen Biologie ist eine implikationsreiche konzeptuelle Linse. Sie unterstützt eine Fokussierung der Forschung auf die gesetzmäßigen Beziehungen zwischen genetischen Teilen und den darauf aufbauenden Funktionen eines Organismus' und den Optionen, diese Funktionen gezielt zu verändern. Gleichzeitig blendet die Maschinenmetapher jedoch systematisch Merkmale von Organismen wie evolutionäre Entwicklung und Veränderung und Wechselwirkungen in Ökosystemen aus. Dies kann dazu führen, dass Auswirkungen synthetischer Organismen auf die Umwelt unterschätzt werden. Aus der Sicht der Maschinenmetapher greift die Beschränkung auf die Herstellung leicht veränderter natürlicher Organismen zudem zu kurz, wenn das volle Potenzial der synthetischen Biologie ausgeschöpft werden soll, das aus dieser Sicht in der Entwicklung neuartiger Organismen besteht (wie z. B. Organismen mit synthetischer DNA, die aus einer Vielzahl natürlicher Vorlagen stammt, und Organismen mit DNA, die auf alternativen Basenpaaren basiert). Wie mögliche Nebenwirkungen solcher neuartiger synthetischer Organismen auf die Umwelt angemessen zu bewerten sind, ist eine offene Frage. Zweitens ist es aus der Perspektive der Maschinenmetapher zweifelhaft, eine Entität als „moral agent" bzw. „moral patient" zu betrachten. Die Eigenschaften von Lebewesen, die die Zuschreibung eines moralischen Status' rechtfertigen, stehen in einem Spannungsverhältnis zu Erklärungen in Form von Teilen, die zuverlässig bestimmte Wirkungen aufeinander und auf das Ganze, das sie formen, haben. Drittens enthält die Maschinenmetapher ein Konzept des wissenschaftlichen Fortschritts und der Stellung der synthetischen Biologie innerhalb dieses Fortschritts. Dieses Konzept betont die Stellung der synthetischen Biologie als Speerspitze der Wissenschaft und Technik und kann dazu führen, dass der potenzielle Beitrag von Anwendungen der synthetischen Biologie zur Lösung gesellschaftlicher und ökologischer Probleme überschätzt wird.

Wenn man sich dieser Implikationen des Maschinenparadigmas bewusst ist, wird man den damit verbundenen ethischen Begrenzungen und Herausforderungen begegnen können. Im Hinblick auf Risiken für Umwelt und Ökosysteme gehört dazu vor allem, die Praxis der multidisziplinären Risikobewertung zu stützen und auszubauen. Ein schrittweises Herstellen zunehmend von natürlichen Vorbildern entfernter Organismen kann eine weitere Maßnahme zur Risikominderung sein. Im Hinblick auf den potenziellen moralischen Status von Organismen kann eine Analyse der Maschinenmetapher dazu beitragen zu verdeutlichen, dass Zuschreibung von moralischen Status auf Eigenschaften rekurriert, die nicht einfach in das Maschinenparadigma zu integrieren sind, und auf die Notwendigkeit anderer Quellen für diese Zuschreibung aufmerksam zu machen. Drittens kann die Kenntnis der inneren Logik der Maschinenmetapher und ihrer epistemischen Hintergrundannahmen davor schützen, das Problemlösungspotential der synthetischen Biologie für gesellschaftliche und ökologische Probleme zu überschätzen und sie kann dazu beitragen, die vielfältigen Verflechtungen zwischen technischen Lösungen und ökonomischen, gesellschaftlichen und sozialen Kontexten angemessen zu berücksichtigen.

Literatur

[1] Janich P. Metaphern in der Genomforschung. Gegenworte. 2001;7:32–5.

[2] Hellsten I, Nerlich B. Synthetic biology: building the language for a new science brick by metaphorical brick. New Genet Soc. 2011;30(4):375–97. doi:10.1080/14636778.2011.592009.

[3] Vincent B. The moral economy of synthetic biology. In: Boldt J, editor. Synthetic biology: metaphors, worldviews, ethics, and law. Wiesbaden: Springer Fachmedien Wiesbaden; 2016. p. 87–100.

[4] Boudry M, Pigliucci M. The mismeasure of machine: synthetic biology and the trouble with engineering metaphors. Stud Hist Philos Sci C. 2013;44(4, Part B):660–8. doi:10.1016/j.shpsc.2013.05.013.

[5] Nicholson DJ. Organisms≠Machines. Stud Hist Philos Sci C. 2013;44(4, Part B):669–78. doi:10.1016/j.shpsc.2013.05.014.

[6] Rosen R. Bionics revisited. In: Haken H, Karlqvist A, Svedin U, editors. The machine as metaphor and tool. Berlin: Springer; 1993. p. 87–100.

[7] iGEM Foundation. iGEM Foundation. 2018 [cited 2018 Feb 28]. Available from: http://www.igem.org

[8] Weiss R, Basu S, Hooshangi S, et al. Genetic circuit building blocks for cellular computation, communications, and signal processing. Nat Comput. 2003;2(1):47–84. doi:10.1023/a:1023307812034.

[9] Roelants SLKW, Saerens KMJ, Derycke T, et al. Candida bombicola as a platform organism for the production of tailor-made biomolecules. Biotechnol Bioeng. 2013;110(9):2494–503. doi:10.1002/bit.24895.

[10] Van Lunteren F. Clocks to computers: a machine-based "big picture" of the history of modern science. Isis. 2016;107(4):762–76. doi:10.1086/689764.

[11] Zaccaria M, Dedrick S, Momeni B. Modeling microbial communities: a call for collaboration between experimentalists and theorists. Processes. 2017;5(4):53.

[12] Köchy K. Philosophische Implikationen der synthetischen Biologie. In: Köchy K, Hümpel A, editors. Synthetische Biologie: Entwicklung einer neuen Ingenieurbiologie? Dornburg: Berlin-Brandenburgische Akademie der Wissenschaften; 2012.

[13] Heinemann M, Panke S. Synthetic biology – putting engineering into biology. Bioinformatics. 2006;22(22):2790–9. doi:10.1093/bioinformatics/btl469.

[14] Schyfter P. How a 'drive to make' shapes synthetic biology. Stud Hist Philos Sci C. 2013;44(4):632–40.

[15] Church GM, Regis E. Regenesis: how synthetic biology will reinvent nature and ourselves. New York: Basic Books; 2012.

[16] Kastenhofer K. Synthetic biology as understanding, control, construction, and creation? Techno-epistemic and socio-political implications of different stances in talking and doing technoscience. Futures. 2013;48:13–22. doi:10.1016/j.futures.2013.02.001.

[17] Boldt J. Life as a technological product: philosophical and ethical aspects of synthetic biology. Biol Theory. 2013;8(4):391–401. doi:10.1007/s13752-013-0138-7.

[18] Wright O, Stan GB, Ellis T. Building-in biosafety for synthetic biology. Microbiology. 2013;159(7):1221–35. doi:10.1099/mic.0.066308-0.

[19] Guo L, He X, Shi W. Intercellular communications in multispecies oral microbial communities. Front Microbiol. 2014;5:328. doi:10.3389/fmicb.2014.00328.

[20] Schmidt M. Xenobiology: a new form of life as the ultimate biosafety tool. Bioessays. 2010;32(4):322–31. doi:10.1002/bies.200900147.

[21] MacIntyre A. After virtue. London: Bloomsbury Publishing; 2013.

[22] Torrance S. Artificial consciousness and artificial ethics: between realism and social relationism. Philos Technol. 2014;27(1):9–29. doi:10.1007/s13347-013-0136-5.

[23] Dar-Nimrod I, Heine SJ. Genetic essentialism: on the deceptive determinism of DNA. Psychol Bull. 2011;137(5):800–18. doi:10.1037/a0021860.

[24] Black JB, Perez-Pinera P, Gersbach CA. Mammalian synthetic biology: engineering biological systems. Annu Rev Biomed Eng. 2017;19:249–77. doi:10.1146/annurev-bioeng-071516-044649.

[25] Markson JS, Elowitz MB. Synthetic biology of multicellular systems: new platforms and applications for animal cells and organisms. ACS Synth Biol. 2014;3(12):875–6. doi: 10.1021/sb500358y.

[26] Basl J. Machines as moral patients we shouldn't care about (yet): the interests and welfare of current machines. Philos Technol. 2014;27(1):79–96. doi: https://doi.org/10.1007/s13347-013-0122-y.

[27] Regan T. The case for animal rights. Berkeley: University of California Press; 1983.

[28] Jonas H. Is God a mathematician? The meaning of metabolism. In: Jonas H, editor. The phenomenon of life: toward a philosophical biology. Evanston, IL: Northwestern University Press; 2001.

[29] Vincent B. Between the possible and the actual: philosophical perspectives on the design of synthetic organisms. Futures. 2013;48:23–31. doi: https://doi.org/10.1016/j.futures.2013.02.006.

[30] ETC Group. Extreme genetic engineering: an introduction to synthetic biology. ETC Group; 2007.

Jonathan Benecke

6 On the problem of epistemic metaphor

Abstract: Traditionally, starting with Aristotle, metaphor has been analyzed in accordance with its functions in rhetoric and poetics. Here, metaphor is understood as a way of *transferring* meaning from one domain to another. This focus on the structure of transfer within metaphor has, however, obscured the productive element of metaphor in the creation of new concepts. With a growing understanding of the role metaphor plays in modern science, the *epistemic* function of metaphor must take center stage. In the following, I will point to some problems of Aristotle's as well as Nietzsche's accounts of metaphor when it comes to its epistemic function and argue that this function cannot be adequately understood without putting the experiment at the center of metaphor's productivity and indeed understanding metaphors as linguistic experiments.

Traditionellerweise, beginnend mit Aristoteles, wurde die Metapher in Bezug auf ihre rhetorischen und poetischen Funktionen analysiert. Hier wird die Metapher als Art des *Transfers* von Bedeutung von einer Domäne zur anderen verstanden. Dieser Fokus auf die Struktur des Transfers in der Metapher hat jedoch ihr produktives Moment in der Erschaffung neuer Konzepte verdeckt. Mit einem wachsenden Bewusstsein für die Rolle der Metapher in der modernen Wissenschaft muss die *epistemische* Funktion in den Vordergrund gerückt werden. Im Weiteren werde ich einige Probleme von Aristoteles und Nietzsches Positionen in Bezug auf die epistemische Funktion aufzeigen und argumentieren, dass sie nicht adäquat verstanden werden kann, ohne das Experiment in das Zentrum der metaphorischen Produktivität zu stellen und Metaphern selbst als linguistische Experimente zu verstehen.

6.1 Introduction

What would it take to provide a precise definition of metaphor or *any* definition for that matter? This question depends on an explication of representation.[1] In the classical picture, which might be best described as *linguistic essentialism*, language represents the world through precise concepts with which it cuts the world into precise categories ("at its joints" some might say), the objects of which form the extension of a concept. Definitions of a concept are then constructed in the form of necessary and sufficient conditions via a listing of applicable predicates in the form "X is Y" – its intension.

1 For an extended treatment of linguistic representation and its critique see the central works of Deleuze and Guattari [1,2,3].

https://doi.org/10.1515/9783112215685-006

Infinite precision, however, can only be achieved under a set of linguistic postulates. Either one supposes the existence of ready-made categories within a closed axiomatic that need no further explication or *cannot* be explicated in any way. These definitions are nothing more than the Platonic ideals of pure language – pure *sense* – and provide meaning without recourse to anything else. Indeed, they impose their meaning on everything else in every act of recognition. Hence representation is always a re-presentation. Or one supposes the capacity (and the necessity) of concepts to achieve infinite intension, which corresponds to an extension = 1. Here, it is possible to precisely describe every individual through a unique concept. As Deleuze has shown, both ways of approaching concepts are not feasible. Concepts conceived in this way will always be blocked from reaching infinite intension [1 chapter 1].

The ideas of the later Wittgenstein [4] further show that a position relying on infinite linguistic precision has become untenable in the case of ordinary language. Categories are always vague and fuzzy, at best they have a center (an exemplar or prototype) and a periphery, but no clear borders. Definitions are pragmatic and meaning is constructed through the use of language itself. The intension of any concept is not merely a listing. Any language system is a network of differentially connected words that mutually depend on each other and are formed by pragmatic speech acts. Indeed, the only "grounding" that seems possible for linguistic categories is the ostensive connection of speech acts to the ecological lifeworld that humans as a shared social collective were formed in and inhabit. This problematizes representation from the side of language, but the side of the world can also be investigated. Here, it is clear that our use of representation language – the structure of the idealized concept – shapes our understanding of the world through *container metaphors* [5]. Classical concepts are containers – objects with a clear boundary – that contain predicates. And presupposing the possibility of precise representation, things in the world must also show this structure. They must be *objects* that *contain* properties. This transposes the idealist or Platonic picture onto reality. In this view, things that do not fit into established categories can only be seen as unspeakable. The fluidity and vagueness of real things become untenable.

Under these accounts of linguistic representation – under linguistic essentialism – the essence of metaphor is considered a *transfer* of meaning. The meaning of one word is poured into the emptied frame of a different one. Metaphor operates on the order of the word; it is a substitution that can always be reversed. Here, metaphor cannot have epistemic value. It is merely poetic, merely rhetoric, or in short: Ornamental [6]. But genuine epistemic metaphors – those that are productively involved in creating scientific concepts – show precisely the limits of this classical picture of language.

While representing (using established concepts to categorize the world) is certainly how ordinary language works on a surface level, metaphor seems to give us a *genetic* account of old concepts and a mechanism for generating new ones. The question I wish to ask in this context is the following: How must one conceptualize specifically *epistemic* metaphor? If transfer and substitution are bound to linguistic representation and historically to poetic and rhetoric metaphor, what concept of metaphor helps us to understand particular metaphors in the context of theory-making and the context of laboratory work or in short: In the process of scientific experimentation? To approach these questions, I will first recapitulate the accounts of Aristotle and Nietzsche. The two writers provide rival accounts that, despite their dissimilarity, both struggle to capture epistemic metaphor. Afterward, I will argue that the productivity of epistemic metaphor can only be conceptualized when one focuses on the role of the experiment in modern scientific inquiry and on epistemic metaphor as a non-representational linguistic experiment that is connected to the epistemic object it purports to describe through the materiality of the respective experimental systems in a recursive praxis.

6.2 Aristotle, Nietzsche and the problem of metaphoric transfer

Since Aristotle organizes concepts into a hierarchy of genera and species lying between the terminal categories and the terminal individuals, metaphors – like messengers – transfer meaning between these linguistic layers vertically, horizontally, or by analogy [7 1457a–1457b]. Aristotle's metaphor of metaphor thus is *Epiphora*. This first concept is what some might call a commonsensical account of metaphor. But what exactly is the function of metaphor in this case? What can we gain from such a transfer? It is instructive in this context, to turn to Aristotle's theory of *mimesis*. He constructs this concept in some contrast to (but still under the influence of) Plato, for whom it consists – briefly – in the connection of the illusory sense-world to the true world of ideas.[2] The former imitates or represents the latter, which structures a hierarchy of Being in which a division of reality/illusion is constructed. Artistic acts – those that produce representations of sensual objects – are removed even further from the "real" thing than the object itself. Even though Aristotle rejects Plato's ontological divide and makes artistic acts a proper *Techne* with its own (natural) rules and objects, he still retains the notion of representation inherent in art – art still copies the natural world. Poetry (which Aristotle restricts to works having at least one whole narrative as its subject) then imitates acting humans through its *Mythos* [7 1450a]. This leveling displaces Plato's concept of mimesis somewhat since poetry does not imitate stories that have really taken place. It imitates stories that are *possible* and *probable* – in short *general* – which idealizes the actual world [7 1448a,1451a–1452a]. The

2 See Plato [8], especially his treatment of poetry in book X, 595a ff. For a more detailed discussion see Potolsky [9].

viewer feels *Katharsis* [7 1449b] in this because they experience a "miraculous surprise" that helps them to *recognize* [7 1448b] the truth and learn something. Art, in Aristotle, is therefore connected to the pursuit of knowledge and human reason whereas in Plato it is mostly placed in opposition to it.

The role of metaphor becomes clearer: The production of *surprise* is why metaphor functions as a poetic device. In the *Rhetoric* as well, metaphor is placed under *Lexis*, under the stylistic uses of speech [10 1403b–6 ff.]. Words, here, are also imitations [10 1404a–20] and metaphors also produce surprise [10 1412a–15] but they serve a different function than in poetic speech since the goal of rhetoric speech is to convince the listeners. Surprise can be used – by the talented orator or poet – to draw the listener's cognition to a previously unnoticed (objectively true) likeness, which may evoke particular feelings or influence the listener towards an argument. These are the first two functions of metaphor, which find their origin in speech. But what of their epistemic value?

In Aristotle's account, metaphor is bound by likeness and truth.[3] Likeness between words is precisely produced by their relationship as species and genera while truth lies in the correspondence of these precise concepts to a world of real and similarly precise objects (representation). Likeness here is a form of semantic nearness and truth is its guarantor [10 1410b–10]. As such, the surprise of a successful metaphor lies in the unexpected likeness of two words in a given context. But once the likeness is recognized, once the surprise fades, so does the metaphor. A substitution of meaning from one word to another is, as Paul Ricoeur has put it, a *rule-violation*:

> Metaphor occurs in an order already constituted in terms of genus and species, and in a game whose relation-rules – subordination, co-ordination, proportionality or equality of relationships – are already given. Second, metaphor consists in a violation of this order and this game [6 p. 21].

Metaphor falls under mimesis; it is a form of mimesis and not much more than a grammatically disguised simile [10 1406b–20]. Its productivity must be fleeting and debased since what is real is the hierarchical structure of words and things (and the likenesses therein). Particular metaphors can always be replaced by the "correct" or rather conventional word [6 p. 85]. The bounds of metaphor are rigid. Epiphora implies reversibility. For Aristotle, metaphor is a little game we play to amuse ourselves or, at best, rid ourselves of cognitive errors. Metaphors are not inherently productive with respect to new concepts. While his account captures the synchronic structure of language, as well as some ordinary usages of metaphor, it does not capture the conceptual uncertainty of a scientist trying to grasp a new phenomenon or diachronic language change in general. It does not capture that unstable moment when previously fixed meanings become untenable and new ones appear from beyond.

While Nietzsche is notoriously difficult to interpret in general – and it is no different in his treatment of metaphor – we can see a general inclination to dynamize met-

3 For further discussion, see Hines [11 pp. 31–55].

aphor in his work that better grasps these moments of instability than Aristotle's account. Nietzsche, however, does not present a "systematic" account but rather performs his understanding of metaphor through his texts. As Sarah Kofman has emphasized, one must differentiate multiple phases in Nietzsche's thought on metaphor [12]. The early phase stands apart as a subversion of the Aristotelian concept of metaphor, while still being beholden to it. Kofman thinks that the early Nietzsche believes in a "secret being of things", which cannot be expressed through language in any way but that he will reject this claim in his later writings [12 pp. 30–31]. This is why I will consider two possible interpretations. On a surface level, Nietzsche could be taken to simply invert the Aristotelian account of metaphor. In this case, metaphor would take primacy over the concept. In a more complicated reading, proposed by Kofman, Nietzsche in fact not only inverts Aristotle's account but simultaneously extremizes metaphor's function and thereby dissolves it into the more general concept of the Will to Power.

In any case, Nietzsche provides us with an account of metaphor that contrasts sharply with Aristotle's, since it is very much intertwined with his anti-metaphysical intentions. Where Aristotle's world was a recognizable one of particulars and general concepts, a world of forms inhering in matter, Nietzsche rages against the representational perspective on the world. In "Über Wahrheit und Lüge im außermoralischen Sinn" (TL), Nietzsche's most direct treatment of metaphor, he emphasizes that the world is made up of entirely singular entities [13 p. 880], while on other occasions he seems to endorse a more Heraclitean picture of the world, that rejects "thingness" as such [14 pp. 799–872]. In both cases, he rejects the possibility of representational structure or law capturing the world accurately [13 p. 878]. Truth and preformed sense are marked as illusory and thus rejected. This is what Nietzsche creates an account of metaphor for, why it is useful to him, and why it differs, so radically, from the prior tradition.

In TL, metaphors are transfers of meaning not between species and genera but through embodied domains.[4] Metaphors reflect the disposition of the singular entities, showing something of their style or taste – their unique connection to the world. As such, they are removed from any generality, they formulate a *perspective*. One must say that the subject *is itself* a metaphor, that it masquerades itself, and transforms the world through its unique metaphor. Metaphor is beyond language, or rather the foundation of all language and thought. Concepts in contrast belong to the order of generality. The concept is a crystallized impression, that cannot capture the original fluid impression from which it originated [13 p. 879–882]. This is because, through metaphor, the impression was connected to other like impressions. For Nietzsche, it is

4 "Ein Nervenreiz zuerst übertragen in ein Bild! erste [sic] Metapher. Das Bild wieder nachgeformt in einem Laut! Zweite Metapher. Und jedesmal vollständiges Ueberspringen der Sphäre, mitten hinein in eine ganz andere und neue." [13 p. 879].

clear that this operation, this generalizing, is in some sense unjustified because no Platonic idea can serve as the guarantor of this process.[5] Like in Aristotle's account, but for very different reasons, metaphor is a mistake. For Nietzsche, however, it is a *necessary* one, insofar as humans must use language. Just as we build analogical metaphors, we build equivalences, in short: Concepts. This is what Nietzsche calls the "drive to metaphor" [13 p. 887]. Humans (and life in general) must form metaphors, and must use them to interpret the world. Here, Nietzsche seems to present an inverted Aristotelian account. Metaphors are the fundamental operations of meaning-making while concepts are simply conventionalized metaphors, the results of a meaning transfer from the singular world to the generalized human subject. Metaphor remains a kind of transfer but is no longer Epiphora since the world is not differentiated into genera and species. The transfer is always a transformation or rather a "formation" (producing a form, pressing the world of singularities into a general form). Since no "world as such" is intelligible [13 p. 879], Nietzsche recognizes that even the attempts to conceptualize (the phenomenon of) metaphor as a transfer are metaphorical.

Nevertheless, humans cannot escape this illusory activity. The power of the drive to make truths relies on an active force of *forgetting*, entailed by the drive [12 p. 44], in which the subjects forget the drive itself [13 p. 883–884]. The concept is nothing more than a *forgotten* metaphor. A metaphor that has been worn out (rather effaced) through habit. As Kofman [12 p. 13] has said, concepts are *condensed* metaphors, restrictions of meaning from the original multiplicity effected through the leveling of the singular into the all-too-human general. The seeming existence of a "true" world and its separation from the perceptible world are only possible through this forgetfulness. The conscious, rational mind can only grasp this drive through itself, through metaphor. Here, Nietzsche articulates the paradox of metaphor, dethrones the Aristotelian "proper" and replaces it with the metaphorical [12 p. 65 ff.].

Again, in some sense we seem to find the reversion of Aristotle's (or Plato's) position here. The order of the world is no longer fundamental, it is not a guarantor of truth or the ground from which metaphor rises as mere wordplay. Metaphor is rather the ground of the world as such. In so far as we still have truths, metaphor produces them. The proper concept is only a more conventional metaphor and new metaphors always relate in their novelty to this conventional properness, not to an absolute truth [13 pp. 880–881]. Such a reversion still entails the relation of this concept of metaphor to the proper. In his later writings, according to Kofman, Nietzsche changed his focus from metaphor to the concepts of the text and its interpretation – the essential aspects of the *Will to Power*.

5 "Jeder Begriff entsteht durch Gleichsetzen des Nicht-Gleichen." [13 p. 880].

In Kofman's view, the later Nietzsche does not pursue an inversion of the Aristotelian account, since it would force him to remain in the realm of metaphysics.[6] He proposes not merely a reversion of Aristotle/Plato, not merely a reversion of concept and metaphor, but a complete leveling of the two. In his affirmation of the perceptible, the "true" world does not subordinate itself to it but *ceases to matter*. The words "imaginary" and "real" lose their meaning, since they are based on a flawed opposition. The proper is entirely dissolved. Or rather it is recognized as what it really is: *Appropriation* of the world by a single perspective [12 p. 125]. This account relies on a shift from the drive to metaphor to the Will to Power which is, according to Kofman, not a metaphysical proposition but an "anhypothesis" [12 p. 139]. Here, the concepts of text and interpretation become central. The world is a text that must be interpreted by life. But it is not a bare text that stands "before" life. Life constitutes *itself as a text* through the act of interpretation. Life interprets only itself. The Thing-in-itself and the "secret being of things" have lost their meaning. The Will to Power has become the beginning and end of all living activity. While Nietzsche emphasizes the illusory products of the drive to metaphor, the Will to Power is not a deficient activity precisely because of its self-constitutivity.

We can see that the shift from Epiphora to this new way of thinking metaphor is profound. The transfer is the original activity and structure of metaphor, but not between two preformed domains. The transfer itself is the process that constitutes both domains – text and interpretation. It is a pure difference that produces two opposing sides that express themselves through it: At first in the form of resemblances and later in the act of forgetting through the reconstitution of a total identity. This is why metaphor dissolves into the Will to Power. The concept of metaphor as transfer is inverted and then taken to its extreme point, where it ceases to exist.

For a concept of epistemic metaphor, it will be useful to briefly consider the impact of Nietzsche's account on his views on scientific inquiry. It is not surprising that Nietzsche's relationship with scientific activity is a strangely ambivalent matter. In "Die Fröhliche Wissenschaft" (GS) we are subjected to some aphorisms that seem particularly in favor of science while others adopt a more critical tone. How should we deal with this? We must keep in mind that Nietzsche's goal is the destruction of the proper as ground. A science that prides itself in having found the proper or being able to find the proper even in principle, a science that values Truth – dogmatically – above all else, must therefore be unjustified because this kind of science remains in the Platonic/Aristotelian paradigm of recognition, the metaphysical belief that nature conforms to an eternal order and the subordination of human activity to this order [15 p. 577]. It is a naive realism that transmits our metaphoric meanings into an objective domain [15 pp. 421–422]. Similarly to Nietzsche's treatment of the world in TL, in

6 "Wenn man den metaphorischen Status des Willens zur Macht vergisst, mag man Nietzsche für den letzten Metaphysiker halten, für denjenigen, der den Platonismus einfach umgekehrt hat." [12 p. 142].

GS it is presented as chaos without any laws [15 pp. 467–468]. Our belief in cause and effect and our explanations of phenomena through mathematics do not adequately capture chaos, since it is a true continuum and we cannot really understand it by slicing it into objects [15 pp. 473,477–478). Nevertheless, as humans, we have no choice but to think in this way and the rigor of science as well as mathematical precision can have benefits for the strength of our minds [15 pp. 514–515,533–534,551]. What Nietzsche doesn't devalue, however, is the experiment.[7] It seems that science is only valuable insofar as it leaves open the future, and always leaves open the possibility of experimentation. Experimentation, however, is not a form of pure discovery. It is a form of creative action [15 p. 422]. It is also itself an "experiment" in a wider sense since its success is never guaranteed [15 p. 471]. The proper reaction towards science and epistemic metaphor is then: Surprise. On Nietzsche's account of metaphor, we must be surprised that science works at all [15 pp. 411–412]. Science conceived in this way cannot proclaim to have found Truth, only ever-preliminary truths that it has created itself, dependent on our present metaphors. Recognition here is only akin to dreaming, to preserving a particular kind of dream – the dream of "reality" [15 p. 417]. It is clear that our scientific activity then only describes ourselves (since our interpretative activity constitutes the text itself). Nietzsche subsumes science under self-discovery [15 p. 473] and his radical perspectivism, believing it to be impossible to ever understand other perspectives while still granting that infinitely many such perspectives must exist, that the world is infinitely interpretable [15 p. 626–627].

In my view, both Aristotle's and Nietzsche's accounts of metaphor are insufficient when one tries to understand the role epistemic metaphors play in modern science. Why is this? On the one hand, Aristotle's account leaves no room for creativity and the novelty of scientific concept creation. His "transfer" is based on a fixed representational structure of genera and species. On the other hand, Nietzsche's "transfer" is either an inversion of the Aristotelian account and thereby still bound to the proper or metaphor is dissolved into the Will to Power, in which case the account leaves too much room for creativity. Here, it becomes impossible to understand why some epistemic metaphors work better than others and it becomes hard to explain how epistemic metaphors evolve and interact with experimental praxis. While Nietzsche is correct in rejecting Aristotle's ontology and non-epistemic account of metaphor, recognizing the importance of metaphoric meaning-making over representational concepts, he underdetermines the connection between metaphor and the experiment and thus does not provide a useful concept of epistemic metaphor. Indeed, the scientific experiment is the missing centerpiece in both accounts of metaphor. Aristotle places no value on the experiment and while Nietzsche does value experimentation as

7 "Ich lobe mir eine jede Skepsis, auf welche mir erlaubt ist zu antworten: "Versuchen wir's!" Aber ich mag von allen Dingen und allen Fragen, welche das Experiment nicht zulassen, Nichts mehr hören. Diess ist die Grenze meines "Wahrheitssinnes": denn dort hat die Tapferkeit ihr Recht verloren." [15 pp. 415–416, see also pp. 526–527].

such, his treatment of the concept is not structured enough to apply to the natural sciences. This is why I will now consider the role experiments play in scientific praxis.

6.3 Experiment and epistemic metaphor

Central to the modern understanding of the experiment is Bachelard's concept of *phenomenotechnique* which he develops in the face of the overwhelming experimental successes of the modern natural sciences. For him, in contrast to the world as pretext, scientific objects – describable phenomena – are constructed within the experimental process, within a controlled and parameterized environment, in the interplay of theoretical deliberations and technical interventions [16]. The objects we perceive are only surface-level effects of our experimental processes.[8]

Ian Hacking, among others,[9] therefore emphasizes the process of *intervention* in experimental praxis. In contrast to theoretical work, experimental scientists must interact with the world, build machines and learn to operate them. They must isolate and stabilize particular phenomena and *cleanse* their experimental systems from unwanted interference because things are only real insofar as they are usable to conduct new experiments (Hacking 2010).

Hans-Jörg Rheinberger expands on Hacking's position. Experimentation is not a kind of hyper-rational engineering of technical systems that are then used to falsify or validate pure hypotheses but rather a form of *bricolage* [19 pp. 229–230]. Experimental scientists are tinkerers who play with the present experimental systems by exploring what they *can do* (and not what the epistemic objects *are*). The recursive relationship of the experimental system and the material enables this process because the reach of the former can potentially be extended by *grafting* new functions onto them or splitting them apart [19 chapter 4]. The goal is always the production of novel phenomena that cannot be adequately grasped with the present experimental system. In this way, the experiment always entails a performative contradiction. It tries to invalidate its foundations while simultaneously opening up further avenues of research. Experimental systems – as long as they are *experimental* – must always be conceived

8 "All identities are only simulated, produced as an optical "effect" by the more profound game of difference and repetition." [1 preface].

9 The importance of the experiment for science in general has only really been acknowledged by philosophers of science in the last century, although one must certainly credit Francis Bacon for his much earlier contributions. Before, like in the much older contemplative tradition of natural philosophy, the role of the *theory* took much of the academic attention. The beginning of the so-called "experimental turn" is often credited to Hacking [17]. While his work has certainly taken a central place in the philosophy of science in the last 40 years, one should not overestimate its novelty, as many authors beforehand have dealt with the nature of the experiment. See Simons and Vagelli [18].

as a socio-technical processes of differentiation. They undergo variations, they split, they fuse, and can even change their epistemic objects [19 pp. 148–149]. A technical assemblage that intervenes but only demonstrates an already known phenomenon or categorizes materials with an always already fixed *method* cannot, therefore, rightly be called an experiment [20].

While intervening in their experimental systems, scientists must have a keen intuition for *traces*. The traces that an experimental system produces in this way are best understood as *encounters* between it and the epistemic thing that come to phenomenological importance as *gaps* or *fissures* – in short problems – in the scientist's perception. Traces are situated in a sub-representational realm, the realm of Derridean *différance*, and therefore in principle not graspable through conceptional thinking. They tell of a certain resistance or absence in the experimental system and are an immediate sign of an epistemic thing that expresses itself but can never be adequately captured. The intervention of the scientist is then an attempt at stabilizing the trace into a phenomenon that can be represented and is open to conceptional thinking as well as description and explanation by tuning into a recursive interaction with the material [19 pp. 19–20]. Rheinberger calls this epistemological procedure *subduction* since the experiment always unpredictably (but in a provoked manner) subducts old knowledge in a serendipitous encounter with the new [19 p. 17]. Experiments bring something into our phenomenological reach, they produce phenomena, they are *phenomenotechniques*. To make the invisible visible, to move from the realm of traces to the realm of *data* or phenomena, requires a form of epistemological "deformation" (although, as before, the term formation seems more apt). Rheinberger distinguishes firstly between spatial (structural) and temporal (processual) deformations and secondly between compressions and dilatations. To deform things that are too small/large or too fast/slow must be an inherent part of the experimental system [19 chapter 3]. The production of data is therefore a movement from entirely singular traces to an arrangement that opens the possibility of comparing multiple events. The results of many experiments (be they experimental series of the same or slightly modified setup or entirely different experimental systems) are conjoined through their supposed similarity into a single data-space in which mathematical and conceptual modeling can occur [19 pp. 33].

A model is therefore only possible through a deforming domain-jump – from the sub-representational trace to the representational datum. It is a structured amalgamation of former traces representing an epistemic object on time- and space-scales we can understand. How exactly a model refers to an epistemic object or what part (function or spatial structure being the two main examples) of the latter it models may differ. Like Nietzsche does for metaphor, however, Rheinberger emphasizes the *illusory* nature of the model in this process. The model purports to present *a whole* and not simply disjointed parts while simultaneously reducing the complexity of the epistemic object. This "reductive synthesis" [19 p. 38] is a form of fabulation that conceals its own inadequacy. Insofar as a model represents a thing, it can never *be* that thing.

More important, however, is the fact that the model allows for interaction with the experimental system and the type of tinkering that is necessary for intervention in the first place. The representational nature of the model is thus not what makes it useful in itself. Only because it provides falsity with a certain power that propels the scientist into recursive epistemic actions can it enable intervention. Here, like the experimental systems themselves, models are not static but always strive to undermine their own foundations. Only when they are removed from scientific praxis (e. g. when models find their way into textbooks), when they are reduced to their representational content, do they become static and take on a veneer of Truth.

For our purposes, the general epistemic structure of the model is of relevance, since both epistemic metaphor and model operate on the order of similarity and resemblance. Epistemic metaphors also try to grasp new phenomena through a construction of likeness and make them accessible to cognitive activity. Are models and metaphors the same thing? This question has been discussed at length in the literature (Compare Black [21], or Hesse [22]). Ultimately, the distinction is not very important either way, since the discussion has mostly focused on the representational aspects of models.[10] In this sense, one can choose to find differences between them by restricting their respective domains – metaphor in the rhetoric/poetic and model in the epistemic – or one can merge them by expanding the scope of either – extending metaphor into the epistemic domain or making concepts in general "small" models.

It seems to be the case that, from an experimental perspective, epistemic metaphors show much of the same capacities as models. At the forefront of research, scientists are grappling with entirely new phenomena that have no designations and – as traces – not even any meaning. Like the conversion of traces into data in the case of models, the conversion of singular experiences into generalized categories makes metaphors possible. Here, similarities become accessible on which the scientist can perform a cognitive domain mapping – a meaning-model – based on past experience. The metaphors that are constructed in this way are always provisional. They provide a certain perspective on the world – just like models – and allow certain interventions to become thinkable. More importantly, epistemic metaphors also react to those interventions. They can change, shift their contexts, and differentiate, which in turn informs different interventions.[11] Models and metaphors also serve, since traces can't be communicated and small amounts of data are not particularly useful, as a way of communication within scientific communities. Both can interact with one another; they can compete and they can merge or split depending on their usefulness which also enables tinkering on the level of data [19 p. 58]. This speaks to the important in-

---

10 See here also the influential account of Lakoff and Johnson [23], in which cognitive metaphor is grounded in bodily experience but the experimental nature of this experience is not recognized.

11 See Brandt [24] for a detailed examination of this recursive relationship in German biological research on viruses.

sight that modern scientific activity happens *in a culture*, that it is a communal activity and necessitates at least the possibility of communication and shared language.

These considerations on experimental praxis show that knowledge is acquired at the edge of the sub-representational and representational domains. At this edge recursive intervention becomes possible. What kind of concept of epistemic metaphor becomes useful here? Must we still rely on the concept of transfer just because we recognize that we trespass between domains? Aristotle's account captures only the representational side of metaphor. Metaphor is subordinated to the fixed concept and lies in the realm of an impotent form of art. It is bound to rhetoric and poetics. Nietzsche's account provides a more comprehensive picture. He indeed recognizes that knowledge – as far as it can exist – is only accessible through a certain kind of falsehood and that metaphor embodies a jump between two domains. It might well be possible to interpret Nietzsche in a way that brings his account of metaphor into agreement with modern scientific praxis, but in my view, his account is too focused on the individual and because of this is too pessimistic with regards to knowledge. His perspectivism (while correctly rejecting naive Realism) seems too strong. It does not properly credit that modern science is a collectivized, intersubjective activity. If metaphors were merely an expression of one's own individual nature, the foundations of communication become dubious. The epistemic function of metaphor depends on the relationship between the sub-representational and the representational domains, the movement from the singular to the general, which Nietzsche's account does not sufficiently explain.

Experimental systems that deal with singular traces are able to transform them into generalities through the *seriality* of the epistemic objects and their traces. Singularities are expressed through difference and repetition [1], which is why an ecological approach that reconciles singularity and generality seems necessary to make sense of intersubjectivity, science, and metaphor. Relatedly, the problems which are posed to the scientist do not seem to come from within. Epistemic metaphors do not merely seem like passive "nerve signals" or *entirely* a response to one's own nature. Quite the opposite, they seem to come from the act of intervention, from tinkering with the natural world through experimental systems.[12] As far as metaphors reflect human embodiment, they extend the individual human into a connection with the world and other humans, they cross the arbitrary nature/culture dichotomy and are signs of our place in a whole ecology of signs.

In a way, metaphors are themselves experiments if we reject the sharp distinction between "theoretical" cognitive work and the "practical" experimental systems that

12 As always, it is possible to deny the world and retreat to a form of idealism. Besides going against Nietzsche's own world-affirming project, such ontological moves are beyond the scope of the present discussion and in any case do not change the phenomenological analysis of the experiment and epistemic metaphors.

instantiate it. Epistemic metaphors are linguistic experiments on the level of the model. But models are always in communion with praxis. This explains why some metaphors are very successful while others feature only briefly in scientific history.[13] The experimental character of a metaphor makes it susceptible to results from interventions that determine its long-term trajectory. What a useful concept of epistemic metaphor must be based on are an ontology of novelty, an epistemology of serendipity, and a phenomenology of surprise.

The question of metaphor being conceptualized as transfer becomes less important. While the transfer of meaning is still happening on the linguistic level, this is not the productive moment of metaphor. The initial transfer of meaning from a conventional domain to a new, at first meaningless, epistemic object – the process of catachresis – is only the starting point of a process of differentiation in which metaphor and experimental system create novel meanings. To stress the importance of the interventive aspect of metaphor rejects both the Aristotelian account and any simple reversion of it. In some way, it acknowledges the dissolution of the proper and a stringent concept of metaphor with it. Metaphors are then only extreme forms of more subtle conceptual shifts that are possible because thinking is in fact a form of acting, of intervening, of experimenting.

As Paul Ricoeur has said, metaphors are *alive* and a form of *world-making* like other narrative structures [6]. Metaphors put us into communication with Being precisely through fabulation. The crystallized meanings we find in our language-systems are always connected to an active language in contact with the world. Here we find the operative capacity of language in its interventive activity. Language is not only used for representational communication but primarily grounds (and perpetually ungrounds) this communication through its embodied and ostensive speech acts.

A metaphor for Ricoeur – like Aristotle and Nietzsche – is indeed a mistake. But crucially it is a mistake with a purpose. Metaphor disrupts the structure of the semiotic field of differences that describes a language-system and transgresses it, which can, from the synchronic perspective, only be perceived as a category-mistake. Metaphor differentiates language-systems wholesale through de- and re-construction [6 p. 22]. In this process the metaphor itself transforms into a new concept or category, obscuring its origin and losing its metaphoricity. Living language, or rather *discourse*, is thus often metaphorical when it comes into contact with the world. It is not trapped in a purely representational mode and it cannot be reduced to structural similarities. Metaphors similarly do not express prior categories, even though they make use of them, but form new ones:

> A significant trait of living language, in this connection, is the power always to push the frontier of non-sense further back. There are probably no words so incompatible that some poet could

13 See e. g. the immensely successful concept of the "cell" and several mostly unsuccessful rival concepts in Reynolds [25].

> not build a bridge between them; the power to create new contextual meanings seems to be truly limitless. Attributions that appear to be 'non-sensical' can make sense in some unexpected context. No speaker ever completely exhausts the connotative possibilities of his world [6 p. 95].

The meaning of an epistemic metaphor (and that necessitates that it is living) relies on experiential – and we can specify experimental – contexts and interventions. Epistemic metaphors are, like the experimental traces they try to capture, events that immediately die a conventionalized death of generalization to *make sense*. They *point* to a phenomenon before any kind of definition is formed. In this way, Ricoeur reintroduces Nietzsche's insight into the interpretative nature of metaphor, although he grounds his hermeneutic approach in a shared Being. Metaphors *make* the world sensible since sense lies prior to any kind of reference.[14] The interpretative series thus complements or even falls together with the recursion at the experimental frontier. Epistemic metaphors construct new references in the process of generalization and thus make truths possible. Literary works also construct worlds and references in this way, which is why Nietzsche rejects any dichotomy between fiction and reality. The crucial difference, that we can now recognize, is again the experiment. Fictional worlds do not present this kind of affordance to us.[15]

6.4 Conclusion

To attempt to say what a metaphor *is* immediately takes one to the heart of the problem of metaphoricity. If one starts from a certain understanding of metaphor that takes the concept of *transfer* as a core part of metaphorical functioning (as most scholarly work since Aristotle has done), we can see that we are either reducing metaphor to nothing at all (an entirely reversible transfer) or that we are in perpetual search for a metaphor of metaphor to cast the metaphoric process, *through itself*, into a strictly defined category of intelligibility. A fixed concept of metaphor requires fixed meanings – the proper – in the process of meaning-making. As such, if metaphor really is a transfer of proper meanings, a *concept of metaphor* is either trivial and an expression of human ignorance, because the former plays no role in constructing concepts at all (Aristotle), or it can never represent the *phenomenon of metaphor* because it perpetually displaces its own nature as a transfer (Nietzsche).

An essentialist approach to the concept of metaphor seems problematic if the constructive role of metaphors in the creation of concepts is taken seriously. Particular metaphors, like particular concepts, have to be *constructed*, they are never ready-

14 See Deleuze's deliberations on the referential circle [2].

15 „The function of literary metaphor is not typically to send the informed reader out on a research project." [26].

made, they have a history and a certain locality. The meanings of concepts themselves shift and flow rhizomatically [3]. And nevertheless, the process of meaning-production is not entirely devoid of order, (meta)stable meanings do exist. Otherwise, all communication would be impossible. That is why metaphor can be thought of as an experiment. This way of talking about metaphor changes its relationship to the concept, rejecting any kind of priority of the one or the other. It refrains from identifying it and rather proceeds by showing what use is made of metaphor in a certain context. It is my view, that this type of non-foreclosedness is descriptive of the actual uses of epistemic metaphor in modern scientific inquiry as a whole. To think of metaphor as an experiment, an experimental way of talking and thinking, an experimental and self-subducting way of meaning-making, is productive. Where metaphor as mere transfer of the proper could only make sense when fixed categories have already been established, metaphor as experimental transformation and as differentiation connects metaphor to more subtle shifts in our conceptual structures and better communicates the recursive relationship between our thoughts and the world.

References

[1] Deleuze G. Difference and Repetition. London, GB, Bloomsbury, 2014.
[2] Deleuze G. The Logic of Sense. London, GB, Bloomsbury, 2015.
[3] Deleuze G, Guattari F. A Thousand Plateaus. London, GB, Bloomsbury, 2013.
[4] Wittgenstein L. Philosophical Investigations. Oxford, GB, Blackwell, 1953.
[5] Reddy MJ. The conduit metaphor: A case of frame conflict in our language about language. In: Ortony A, editor. Metaphor and Thought. Cambridge, GB, Cambridge University Press, 1993.
[6] Ricoeur P. The Rule of Metaphor. Multi-disciplinary studies of the creation of meaning in language. Toronto, CA, University of Toronto Press, 1977.
[7] Aristoteles. Poetik. Fuhrmann M, translator. Reclam, DE, Ditzingen, 2022.
[8] Platon. Politeia. Krapinger G, translator. Reclam, DE, Ditzingen, 2023.
[9] Potolsky M. Mimesis. New York, USA, Routledge, 2006.
[10] Aristoteles. Rhetorik. Krapinger G, translator. Reclam, DE, Ditzingen, 2020.
[11] Hines A. Metaphor in European Philosophy after Nietzsche. Cambridge, GB, Legenda, 2020.
[12] Kofman S. Nietzsche und die Metapher. Berlin, DE, Wolff Verlag, 2014.
[13] Nietzsche F. Über Wahrheit und Lüge im außermoralischen Sinne. In: Giorgio C, Mazzino M, editors. Sämtliche Werke. Kritische Studienausgabe (KSA). Vol. 1. 2. Ed. Berlin, DE, De Gruyter, 1988.
[14] Nietzsche F. Die Philosophie im tragischen Zeitalter der Griechen. In: Giorgio C, Mazzino M, editors. Sämtliche Werke. Kritische Studienausgabe (KSA). Vol. 1, 2. Ed. Berlin, DE, De Gruyter, 1988.
[15] Nietzsche, F. Die Fröhliche Wissenschaft. In: Giorgio C, Mazzino M, editors. Sämtliche Werke. Kritische Studienausgabe (KSA). Vol. 3, 2. Ed. Berlin, DE, De Gruyter, 1988.
[16] Bachelard G. Noumenon and Microphysics. The Philosophical Forum 2006,37,75–84.
[17] Hacking I. Representing and Intervening. Cambridge, GB, Cambridge University Press, 2010.
[18] Simons M, Vagelli M. Were experiments ever neglected? Ian Hacking and the history of philosophy of experiment. Philosophical Inquiries 2021,9(1),167–188.
[19] Rheinberger HJ. Spalt und Fuge. Eine Phänomenologie des Experiments. Berlin, DE, Suhrkamp, 2021.
[20] Feyerabend P. Against method. London, GB, Verso, 1993.

[21] Black M. Models and metaphors. Studies in language and philosophy. Ithaca, USA, Cornell University Press, 1962.
[22] Hesse, MB. Models, Metaphors and Truth. In: Radman Z, editor. From a Metaphorical Point of View: A Multidisciplinary Approach to the Cognitive Content of Metaphor. Berlin, DE, De Gruyter, 1995.
[23] Lakoff G, Johnson M. Metaphors we live by. Chicago, USA, The University of Chicago Press, 2003.
[24] Brandt C. Metapher und Experiment. Von der Virusforschung zum genetischen Code. Göttingen, DE, Wallstein, 2004.
[25] Reynolds AS. The Third Lens. Chicago, USA, The University of Chicago Press, 2018.
[26] Boyd R. Metaphor and theory change. What is "metaphor" a metaphor for? In: Ortony A. editor. Metaphor and Thought. Cambridge, GB, Cambridge University Press, 1993.

Stefan Heuser

7 Metaphors in ELSA research: Bridging the gap between the laboratory and the life-world

7.1 Key features and critique of ELSA research

Since the inception of the Human Genome Project, interdisciplinary discussions between the natural and social sciences have often been conceptualized as ELSI (in the United States) or ELSA (in Europe). The acronym ELSA/I refers to the ethical, legal, and social aspects or implications of research in the life sciences [1] and has been extended to other fields of technological development, such as AI research [2]. Situated at the boundary of science and society, ELSA research has since then been designed and funded primarily to improve the acceptability of biomedical and biotechnological innovations and to strengthen the overall trustworthiness of science [3].

The integration of ELSA programs into scientific research funding has led to the emergence of a distinct and influential branch of research in bioethics and medical ethics, which encompasses additional initiatives such as "responsible research and innovation" (RRI) and "integrated research" [4–6]. Hub Zwart and Annemiek Nelis have identified four features that are characteristic of ELSA research, namely: „embeddedness in scientific programmes; early anticipation of issues, publics and those responsible for dealing with these issues; interactivity, to encourage stakeholders and publics to assume a more active role in co-designing research agendas; and interdisciplinarity, to bridge the boundaries between research communities such as bioethics and STS" [1, p. 543].[1]

The close interconnection of science policy funding with the bio-industry has, however, raised concerns about the independence of ELSA research [7]. Problems related to joint project funding and the pursuit of economic interests, the emphasis on merely legitimizing science, and the reduction of ethical reflection to a box-ticking exercise – among other potential and actual limitations and biases – were already articulated and criticized in the early stages of ELSA's development [8]. This critique culminates in the suspicion that ELSA research serves merely as a fig leaf for other research interests [9–11]. Ethical research accompanying biotechnological and biomedical innovations faces several challenges.

First, it depends on a general willingness to cooperate across disciplines as well as on third-party funding within ELSA programs.

1 STS = Science and Technology Studies.

https://doi.org/10.1515/9783112215685-007

Second, it is caught between the suspicion that it restricts the freedom of research and the assumption that it acts solely as a lubricant for introducing biotechnological innovations – or as a fig leaf that conceals underlying economic interests and the true scope and risks of research and interventions in order to increase their social acceptability. Critiques of ELSA hold that it has a „facilitative mission (. . .) never to challenge genetic science but to enable its advance“ [12, p. 4].

Despite this critique, it has also become clear that ELSA research is indeed necessary – not only to reduce risks and potential harms arising from translating basic research into clinical applications, but also to ensure that life science research as well as bio- and health technology development are critically and constructively aligned with society's interests, values, and needs [5, 13, 14]. In this context, researchers, institutions, and companies in bio- and medical technologies need to be sufficiently grounded in social and cultural contexts to foster trustworthiness and widespread acceptance of innovative technologies and applications, while also reducing transaction costs and minimizing poor investments.

Critiques of ELSA research limitations and the articulation of further requirements have influenced the evolution of collaborations between science and ethics toward "post-ELSI" frameworks [15] and "integrated" forms of collaborative research [6]. These approaches aim to position ethics and social science research "upstream" in the overall research and technological development process.

In this article, I will explore how metaphors, along with collective interdisciplinary and participatory engagement, can facilitate the early integration of ethical, social, and cultural considerations into biotechnological research, while also encouraging societal stakeholders to help shape relevant research questions and objectives.

7.2 Towards upstream engagement of ELSA and integrated research

Upstream engagement is intended to bring together science and society at an early stage of biotechnological development, aiming to generate knowledge concurrently while integrating ethical and social considerations into scientific innovations and research processes [16]. In an influential article on interdisciplinary collaboration between the natural and social sciences, Balmer et al. propose five "rules of thumb" for establishing a "post-ELSI collaborative space", including „collaborative experimentation, taking risks, collaborative reflexivity, opening-up discussions of unshared goals and neighbourliness“ [15, p. 73]. Such programmes emphasise the importance of collaborative research practices, and also call for shifts in data policy for biomedical research [17]. Additionally, they call for a new understanding of users as active contributors to development [18], the establishment of new governance approaches for handling scientific innovations [19], and the reinforcement of both societal scientific literacy and scientists' communication skills. If research and development are to avoid evolving in a haphazard manner or serving purely economic or special interests, citizens must have opportunities to participate through frameworks that embed ELSA into research.

It remains contested, however, whether and how this procedural integration – across the natural sciences, social sciences, and society; among developers and users; and between basic and applied research – can be successfully achieved [20]. Various barriers stand in the way, such as the vulnerability of participatory processes, stakeholders' lack of interest in engaging, the limited capacity of non-experts to tackle complex scientific issues, the tendency to defer such matters to experts, insufficient insight into laboratory practices and requirements, and, not least, time constraints.

It also remains disputed which factors related to participation and integration ultimately contribute to successful governance processes and how to measure and evaluate the benefits of such efforts for science and society. It is not self-evident that collaborative work on social needs and technological solutions – carried out by groups as diverse as potential users, researchers, and developers, all with different skills and perspectives – will automatically result in more suitable or even groundbreaking solutions, although tensions among participants may stimulate creativity [21]. A longstanding gap exists between the laboratory and the life-world, widened by the abstractness and intangibility of biotechnological research (and its objects) to the public and by the lack of opportunities to gain insight into laboratory processes. For research itself, for science communication, and for integrating society and science, it is therefore essential to visualize and give substance to the often abstract and largely invisible world of molecular biology, with metaphors playing a central role in this endeavor.

At the same time, the perspective of "integrated research" can draw on insights from Science and Technology Studies (STS), which underscore that any research and technology development is already embedded in "socio-technological constellations" and thus interwoven with social practices and institutions, socio-technical visions of future developments, legal frameworks, normative orientations, and policymaking [22–26]. In the relationship between science and society, alienating and integrating effects occur simultaneously. For both sides, it seems advisable not to leave this relationship to chance but to establish parameters for a shared governance of society and science in the development of technological innovations [3, p. 60].

7.3 The gap between the laboratory and the life-world

While STS emphasize the interdependence of science and society, a substantial gap remains – and may even be growing – between the laboratory and the life-world, involving different kinds of knowledge, perceptions, attitudes, practices, and interests.

The evolution of biology into a form of engineering can be interpreted as extending the alienation between the life-world and the laboratory, a phenomenon identified by Husserl nearly a century ago.

In his final, unfinished work, *The Crisis of the European Sciences and Transcendental Phenomenology* [27], which builds on lectures he gave in 1935, Husserl contends that modern science, by devoting itself to abstraction, objectivism, and mere facticity, has become estranged from its original roots in the life-world, and thus severed from its sources of meaning and orientation. Here, he characterizes the life-world as a pre-scientific, everyday sphere of experience that forms the basis for all scientific knowledge. Husserl argues that our concepts of science and knowledge must be revised to account for the importance of subjective perception and the intentional structures of consciousness. To establish a more robust foundation for a science that acknowledges both the objective and subjective dimensions of knowledge, he proposes developing a "transcendental phenomenology" that investigates the fundamental structures of consciousness and experience.

While one need not fully embrace Husserl's transcendental approach to address the alienation between humanity and the world, his diagnosis continues to inspire critical thinking about the relationship between science and society. In light of contemporary biotechnological developments, one might refer to Jürgen Mittelstraß' argument that modern societies develop technical cultures to such an extent that they create what he calls a "Leonardo world" [28], yet still rely on traditional – and specifically Aristotelian – concepts of "nature" to guide the perception of biological processes and biotechnologies.

Mittelstraß' perspective on different types of life-related knowledge, presented in his work „Der Flug der Eule“ [29], offers a distinct view of the intricate interdependence between science and socio-cultural settings and practices. For the time being, it reveals how classical distinctions between nature and technology remain operative. In everyday language, "nature" is still used ontologically as a category of entities possessing their own principles of origin and motion. For the moment, this Aristotelian perspective promotes a contrast between "nature" and the products of "culture" and "technology," which do not contain their origin or *telos* within themselves but rather in an artist or engineer. Such distinctions – between the natural and the technical or artificial, or between things that are "given" and those that are "made" – are not only central elements of intellectual history and culture (particularly in Western societies) but also continue to provide orientation in everyday life.

Recent biotechnological innovations – particularly in synthetic biology – challenge this long-standing distinction between nature and technology. By applying engineering principles to living organisms in an effort to create "artificial life" or "life 2.0", these developments appear to close the gap between life and technology. During this debate, the metaphor of "playing God" has been invoked, yet it has primarily been dismissed as mythological, including by theologians [30]. From their perspective, modern bioengineers are merely working with "natural" forces, "natural" laws, and existing "natural" elements.

Ironically, even if "synthetic" biology succeeds in creating living systems entirely from scratch, determining whether such entities are truly "living" still depends on categories derived from everyday experience. Once we recognize something as living, it ceases to be considered "artificial" life [31]. Consequently, the question is not whether something "is" natural, but whether we perceive and accept it as "natural" [32, 33].

Since biotechnologies appear to shift – or even dissolve – the traditional boundary between "nature" and "technology" in everyday language, the categories by which we perceive and classify something remain in constant flux. This reevaluation is not new. From the earliest forms of plant breeding and animal domestication to modern biotechnology, humans have always intervened in what is considered "natural" or "given" life. In line with scientific progress, these interventions continually reduce aspects of nature that elude human knowledge and control – elements that must nonetheless be acknowledged, however reluctantly [34].

Still, the metaphor "nature" persists as a way of reminding us that there is an order of things that human planning and action cannot simply ignore. We must respond and adapt to this order to avoid becoming "worldless." Through this metaphor, human beings appear as integral parts of a larger framework. Their intentions, desires, and ideas are both shaped by it and motivated to transform it. The concept of "nature" also underscores that much of existence lies beyond human choice – subject instead to chance. Thus, "nature" reminds us that the boundary between what is beyond human control and what can be technically manipulated or bioengineered remains in continual motion, as do the concepts, orientations and guiding principles of science and society.

The crucial question is whether and how we actively engage with these concepts. The gap between the world as portrayed through scientific metaphors and the life-world, where those same metaphors may imply entirely different perspectives and evaluations, can be larger or smaller but remains a vital consideration for science communication. Specifically, we must pay attention to the role a particular metaphor may play within a given context. As Domenico Schneider discusses in this volume, building on Boyd [35] and Hacking [36], the instrumental and interventionist nature of much scientific work generates specific modes of expression and metaphors that are essential for scientific theories but are almost impossible to integrate into the "sensus communis" of public discourse.

It follows that science is neither wholly detached from the life-world nor fully immersed in it – it is both, to varying degrees. Metaphors like "nature," "life," "technology," and "system" significantly shape the cognitive and affective foundations on which scientists and citizens base their understanding of the world, their attitudes toward research practices, and their judgments about trustworthiness, acceptability, and risk [37].

A telling example is the metaphor of "life," which opens up an entire sphere of orientations in which scientific inquiry is conceived and carried out. Scientific research must tie its novel findings back to these orientations in order to communicate effectively. Drawing on Hans Blumenberg, we might even consider "life" an "absolute" metaphor [38] – one that cannot be fully converted into more straightforward terms because it continuously conveys meaning that either awaits discovery or cannot be exhaustively captured by language. In this sense, metaphors help position the methods, observations, and results of scientific research within various orientations, worldviews, and systems of knowledge, while also exceeding those very boundaries in both scientific and everyday contexts. Reflecting on such metaphors can therefore contribute to bridging the gap between the laboratory and the life-world by bringing knowledge and understanding closer together.

7.4 Bridging the gap with metaphors

In the course of the project "How Metaphors Shape Biotechnology" – the results of which are presented in this volume – it proved illuminating to treat metaphors metaphorically as "links," or even as "thought-taxis"[2] that help us "bridge the gap" between the laboratory and the life-world. As Lakoff and Johnson demonstrated in their seminal work *Metaphors We Live By* [39], metaphors are not mere rhetorical devices; rather, they play a fundamental role in structuring human thought processes, shaping perceptions, and informing our understanding of the world we inhabit and navigate.

According to Lakoff and Johnson, we use "conceptual metaphors" to comprehend abstract ideas by relating them to more concrete and tangible experiences. These conceptual metaphors work by mapping one domain (the concrete source domain) onto another (the abstract target domain), allowing us to approach and interpret complex or intangible concepts through familiar ones, which are largely informed by culturally embedded experiences, practices, and values. Metaphors thus function not only as tools of language but also as structures of thought that help us make sense of abstract concepts and facts. To illustrate, in seeking to understand the abstract notion of "life," we might correlate it to metaphors such as a "container" or a "gambling game" [39, p. 51]. For Lakoff and Johnson, "the essence of metaphor is understanding and experiencing one kind of thing in terms of another" [39, p. 5].

Other examples include conceptualizing "argument as war" [39, p. 4] or "time is money" [39, p. 7]. By employing such metaphors, we import elements of the concrete source domain (e.g., money) to the target domain of "time," thereby making this abstract concept more readily graspable and shaping our interpretation of the related experiences. With this conceptual metaphor theory, Lakoff and Johnson influenced

2 I am indebted to Bettina Wahrig, Professor of the History of Pharmacy and Science at TU Braunschweig, for suggesting this term.

subsequent research initiatives that have effectively revealed the conceptual foundations of everyday language [40, 41].

Research on metaphors has also shown that conceptual metaphors function differently depending on their degree of conventionalization [42]. As metaphors become more conventional, the mode of metaphor mapping shifts from comparison to categorization [43]. Eventually, when a metaphor reaches the end of its "career," its literal meaning ceases to be recognized, rendering it "dead." This phenomenon is crucial for both internal and external science communication: previously novel metaphors may no longer be consciously noticed by scientists, yet they may still influence thought processes and guide research. The metaphor of the "genetic code" is a well-known example [44]. Metaphors may be "dead" to scientists but appear novel and groundbreaking to non-experts – or vice versa – causing potential confusion or misunderstanding [45].

Some metaphors, such as "life," may even function as an "absolute" metaphor, as Hans Blumenberg suggests. According to Blumenberg, "absolute" metaphors govern our perception and theorizing of target domains that elude direct observation and sensory access – domains like "world", "truth", "history", or "liberty" [38]. Crucially, however, these metaphors cannot be fully translated into terms and technical vocabulary or reduced to well-defined concepts. Their use in science thus involves ongoing association and interpretation, which can risk sliding into mythological thinking [46] but may also spur innovative methods and ideas. When venturing into life science's central domain – "life" – which cannot be fully captured by terminology and definitions, new metaphors and fresh insights become necessary. Here, a hermeneutic approach to metaphors can serve as a guiding principle. Where terminology is lacking for novel phenomena observed in living systems, we must resort to imagination [46, p. 74], however provisional this may be. In so doing, we push beyond the limits of strictly objective science to make new discoveries, yet we must still return to precise terminology to integrate these insights into our existing knowledge framework.

For this approach to scientific discovery, which frequently surpasses the confines of established methods, we must draw on every socio-cultural and linguistic resource at our disposal. In this context, metaphors function as navigational aids, guiding us into the unknown while linking the realm of scientific exploration – and the acquisition of new knowledge – with familiar concepts and richer modes of understanding. Adding to this complexity, metaphors invoked in emerging fields of biotechnology – such as synthetic biology or gene editing techniques like CRISPR-Cas9 – should undergo political deliberation and democratic decision-making about the futures societies may adopt, regulate, or attempt to prevent [47, 48]. Because the acceptability of new technologies strongly depends on how seamlessly potential users can integrate them into their life-world – without disrupting existing practices, language, or values [49] – it is logical to align research in bio- and health technologies with the lived realities of those who might eventually use them. At the same time, bioscientific research can challenge and reshape these realities by providing new insights into the biological foundations of life, thereby prompting a re-evaluation of commonly accepted but potentially detrimental social habits.

In order to clarify and elaborate the critical potential of metaphors, bridging the gap between the laboratory and the lifeworld is just as an important task for ELSA research as maintaining it. Accordingly, interdisciplinary as well as integrated engagement with metaphors can offer critical perspectives on both science and society. The views, attitudes, understanding, and language games of the lifeworld may serve as a basis for critiquing purely instrumental or technical metaphors produced by research – and vice versa. At the same time, we should remain prepared for the possibility that the very process of metaphor production – within the interdependence of science and society – might generate exactly those metaphors that mislead us and foster problematic orientations, precisely because they fit seamlessly into both spheres. Consequently, our metaphors may deceive us about ourselves and about the reality we aim to investigate, by virtue of their very coherence.

It is not uncommon for ELSA research to be caught between observing biotechnological developments and actively participating in their progression. At times, ethics is reduced to a mere legitimization process, as if the only task were to introduce normative orientations from society to either justify technological advances or deny them moral legitimacy. This perspective overlooks the fact that both scientists and non-experts live within particular life-forms, each defined by language games, practices, social relations, and social structures that nurture their ethical decisions. Metaphors are a key element of these life-forms – and of research itself. They can, if all goes well, act as bridges that bring the ethical grammar of the life-world into laboratories, and conversely, they carry biotechnological concepts back into everyday frameworks of understanding. The added dimension of meaning carried by metaphors – one might describe it as their terminological "fuzziness" – can foster curiosity and imagination that extend beyond our usual limits of perception and comprehension.

In these multifaceted processes of "μεταφορά" (literally "carrying over"), the need to embed knowledge in understanding, to involve citizens in science, and thus to implement ELSA practices comes clearly into view. This is, of course, related to increasing the legitimacy or social acceptability of research, raising the likelihood that biotechnological and biomedical innovations will find their way into the life-world, empowering society to engage in the governance of scientific innovation, and aligning research objectives with the genuine needs and issues of stakeholders [3]. This embedding, however, is also an integral part of scientific invention and innovation itself [48]. Integrating ELSA into research practices and objectives may therefore benefit both society and science.

By supplying metaphors, narratives, imagination, visions, values, emotions, and social practices, the life-world in fact inspires and guides research in directions that continually expand the boundaries of knowledge. This happens by testing how well conceptual metaphors can reveal new insights. Yet it is crucial that these transfer processes be carried out intentionally and reflectively, rather than randomly or without oversight. ELSA research can contribute to better aligning scientific goals with real-world concerns and to merging scientific knowledge with life-worldly understanding. On a more conceptual level, it can facilitate the evaluation of ethical implications and the heuristic value of established metaphors, as well as encourage the exploration of alternatives.

References

[1] Zwart H, Nelis A. "What is ELSA Genomics?" *EMBO Reports* 10 (6), 2009: 540–544. DOI: 10.1038/embor.2009.115.

[2] Van Veenstra A F, van Zoonen E A, Helberger N. ELSA Labs for Human Centric Innovation in AI, 2021. Online: https://nlaic.com/wp-content/uploads/2022/02/ELSA-Labs-for-Human-Centric-Innovation-in-AI.pdf.

[3] Rehmann-Sutter C. Gesellschaftliche, rechtliche und ethische Implikationen der Biomedizin. Zu der Rolle und den Aufgaben von ELSI-Begleitforschung. In Herausforderung Biomedizin. Gesellschaftliche Deutung und soziale Praxis, Dickel S, Franzen M, Kehl C. Bielefeld: Transcript, 2011: 49–66.

[4] Von Schomberg R. "A Vision of Responsible Research and Innovation." In *Responsible Innovation: Managing the Responsible Emergence of Science and Innovation in Society*, Owen R, Bessant J R, Heintz M (Ed.). West Sussex: John Wiley & Sons, 2013: 51–74.

[5] Stilgoe J, Owen R, Macnaghten P. "Developing a Framework for Responsible Innovation." *Research Policy* 42 (9), 2013: 1568–1580. doi:10.1016/j.respol.2013.05.008.

[6] Manzeschke A, Gransche B. Das geteilte Ganze. Horizonte integrierter Forschung für künftige Mensch-Tehcnik-Verhältnisse, Wiesbaden: Springer VS, 2020. https://doi.org/10.1007/978-3-658-26342-3

[7] Dolan D D, Lee, S S-J, Cho M K. Three decades of ethical, legal, and social implications research: Looking back to chart a path forward. In: Cell Genomics, *2* (7), 2022, 100150. https://doi.org/10.1016/j.xgen.2022.100150.

[8] Bauer, M W (Ed.). Resistance to New Technology. Nuclear Power, Information Technology and Biotechnology. Cambridge: CUP, 1995/2010. DOI: https://doi.org/10.1017/CBO9780511563706.

[9] Jasanoff S. Designs on Nature: Science and Democracy in Europe and the United States. Princeton, NJ: Princeton University Press, 2007.

[10] Dickel S, Franzen M, Kehl C (Ed.). Herausforderung Biomedizin: Gesellschaftliche Deutung und soziale Praxis. Bielefeld: transcript, 2011.

[11] Maring M. Vom Praktisch-Werden der Ethik in interdisziplinärer Sicht: Ansätze und Beispiele der Institutionalisierung, Konkretisierung und Implementierung der Ethik. Karlsruhe: KIT Scientific Publishing, 2015.

[12] Yesley M S. What's ELSI got to do with it? Bioethics and the Human Genome Project, New Genetics and Society, 27:1, 2008: 1–6. DOI: 10.1080/14636770701843527.

[13] Owen R, Macnaghten P, Stilgoe J. "Responsible Research and Innovation: From Science in Society to Science for Society, with Society." In: *Emerging Technologies: Ethics, Law and Governance*, edited by Gary E. Marchant, and Wendell Wallach. New York: Routledge, 2020: 117–126.

[14] Ryan M, Blok V. Stop re-inventing the wheel: Or how ELSA and RRI can align. Journal of Responsible Innovation, 10(1), 2023, 2196151. https://doi.org/10.1080/23299460.2023.2196151.

[15] Balmer A S, Calvert J, Marris C, Molyneux-Hodgson S, Frow E, Kearnes M, Martin, P. Five rules of thumb for post-ELSI interdisciplinary collaborations. Journal of Responsible Innovation, 3(1), 2016: 73–80. https://doi.org/10.1080/23299460.2016.1177867.
[16] Rabinow P, Bennett G. Designing Human Practices: An Experiment with Synthetic Biology. Chicago, IL: University of Chicago Press, 2012.
[17] Woolley, J P. Towards coherent data policy for biomedical research with ELSI 2.0: orchestrating ethical, legal and social strategies. Journal of medical ethics 43 (11), 2017: 741–743. doi:10.1136/medethics-2015–103068.
[18] Hölsgens R, Schubert C (Ed.). Popular users: why and how innovation research started to consider users in the innovation process. NOvation – Critical Studies of Innovation, Issue III., 2021. Online: https://revistas.ufpr.br/novation/issue/view/3515.
[19] Braun M, Schickl H, Dabrock P (Ed.). Between Moral Hazard and Legal Uncertainty. Technikzukünfte, Wissenschaft und Gesellschaft / Futures of Technology, Science and Society. Springer VS, Wiesbaden, 2018. https://doi.org/10.1007/978-3-658-22660-2_1.
[20] Myskaja B K, Nydal R, Myhr A I. We Have Never Been ELSI Researchers – There Is No Need for a Post-ELSI Shift. Life Sciences, Society and Policy 10(9), 2014. https://www.ncbi.nlm.nih.gov/pmc/articles/PMC4648827/.
[21] Stark D. The Sense of Dissonance. Accounts of Worth in Economic Life. Princeton: Princeton University Press, 2009.
[22] Rammert W. Technik – Handeln – Wissen. Zu einer pragmatistischen Technik und Sozialtheorie. Wiesbaden: VS Verlag für Sozialwissenschaften, 2007.
[23] Kaiser M, Kurath M, Maasen S, Rehmann-Sutter C (Eds.). Governing future technologies; Nanotechnology and the rise of an assessment regime. Dordrecht: Springer, 2010.
[24] Lindemann G. Weltzugänge: Die mehrdimensionale Ordnung des Sozialen. Weilerswist: Velbrück, 2014.
[25] Felt, U, Fouché R, Miller C A, Smith-Doerr L (Ed.). The handbook of science and technology studies (4th ed.). Cambridge: MIT Press, 2017.
[26] Lösch A, Grunwald A, Meister M, Schulz-Schaeffer I. (Ed.). Socio-Technical Futures Shaping the Present. Technikzukünfte, Wissenschaft und Gesellschaft / Futures of Technology, Science and Society. Springer VS, Wiesbaden, 2019. https://doi.org/10.1007/978-3-658-27155-8_1.
[27] Husserl E. Die Krisis der europäischen Wissenschaften und die transzendentale Phänomenologie. Eine Einleitung in die phänomenologische Philosophie, Ströker E (Ed.), Hamburg: Felix Meiner, 1936/2012.
[28] Mittelstraß J. Leonardo-Welt. Über Wissenschaft, Forschung und Verantwortung. Frankfurt/Main: Suhrkamp, 1992.
[29] Mittelstraß J. Der Flug der Eule: Von der Vernunft der Wissenschaft und der Aufgabe der Philosophie, Frankfurt/Main: Suhrkamp, 1989.
[30] Ried J, Dabrock P. Weder Schöpfer noch Plagiator. Theologisch-ethische Überlegungen zur Synthetischen Biologie zwischen Genesis und Hybris. In: Zeitschrift für Evangelische Ethik, 55 (3), 2011: 179–191.
[31] Moos T. Künstliches Leben gibt es nicht. Anmerkungen zur Ethik der synthetischen Biologie. In: systembiologie.de (Magazin für systembiologische Forschung, deutsche Ausgabe), 8. Mai 2014: 16–18. Online: https://www.systembiologie.de/lw_resource/datapool/_items/item_14/frs-13014_systembiologie_8_2014.pdf.
[32] Rehmann-Sutter C. Das „Leben" synthetischer Zellen. In: Deutscher Ethikrat (Ed.): Werkstatt Leben. Bedeutung der Synthetischen Biologie für Wissenschaft und Gesellschaft, Berlin, 2013: 75–88.
[33] Rehmann-Sutter C. How do we see that something is living? Synthetic creatures and phenomenology of perception. In: Worldviews 17 (1), 2013: 9–24.

[34] Grunwald A. Synthetische Biologie zwischen Durchbruch und Hype. In: Deutscher Ethikrat (Ed.): Werkstatt Leben. Bedeutung der Synthetischen Biologie für Wissenschaft und Gesellschaft, Berlin, 2013: 51-65.

[35] Boyd R. Metaphor and theory change: What is "metaphor" a metaphor for? In: Ortony A (Ed.): Metaphor and Thought. 2nd edition. Cambridge: CUP, 1998: 481-532.

[36] Hacking I. Einführung in die Philosophie der Naturwissenschaften. Stuttgart: Reclam, 1995.

[37] Douglas H E. Science, Policy, and the Value-Free Ideal. Pittsburgh: University of Pittsburgh Press, 2009. https://doi.org/10.2307/j.ctt6wrc78.

[38] Blumenberg H. Paradigmen zu einer Metaphorologie, Frankfurt/Main: Suhrkamp, 1997.

[39] Lakoff G, Johnson M. Metaphors we live by. Chicago: The University of Chicago Press, 1980.

[40] Lakoff G. The contemporary theory of metaphor. In Ortony, A. (Ed.), Metaphor and thought (2nd edition). Cambridge: Cambridge University Press, 1993: 202-251.

[41] Schmitt R, Schröder J, Pfaller L. Systematische Metaphernanalyse. Eine Einführung. Wiesbaden, Springer VS, 2018.

[42] Gentner D, Bowdle B F. Psychology of metaphor processing. In Nadel L (Ed.). The encyclopedia of cognitive science. New York: Macmillan, 2006. https://doi.org/10.1002/0470018860.s00579.

[43] Bowdle B F., Gentner D. The Career of Metaphor. In: Psychological Review, 112 (1), 2005: 193–216. https://doi.org/10.1037/0033-295X.112.1.193.

[44] Knudsen S. Communicating novel and conventional scientific metaphors: A study of the development of the metaphor of genetic code. Public Understanding of Science, 14(4), 2005: 373–392. https://doi.org/10.1075/milcc.4.08knu?locatt=mode:legacy.

[45] Beger A, Smith, T H. Introduction. In: (ibid. ed.): How Metaphors Guide, Teach and Popularize Science. Amsterdam / Philadelphia: John Benjamins Publishing Company, 2020: 1–37.

[46] Blumenberg H. Theorie der Unbegrifflichkeit. Aus dem Nachlaß herausgegeben und mit einem Nachwort von Haverkamp A, Frankfurt/Main: Suhrkamp, 2007.

[47] Jasanoff S, Hurlbut JB, Saha K. CRISPR democracy: Gene editing and the need for inclusive deliberation. Issues in Science and Technology 32(1), 2015: 37.

[48] Kearnes M, Kuch D, Johnston A. How to do things with metaphors: engineering life as hodgepodge. Life Sci Soc Policy, Sep 17; 14 (1), 2018: 22. Doi: 10.1186/s40504-018-0084-z.

[49] Renn O. Technikakzeptanz: Lehren und Rückschlüsse der Akzeptanzforschung für die Bewältigung des technischen Wandels. *Theorie und Praxis* 3 (14), 2005: 29–38.

Daniel Keck

8 Das bedrohte Gleichgewicht. Der Begriff der Krankheit in Pflege und Medizin. Eine historisch-vergleichende Metaphernanalyse

Abstract: Introduction: The aim of this article is to add a metaphorological perspective to the debate on the concept of illness. It focuses on the epistemological question of which metaphors are used by the authors of medical and nursing textbooks and how this metaphorology affects the practice of healthcare professionals.

Method: Eleven texts from textbooks from the 1950s and 2015s as well as trivial comparison texts are analysed in order to investigate the use of metaphors. The theoretical approaches of Lakoff and Johnson as well as the method of systematic metaphor analysis according to Schmitt et al. are used for this purpose. The work of Lakoff and Johnson offers a fundamental perspective on the cognitive function of metaphors, while the methodological approaches of Schmitt et al. enable a structured analysis of metaphorical concepts.

Results: The texts of the 1950s contain expressive and striking metaphors that primarily originate from the source area of spatial experience, technical apparatus and war. A machine-like organism must defend itself against external and internal attacks that threaten to disturb the balance of physical processes. In the more recent texts, the number of metaphors of technology and war decreases sharply and the metaphor of equilibrium gains in importance.

Keywords: systematic metaphor analysis, Lakoff and Johnson, concepts of health and illness, historical comparison

8.1 Krankheit und ihre Metaphern

Fragen um Gesundheit und Krankheit sind nicht erst seit den Pandemiejahren fester Bestandteil des gesellschaftlichen Diskurses. In Zeiten des Umbruchs verengt sich die Diskussion schnell auf Aspekte der Bezahlbarkeit von Leistungen im Angesicht sich verknappender öffentlicher Mittel. Dabei tritt in den Hintergrund, dass sich die so selbstverständlich gebrauchten Begriffe *Gesundheit* und *Krankheit* einer inhaltlichen Bestimmung weitestgehend entziehen. Seit den 1970er-Jahren lassen sich in der Medizinphilosophie eine Vielzahl von Bestrebungen beobachten, einen umfassenden Krankheitsbegriff zu entwickeln, der sich letztlich aber in einem Schulenstreit zwischen naturalistischen und normatavistischen Theoriepositionen festgefahren zu haben scheint. Naturalistische Krankheitstheorien versuchen, Krankheit auf objektive, biologische und wertfreie Weise zu definieren. Eine der bekanntesten und ein-

https://doi.org/10.1515/9783112215685-008

flussreichsten Theorien ist die von Christopher Boorse entwickelte biostatistische Theorie der Krankheit [1]. Krankheiten werden in ihr als signifikante Abweichungen von der *normalen* Funktionsweise biologischer Systeme definiert. Normalität begegnet uns in der biostatistischen Theorie als der Zustand, bei dem ein Individuum in der Lage ist, seine spezies-typischen biologischen Funktionen in einem statistischen Durchschnitt zu erfüllen. Boorses Ansatz zielt darauf ab, Krankheiten in rein biologischen und funktionalen Begriffen zu definieren, ohne auf soziale oder subjektive Bewertungen zurückzugreifen. Dies steht im Gegensatz zu normativistischen Theorien von Krankheit, die den Krankheitsbegriff auf der Grundlage von Werturteilen und sozialen Normen definieren. Normativistische Krankheitstheorien lehnen bereits die Möglichkeit einer wertfreien Betrachtung ab. Sie gehen davon aus, dass die Begriffe *Gesundheit* und *Krankheit* nicht rein objektiv bestimmt werden können, sondern immer auch normative, also wertende, Elemente enthalten [2].[1]

Ziel meines Beitrags ist es, die Auseinandersetzung um den Krankheitsbegriff um eine metaphorologische Perspektive zu erweitern. Vor dem thematischen Hintergrund des Tagungsbandes soll die erkenntnisleitende Frage im Vordergrund stehen, welcher Metaphern sich die Autor*innen medizinischer und pflegerischer Lehrwerke bedienen und wie sich diese Metaphorik auf die Handlungspraxis von Gesundheitsprofessionellen auswirkt. Ein weiteres Ziel ist es, durch die Analyse von Metaphern mögliche Veränderungsprozesse in den Denkstrukturen zu identifizieren und zu verstehen, wie sich bestimmte Narrative im Laufe der Zeit gewandelt haben.

Die Vorstellung, dass sich Metaphern auf das Denken und Handeln von Gesundheitsprofessionellen auswirken, ist kein neuer Gedanke. Das bereits 1977 erschiene Essay der amerikanischen Publizistin Susan Sonntag *Krankheit als Metapher* und der darauf aufbauende Text *Aids und seine Metaphern* haben mit beachtlicher Wirkmacht auf diesen Umstand hingewiesen. Sonntag zeigt, dass Krankheiten mit bestimmten Metaphern in Verbindung gebracht werden. So lassen sich in der Romantik Deutungsmuster erkennen, in denen Tuberkulose mit künstlerischer Schaffenskraft assoziiert wurde: Tuberkulose habe zu einer Vergeistigung der kranken Person geführt, *indem* sie den Körper auflöste [6:21]. Für ihre Zeit stellt Sonntag in Bezug auf Krebs fest, dass die Krankheit das Unvermögen des kranken Menschen widerspiegele, Gefühle auszudrücken und auszuleben, was letztlich die Erkrankung verursache. Sie zeigt deutlich, dass Diagnosen neben einer deskriptiv biologischen auch eine narrative Ebene besitzen, die mit einer Vielzahl von Bedeutungen und impliziten, teils moralischen Zuschreibungen ausgestattet ist. Krebs, so rekapituliert sie das gesellschaftliche Narrativ eindrücklich, sei letztlich selbst verschuldet, weil er mit einer Charakterschwäche einhergehe.

1 Zwei Veröffentlichungen der letzten Jahre setzen sich mitunter recht amüsant mit diesem Hiatus auseinander [3,4]). Zwar gibt es durchaus Synthesevorschläge zwischen den beiden Theoriepositionen, doch auch deren Konsensfähigkeit scheint begrenzt. Zu hybriden Konzepten siehe unlängst erschienen [5].

8.2 Umrisse einer metaphorologischen Perspektive

Um die Rolle von Metaphern für das Verständnis von Krankheit zu rekonstruieren, werde ich mich im Folgenden an den Arbeiten von George Lakoff und Mark Johnson orientieren, die mit *Metaphors We Live By* [7] und nachfolgenden Veröffentlichungen einen grundlegenden Beitrag zur kognitiv orientierten Metaphernforschung geleistet haben. Lakoff und Johnson gehen in ihrer Theorie der „konzeptuellen Metaphern" davon aus, dass sprachliche Metaphern nicht nur rhetorische Figuren sind, sondern tief verankerte und grundlegende Bestandteile unseres Denkens und unserer Wahrnehmung. Als eine Art kognitive Struktur prägen Metaphern unser Verständnis der Welt und wirken sich dabei gleichermaßen auf unsere Handlungen aus [7:11]. Die Autoren stellen fest: „Unser alltägliches Konzeptsystem, nach dem wir sowohl denken als auch handeln, ist im Kern und grundsätzlich metaphorisch." [7:11] Metaphern helfen uns dabei, komplexe Ideen besser zu verstehen, indem sie sie in Beziehung zu konkreteren und greifbareren Dingen setzen. Lakoff und Johnsen zeigen das am Beispiel „Argumentieren ist Krieg", indem sie auf die Kriegsmetaphorik hinweisen, die sich in der Betrachtung von verbalen Auseinandersetzungen zeigt. Als Diskussionsteilnehmer*in kann man z. B. eine Position einnehmen, eine Position verteidigen, der eigene Standpunkt kann angegriffen werden, man kann verschiedene Strategien anwenden und einen Streit gewinnen oder verlieren [7:12]. Die Autoren stellen die Überlegung an, was sich ändern könnte, wenn es eine Gesellschaft gäbe, in der Argumente nicht wie ein Krieg, sondern wie ein Tanz strukturiert wären: Sie gehen davon aus, dass Argumentationshandlungen grundsätzlich anderen Charakter hätten und wir diese Interaktionen wohl gar nicht als Argumentieren erkennen würden [7:12].

Lakoff und Johnson verwenden einen weiten Metaphernbegriff, der sich von dem anderer Autor*innen unterscheidet. Für sie sind alle sprachlichen Figuren oder Wendungen, in denen eine Bedeutungsübertragung von einem Bedeutungsbereich (Quellbereich) in einen anderen (Zielbereich) stattfindet, Metaphern: „Das Wesen der Metapher besteht darin, daß wir durch sie eine Sache oder einen Vorgang in Begriffen einer anderen Sache bzw. eines anderen Vorgangs verstehen und erfahren können". [7:13] In vielen Fällen wird es sich dabei um die Übertragung früher und einfacher Erfahrungen in einen komplexeren Zielbereich handeln [8:26]. Für Lakoff und Johnson gibt es unterschiedliche Arten von Metaphern, von denen einige wichtige an dieser Stelle kurz erläutert seien. Bei *Orientierungsmetaphern* handelt es sich um Metaphern, die auf grundlegende sensormotorische Erfahrungen zurückgehen. Sie beziehen sich auf räumliche Orientierung.[2] Beispiele sind „hoch" und „niedrig", „in" und „aus", „vorne" und „hinten".

2 Räumliche Erfahrungen dienen als metapherngenerierende Schemata, das sind basale Muster hinter den Metaphern, die selbst noch keinen bildhaften Charakter besitzen und der Vergegenständlichung komplexer psychischer oder sozialer Phänomene dienen. Schmitt et al. [8:15–20] bieten eine gute Darstellung metapherngenerierender Schemata. Sie führen neben dem Raum noch Objekt, Substanz, Behälter und Person auf.

Sie strukturieren unser Verständnis von Konzepten in Bezug auf die Orientierung im Raum. „Hoch“ wird oft mit positiven Zuständen assoziiert („hohe Standards“), während „niedrig“ negative Konnotationen hat („niedergeschlagen“, „niedrige Moral“ [7:22–26].[3] “Das Gehirn ist eine Maschine”, “Der Verstand ist ein Behälter”, “Zeit ist Geld“ sind Beispiele für *ontologische Metaphern*. Durch sie gelingt es, abstrakte oder nicht greifbare Erfahrungen so zu gestalten, dass wir sie als Objekte, Substanzen oder Entitäten betrachten können [7:35–39]. Durch *Strukturmetaphern* schließlich werden komplexe oder abstrakte Konzepte durch strukturierte, bekannte Phänomene erklärt [7:75]. Das bereits erwähnte metaphorische Konzept „Argumentieren ist Krieg“ steht beispielhaft für solche Metaphern: Die Erfahrung des Krieges wird auf den Austausch von Argumenten übertragen. Lakoff und Johnson führen die Idee des *Hervorhebens* und *Verbergens* ein, um eine Vorstellung davon zu entwickeln, wie Menschen Strukturmetaphern nutzen. In der Verwendung konzentrieren sich Menschen auf einen Teil der Quellerfahrung zur Entwicklung einer Metapher, blenden aber andere Aspekte der Erfahrung aus [7:18–21] – ein Umstand, der im weiteren Verlauf dieser Untersuchung noch von Bedeutung sein wird.

Schmitt hebt hervor, dass die wesentliche Innovation des Konzepts von Lakoff und Johnson in der Erkenntnis bestehe, dass Metaphern nicht für sich alleine stehen, sondern in metaphorischen Konzepten organisiert sind, also einem System, das auf einer Subkategorisierung beruht [11]. Lakoff und Johnson illustrieren die Vielschichtigkeit solcher metaphorischer Konzepte am Beispiel von „Zeit ist Geld“ [7:15–17]. Der Quellbereich der ökonomischen Ressourcen wird auf den Zielbereich der zeitlichen Struktur übertragen, um Zeit als eine wertvolle, begrenzte Ressource zu verstehen. Wie Geld wollen wir Zeit sparen; man kann Zeit wie Geld investieren oder unter Zeitmangel leiden. In einer Durchsicht der verschiedenen Verwendungsweisen dieser Metapher werden mögliche Subkategorien deutlich, so z. B. unterschiedliche Vergügbarkeits-, Kostbarkeits- oder Managementmetaphern.

8.3 Methodik

Lakoff und Johnson ist es in ihrem Œuvre gelungen zu zeigen, dass viele unserer alltäglichen Begriffe und Konzepte metaphorischer Natur sind und tief in unseren kognitiven Prozessen wurzeln. Sie zeigen, wie Metaphern unsere Wahrnehmung und unser Verständnis der Welt beeinflussen, indem sie konzeptionelle Strukturen in unserem

---

3 Die Arbeiten von Lakoff und Johnson zeigen sich anschlussfähig zu unterschiedlichen Wissenschaftstraditionen. Das Rekurrieren auf die gelebte Erfahrung des Raums hat u. a. den Brückenschlag zu leibphänomenologischen Ansätzen ermöglicht. Beispielhaft sind die Arbeiten von Shaun Gallagher [9, 10] zu nennen, in denen er die Wechselbeziehungen zwischen Sprache, Körpererfahrungen und phänomenologischem Bewusstsein herausarbeitet.

Gehirn widerspiegeln und formen. Darüber hinaus geben sie wertvolle Hinweise, wie Metaphern analysiert werden können. Ihre methodischen Implikationen bleiben allerdings aus einer sozialwissenschaftlichen Perspektive rudimentär und sind für Forschungsvorhaben dieser Art um ein konkretes methodisches Vorgehen zu erweitern. Dafür soll im Folgenden auf die Arbeiten von Rudolf Schmitt und Kolleg*innen aufgebaut werden, die sich in zahlreichen Veröffentlichungen um eine Integration der Konzepte von Lakoff und Johnson in den sozialwissenschaftlichen Methodenkanon verdient gemacht haben. Wie andere Methoden der qualitativen Sozialforschung ist auch die *Systematische Metaphernanalyse* geeignet, die subjektiven Bedeutungen und Interpretationen zu verstehen, die Individuen und Gruppen ihren sozialen Handlungen, Interaktionen und Kontexten beimessen. Damit diese Rekonstruktionen sozialen Sinns aber valide sind, muss eine Metaphernanalyse methodisch sicherstellen, dass sie sich nicht auf die Analyse auffälliger oder plakativer Metaphern beschränkt, sondern die Breite und Fülle der gesamten Metaphorik berücksichtigt wird [8:30]. Zugleich muss der spezifische Gebrauch von Metaphern durch einen Vergleichshorizont aus anderen Quellen sichtbar gemacht werden [8:34]. Schließlich hat eine Metaphernanalyse sicherzustellen, dass der soziale, gesellschaftliche und kulturelle Kontext Berücksichtigung findet und in die Auswertung einbezogen wird [8:37]. Die *Systeamtische Metaphernanalyse* nach Schmitt ist in sieben Schritte gegliedert, die im Folgenden nur deutlich verkürzt wiedergegeben werden:

Tab. 8.1: Schritte der Systematischen Metaphernanalyse nach Schmitt.

1. Indikation klären, Zielbereiche identifizieren Überprüfen, ob die Metaphernanalyse als Methode zur Forschungsfrage und dem Phänomen passt. Die Bestimmung des zu untersuchenden Phänomens definiert die Zielbereiche der Metaphorisierung.	**2. Der kontrastierende Hintergrund und die Eigenanalyse** Die kulturell üblichen Metaphorisierungen werden durch Sammlung verschiedener Materialien (Lexika, Zeitungen, Publikationen etc.) als Vergleichshorizont erfasst. Eigene Metaphern der Forschenden werden durch Eigeninterviews und Publikationen identifiziert, um Reflexion und Sensibilisierung zu fördern.
3. Erhebung des Materials Aufgrund des Aufwands der Metaphernanalyse wird sparsames Sampling im Sinne des Theoretical Samplings der Grounded Theory Methode empfohlen, wobei eine möglichst große Variation des Textkorpus empfohlen ist.	**4. Systematische Analyse einer Gruppe/eines Einzelfalls** Die Texte werde durch Wort-für-Wort-Zergliederung in ihre metaphorischen Bestandteile zerlegt und eine Liste metaphorischer Wendungen erstellt. In einem zweiten Schritt werden metaphorische Konzepte aus dieser Liste durch stetige Vergleiche rekonstruiert und dienen im weiteren Verlauf der Untersuchung als Grundlage der Interpretation.

Tab. 8.1 (fortgesetzt)

5. Interpretation mithilfe einer Heuristik Zur Rekonstruktion der in den metaphorischen Konzepten enthaltenen Implikationen kommt schließlich eine Heuristik zur Anwendung, in der insbesondere die aufmerksamkeitsfokussierenden und -ausblendenden Funktionen des jeweiligen metaphorischen Konzepts sichtbar gemacht werden.	**6. Triangulation, Gütekriterien und Verallgemeinerung** Abhängig vom Einzelfall ist zu prüfen, ob Triangulation mit anderen Auswertungsmethoden die Ergebnisqualiät verbessern kann.
7. Darstellung Die metaphorischen Konzepte und Ihre Implikationen werden in dargestellt.	[8:57–94]

8.4 Verwendetes Datenmaterial

Grundlage der Metaphernanalyse bildet ein Textkorpus von elf Texten aus verschiedenen Jahrzehnten und Fachbereichen (Tab. 8.2). Neben je zwei Lehrbüchern aus Krankenpflege und Medizin der 1950er- und 2015er-Jahre, werden aus beiden Jahrzehnten je ein bzw. zwei Vergleichstexte in die Betrachtung einbezogen. Dieser Vergleichshorizont dient der Kontextualisierung von Metaphern, wodurch präzisere und nuanciertere Analysen möglich werden [8:34]. Für die 1950er-Jahre wird das *Bertelsmann Volkslexikon* herangezogen, das in erster Linie Erwachsene mit Interesse an Allgemeinwissen adressierte. Es wurden die Lemmata „Gesundheit", „Gesundheitswesen", „Herz", „Herzgeräusche", „Herzkrankheiten" und „Krankheit" in die Analyse einbezogen, die sich durch inhaltliche Nähe zum Ausgangsmaterial auszeichnen. Da das Lexikon sich nicht an ein Fachpublikum richtet, kann es darüber Aufschluss geben, ob sich die Metaphorik der Fachsprache von der Alltagssprache abgehoben hat. Die zeitliche Staffelung einerseits und die verschiedenen fachlichen Perspektiven andererseits eröffnen eine Vielzahl von Dimensionen für kontinuierliches und systematisches Vergleichen von Daten, wodurch kontextuelle Unterschiede und Ähnlichkeiten sichtbar gemacht werden können, die der Identifizierung von Mustern dienen [12:1].[4] Aus den vorliegenden Lehrwerken werden Textpassagen ausgewählt, die Krankheitsgeschehen in möglichst allgemeiner Form beschreiben.[5]

4 Aus forschungspraktischen Gründen werden in die Auswertung nur historische Lehrbücher Westdeutschlands einbezogen. Eine spätere Untersuchung aus einer gesamtdeutschen Perspektive scheint aber äußerst lohnenswert.

5 Lehrwerken wurde in dieser Untersuchung der Vorzug gegeben, da sie nicht nur Aufschluss über die Sprachpraxis geben können, sondern auch starken Einfluss auf die nachfolgende klinische Generation haben dürften.

Als heutiger Vergleichstext wird ein „Gespräch“ mit ChatGPT 4 über Krankheit genutzt. Textgenerierungssysteme dieser Art stehen in dem Ruf, als *stochastische Papageien* das nachzuplappern, was sie in Quellen vorfinden. Diese allgemeine Kritik ist sicherlich verkürzend und sollte nicht darüber hinwegtäuschen, dass solche Chatbots helfen können, häufige Muster des Sprachgebrauchs zu identifizieren, da sie die Antworten geben, die auf Basis der Trainingsdaten am wahrscheinlichsten sind. Es ist aber wichtig zu verstehen, dass *wahrscheinlich* in diesem Kontext nicht *am häufigsten vorkommend* bedeutet. Es bedeutet vielmehr *konsistent mit den Mustern, die das Modell in den Trainingsdaten gelernt hat* [13:266–270]. Die genaue Formulierung der Antwort hängt von vielen Variablen ab, einschließlich der konkreten Eingabeaufforderung und kann jedes Mal ein wenig variieren [14]. Bei der Ausgabe von ChatGPT 4 handelt es sich daher nicht um einen repräsentativen Querschnitt des aktuellen Sprachgebrauchs, es spricht aber vieles dafür, dass die heute gebräuchliche Metaphorik in einer für den Zweck dieser Arbeit ausreichenden Form durch ChatGPT wiedergegeben wird. Darüber hinaus fließt ein medizinnaher Aufklärungstext aus der *Apothekenumschau* in die Auswertung ein.

Der Vergleich zwischen den 1950er-Jahren und der Zeit seit 2015 scheint besonders gewinnbringend, da es sich bei den Nachkriegsjahren um eine Phase des Umbruchs handelt, die eng mit einem bürgerlich-konservativen Rollen- und Geschlechterverhältnis vergesellschaftet war. Gerade im Kontrast zur heutigen Zeit scheint es daher möglich, zu untersuchen, wie sich Metaphern entlang gesamtgesellschaftlicher Diskussionslinien entwickelt haben. Allerdings bringt die Breite des Datensamples auch Herausforderungen mit sich: Der Professionalisierungsgrad der Krankenpflege muss für die 1950er-Jahre als ausgesprochen niedrig eingeschätzt werden. Die eingeschränkte berufliche Autonomie und Selbstregulierung der Pflegeberufe in der frühen Bundesrepublik lässt sich auch daran festmachen, dass ihre Standardlehrwerke nicht von Pflegekräften, sondern von (männlichen) Medizinern verfasst wurden.

Tab. 8.2: Übersicht über das verwendete Datenmaterial A.

1950er-Jahre
Pflegelehrbücher
HP1: Georg Thieme Verlag (Hrsg.) (1953): Einführung in die Krankenpflege. Thieme, Leipzig, S. 95–98.
HP2: Fischer et al. (1950): Hand- und Lehrbuch der Krankenpflege. Praktische Krankenpflege. Franckhische Verlagshandlung Stuttgart
Medizinlehrbücher
HM1: Bürger, M. (1952): Der Kliniker. Einführung in die Innere Medizin. De Gruyter, Berlin.
HM2: Heilmeyer, L. (Hrsg.): (1955): Lehrbuch der inneren Medizin. Springer Verlag: Berlin, Göttingen, Heidelberg, S. 421–428 448–450.

Tab. 8.2 (fortgesetzt)

Historische Vergleichsliteratur
HZ: Bertelsmann (Hg.) (1956): Bertelsmann Volkslexikon. Bertelsmann, Gütersloh.
2015er-Jahre
Pflegelehrbücher
GP1: Haider-Sturtz, I. (2022): Allgemeine Pathologie. Ein Lehrbuch für Pflege- und andere Gesundheitsberufe, 3. Aufl., Wien: Facultas, S. 61–64.
GP2: Thieme Verlag (Hrsg.) (2015): I care Pflege. 2. Aufl., Thieme, Stuttgart, S. 103–105.
Medizinlehrbücher
GM1: Weber, Paul (2023): Grundwissen Krankheitslehre: zum Einstieg in Studium und Praxis.: UTB, Stuttgart S. 19–25.
GM2: Anton, L. et al. (2018): Innere Medizin. Symptome und klinische Probleme. 9. Aufl., Facultas, Wien S. 134–145.
Heutige Vergleichsliteratur
GZ: Apothekenumschau (Hg.) (2019): Herzinfarkt erkennen und behandeln. Im Internet: https://www.apotheken-umschau.de/krankheiten-symptome/herz-kreislauf-erkrankungen/herzinfarkt-erkennen-und-behandeln-734303.html
ChatGPT 4: „Gespräch" über Gesundheit und Krankheit.

8.5 Auswertung I: Krankheitsmetaphern in Texten der 1950er Jahre

Die Untersuchung von Krankheitsmetaphern gestaltet sich vor dem Hintergrund herausfordernd, dass *Krankheit* in den vorliegenden Texten nicht als isoliertes Phänomen konzipiert wird, sondern – analog zum Sprachgebrauch – in vielen Fällen über das Antonym hergeleitet wird. Zwischen Gesundheit und Krankheit gibt es eine enge sprachliche Verbindung. Daher werden Gesundheitsmetaphern dort, wo sie der Beantwortung der Forschungsfrage dienen, in der Auswertung berücksichtigt. Im folgenden werden nicht alle metaphorischen Konzepte im Detail dargestellt, sondern lediglich die quantitativ bedeutsamsten.[6]

6 So finden sich z. B. im Material immer wieder Metaphern aus dem Quellbereich des Theaters, beispielsweise *spielen* sich die Lebensvorgänge in einer bestimmten Weise ab oder bestimmte Faktoren *spielen eine begrenzte Rolle* in der Krankheitsentstehung. Vereinzelt lassen sich zudem Metaphern aus dem Quellbereich des *Gewichts* und der *physischen Erfahrung identifizieren,* die oft mit körperlichen

8.5.1 Krankheit kommt von außen (oder innen)

In den vorliegenden Texten gibt es eine Vielzahl von Orientierungsmetaphern, die verbindet, dass sie das Krankheitsgeschehen über räumliche Bezüge konzeptualisieren. Krankheiten werden als Orte vorgestellt, die wir besuchen, verlassen oder durchqueren können, die aber auch Grenzen besitzen und die Differenzierung zwischen dem Selbst und dem Anderen ermöglichen.

> [das] Verhalten gegenüber den Reizen aus der äußeren und inneren Umwelt (HP1:96)

Gesundheit begegnet den Lesenden als normgerechter innerer physiologischer Ablauf, der in steter Auseinandersetzung mit den Einflüssen einer potenziell feindlichen Umgebung steht und auf diese reagieren muss. Das verlangt vom Organismus ein aktives Gegensteuern, das sich in einigen Herstellungsmetaphern zeigt. Gesundheit ist demnach nichts, was dem Menschen zufällt, sie ist brüchig und ihr Erhalt benötigt viele Ressourcen sowie aktives Zutun. Die in weiten Teilen, insbesondere aber in den medizinischen Texten biologistisch geprägte Wortwahl ist auffallend: Krankheit ist ein Zustand des *Orgnismus*, der einerseits sprachlich anthropomorphisiert wird, d. h. die Krankheit tritt als eigenständig handelnde Akteurin auf, andererseits wird der *Mensch* hinter den biologische Abläufen kaum in den Blick genommen.

> Unter- und Überfunktion sind wichtige Faktoren bei der Entstehung zahlreicher Krankheitszustände. (HP2:48)

Eine weitere raumbezogene Dimension stellen Metaphern dar, die auf den Präpositionen „unter" und „über" basieren. Im Allgemeinen beziehen sich diese Metaphern auf eine räumliche Orientierung in Bezug auf eine aufrechte Körperhaltung und stehen in Verbindung mit Dualismen wie "gut" und "schlecht" oder "mächtig" und „ohnmächtig". In den vorliegenden Fällen folgt die metaphorische Bedeutung nicht den üblichen konzeptuellen Mustern und repräsentiert eine Abweichung von dem, was zu erwarten wäre. Eine *Überfunktion* stellt sich gerade nicht als herausragende Erfüllung der biologischen Anforderungen dar, sondern, wie auch die Unterfunktion, als funktionelle Fehlleistung.

> [...] das Absterben mehr oder weniger begrenzter Gebiete des Herzmuskels (HV:HerzInf)
> [...] durch Blutverluste nach außen, oder durch Liegenbleiben größerer Blutmengen in erweiterten Gefäßprovinzen (HM1:25)

Die bereits eingeführte Differenzierung zwischen „Innen" und „Außen" wird durch verschiedene Formen der Grenzmetaphern erweitert. Grenzen trennen zwei unter-

---

Empfindungen und physischen Interaktionen mit der Welt verbunden sind. Beispiele hierfür sind *leichte* oder *schwere* Erkrankungen. Auch Anthropomorphismen lassen sich vorfinden, so hat der „Blutkreislauf hat für rechtzeitige [...] Versorgung der Organe mit Sauerstoff [...] zu sorgen" (HM1).

schiedliche Dinge oder Orte, z. B. zwei Länder. Sie markieren den Übergang von einem ins andere und vermitteln die Vorstellung von Gesundheit und Krankheit als dichotome Zustände die sich gegenseitig ausschließen. Gleichzeitig bieten Formulierungen mit starken geographischem Bezug (z. B. Gefäßprovinzen) Anschluss zu Reisemetaphern, die das Gesunde als zu gehenden Weg verstehen. Eine solche Metaphorik lässt sich aber aufgrund des begrenzenden Datenmaterials nicht hinreichend verdichten.

8.5.2 Krankheit ist verlorenes Gleichgewicht

> Der Mensch ist gesund, so lange er sich mit der ihn *umgebenden Außenwelt* im Gleichgewicht zu halten vermag. (HP1:95)
>
> Das Wesentliche eines jeden Krankheitsgeschehens ist eine Gleichgewichtsstörung im Zusammenspiel aller Kräfte und Organfunktionen. Einzelne Organe können zu wenig oder zu viel leisten; (HP2:48)

Auch bei Gleichgewichtsmetaphern handelt es sich um Orientierungsmetaphern, denen individualentwicklungsgeschichtlich frühe räumliche Erfahrungen zugrundeliegen. Die Vorstellung von Gesundheit als Gleichgewicht suggeriert, dass unser Körper ein komplexes System ist, das durch eine fein abgestimmte Balance verschiedener Faktoren funktioniert – wie beispielsweise Stoffwechselprozesse, Hormone, körperliche Aktivität und Ruhe und so weiter.[7] Wenn alle diese Faktoren im Gleichgewicht sind, so impliziert die Metapher, sind wir gesund. Die Gleichgewichtsmetapher findet sich prominent in allen Texten und kann als integrative Metapher verstanden werden, die verschiedene untergeordnete metaphorische Konzepte zusammenführt: Das Verhältnis zwischen innen und außen, Über- und Unterfunktion, zu viel und zu wenig von etwas kumulieren in dieser Metapher als Mittlerin der zentralen Vorstellung eines physiologischen Sollzustands. Das Gleichgewicht begegnet den Lesenden auch in der Metapher der „Norm" und des „Normalen", als Erfüllungszustand des angestrebten Gleichgewichts. Ein solches Konzept von Gesundheit ist nicht statisch, sondern dynamisch. Es betont, dass ständige Anpassungen und Regulationen notwendig sind, um die Homöostase im Körper aufrechtzuerhalten. Dadurch bleibt die Gleichgewichtsmetapher anschlussfähig zum aktiven Handeln der Herstellungsmetaphern. Der mitunter technisch anmutende Begriff der „Norm" kennt schon eine gewisse Nähe zu den weiter unten zu besprechenden Maschinenmetaphern. Krankheit wird

7 Die Gleichgewichtsmetapher lässt sich bis in zahlreiche antike Traditionen zurückverfolgen so z. B. das „mesotes", das *rechte Maß*, als Kristallisationspunkt aristotelischer Ethik [15:149], aber auch die Figur der Justitia, die auf die altägyptische Seelenwaage rekurriert [16:337]. Aufbauend auf die Vier-Elemente-Lehre findet sich kaum ein antiker Denkraum, für den der Gedanke des Gleichgewichts nicht von essenzieller Bedeutung wäre. Einleitend und lesenswert Schmitt [17], zur Humoralpathologie siehe Kapitel 7.

im Gegenzug oft als das Ergebnis eines Ungleichgewichts betrachtet. Irgendetwas ist aus der Balance geraten, sei es durch einen äußeren Angriff, innere Zustände (wie Krebs oder Autoimmunerkrankungen) oder eine Kombination von beidem. Das Ziel einer Behandlung ist es dann, das Gleichgewicht wiederherzustellen.

8.5.3 Wenn die Maschine aus dem Takt gerät: Maschinen- und Apparatemetaphern

Handelte es sich bei Raum- bzw. Gleichgewichtsmetaphern um Orientierungsmetaphern, müssen die Maschinenmetaphern den Strukturmetaphern zugerechnet werden. Strukturmetaphern sind metaphorische Ausdrücke, die das Verständnis komplexer Zusammenhänge oder abstrakter Konzepte erleichtern, indem sie konkrete Erfahrungsstrukturen eines Quellbereichs (Maschine) auf einen abstrakten Zielbereich (Krankheit) übertragen. In den ausgewählten Texten lassen sich insgesamt drei unterschiedliche Typen solcher Metaphern unterscheiden:

> [...] trennen wir die Kreislaufstörungen in kardiogene, vasogene und kombinierte (HM1:25)

Zunächst lassen sich Störungsmetaphern identifizieren, die auf die Vorstellung eines menschlichen Körpers als Maschine rekurrieren, der gut *funktioniert* oder *defekt* ist. Hier dienen spezifische Kenntnisse über Maschinen – ihre Funktion, ihre Struktur, ihre Wartung und Reparatur – dazu, das abstrakte und komplexe Konzept der menschlichen Gesundheit und Krankheit zu strukturieren. Das wird beispielsweise deutlich, wenn Gesundheit als „ungestörte[r] Ablauf der Lebensvorgänge (HP1:98)“ beschrieben wird. Auch historisch betrachtet ist der menschliche Körper im wissenschaftlichen Diskurs oft als Maschine verstanden und beschrieben worden.[8]

> [...] und die Reaktionsweise des vegetativen Systems beeinträchtigt, wird die Funktion einzelner Kreislauforgane und ihr Zusammenspiel zueinander gestört. (HM2:448)

Der menschliche Körper wird nicht als einheitliches Ganzes verstanden, sondern ist wie eine Maschine aus unterschiedlichen Teilen und Teilsystemen zusammengesetzt, die funktionell ineinandergreifen. Die Metapher des *Körpers als Maschine* suggeriert, dass der menschliche Körper als integriertes, koordiniertes System funktioniert. Jeder Teil ist notwendig, und das Versagen eines Teils kann das gesamte System beeinträchtigen. Paradoxerweise impliziert das aber auch ein Auseinanderfallen des menschlichen Funktionsganzen in einzelne Teile, wodurch der Körper als etwas dargestellt wird, das partiell repariert werden kann, wenn es *kaputt* geht, ähnlich wie man ein

8 Als herausragendes Beispiel kann sicherlich René Descartes gelten, der in seine mechanistische Weltsicht auch den Menschen einbezieht. In seinem Werk *Die Leidenschaften der Seele* beschreibt er den Körper als mechanisches System, das von Geist und Selbst „bewohnt“ wird. [18].

Auto oder eine andere Maschine reparieren würde. Durch Apparatemetaphern findet die Technisierung der Sprachbilder nochmals eine Steigerung. Das Herz wird als *zentraler Motor* verstanden, an den ein *Gefäßsystem angeschlossen* ist. Im *Kreislauf* befindet sich ein *Druckgefälle*, der Herzmuskel ist das *Triebwerk* des gesamten Systems usw. Durch die enorme Plakativität der Metaphorik drängen sich die Maschinenbilder für die Rezipient*innen, so muss vermutet werden, in besonderer Weise vordergründig auf. Die Dominanz der Maschinenmetaphern, insbesondere in den medizinischen Publikationen wird aus der historischen Perspektive verständlich: Durch Wirtschaftswunder und Technisierung vieler Lebensbereich setzte eine enorme Fortschrittsgläubigkeit ein: Die Zukunft verhieß Gutes, gerade auch, weil sie technische Lösungen versprach.

> der Gesunde ist daher in der Lage, körperliche Arbeitsleistungen verschiedenster Art zu verrichten (HP2:48)

Schließlich finden sich Metaphern, die die Leistungsfähigkeit des Körpers als zentrales Merkmal der Gesundheit in den Vordergrund stellen und dadurch den konzeptuellen Zugang zu einer Unterwerfung des Körpers unter einer Ausbeutungslogik ermöglichen. Für diese Annahme spricht auch, dass sich Leistungsmetaphern an marktwirtschaftlich orientierte Metaphernkonzepte anschlussfähig zeigen, die den Körper als eine Ressource betrachten. Gerade die Betonung der apparateartigen Konstitution des Körpers dürfte solchen Konzepten Vorschub geleistet haben.

8.5.4 Im Krieg mit dem Körper

Kriegsmetaphern gehören zu den Klassikern der Krankheitsmetaphern. Schon Susan Sonntag setzt sich in *Krankheit als Metapher* umfangreich mit dieser Art der Metaphorik auseinander. *Patient*innen kämpfen einen Kampf*; *der Krebs soll besiegt werden*; *die Behandlung wird als aggressive Schlacht* dargestellt. Und auch die Kritik an solchen Metaphern verwundert nicht: Wenn der Kampf verloren geht – das heißt, wenn der*die Patient*in stirbt – suggeriert die Metapher, dass nicht hart genug gekämpft worden sei [6].

> Der Körper reagiert einmal durch [...] Abwehr der Schädigungen, die ihn getroffen haben. (HP2:49)

Zunächst lassen sich eine Vielzahl von Abwehr- und Widerstandsmetaphern identifizieren. Sie sehen analog zu den Orientierungsmetaphern den Körper im Belagerungszustand von äußeren Feinden wie Reizen oder Krankheitserregern, gegen die sich der Organismus verteidigen muss. Es mag erstaunen, dass sich der Körper darüber hinaus auch mit inneren Feinden konfrontiert sieht, so z. B. bestimmten Krankheitsdispositionen, wodurch strukturell die Nähe zu einer Art „Dolchstoßlegende“ hergestellt wird.

> Menschen einer bestimmten Konstitution werden häufig auch von bestimmten Krankheiten befallen, wenn die dazu notwendigen Umweltbedingungen gegeben sind. (HP1:96)

Diese umfassende Bedrohungs- und Unsicherheitssituation zeigt sich auch durch die spezifische Metaphorik, in der die Angriffe konzipiert werden. Sie ereignen sich in vielen Passagen nicht aus der zuvor dargelegten Belagerungssituation, sondern überfallartig. Das Sprachbild impliziert weniger geordnete militärische Aktionen denn asymmetrische Angriffe, gegenüber denen man sich in besonderem Maße wehrlos sieht. Krankheit erweist sich hier als hinterhältig, die Angriffe erfolgen unerwartet und, so scheint es die Metaphorik aussagen zu wollen, treffen den Organismus unvorbereitet.

> [...] die Krankheitsursache selbst [...] zu beseitigen, [...] durch Kampf gegen die eingedrungenen Erreger (HP2:49)

Angriffsmetaphern sind weit verbreitet, wenn es um die Behandlung von Krankheiten geht. Diese Art von Metaphern beinhaltet das Konzept eines aktiven, oft aggressiven Vorgehens gegen die Krankheit. Dies wird häufig in Begriffen wie "Kampf gegen Krebs" oder "Angriff auf das Virus" zum Ausdruck gebracht.

8.6 Auswertung II: Krankheitsmetaphern in heutigen Quellen

Im Gegensatz zur ersten Gruppe, die sich durch eine ausdrucksstarke und plakative Verwendung von Metaphern auszeichnet, lässt sich in der Zweiten ein zurückhaltenderer und weniger auffälliger Einsatz beobachten. Das kann insbesondere an den Maschinenmetaphern festgemacht werden. Metaphern, die Apparaturen als Quellbereich besitzen finden keinerlei Verwendung mehr, gleiches gilt für Sprachbilder, die auf Leistungsfähigkeit rekurrieren. Zudem tritt die Vorstellung eines Gesamtorganismus in den Hintergrund, der sich aus verschiedenen Teilen zusammensetzt. Dieser, als biomedizinisches Modell bekannte Ansatz, nach dem Krankheiten ausschließlich auf biologische Ursachen zurückzuführen sind, und der den menschlichen Körper als eine Art komplexen Mechanismus versteht, ist in den letzten Jahrzehnten zunehmend in Kritik geraten und hat seine Bindungskraft verloren. Ein Ausbleiben entsprechender Metaphern kann also nicht verwundern. Maschinenmetaphern finden sich aber noch dort, wo Störungen im Ablauf zur Darstellung gebracht werden sollen:

> Einige Krankheiten entstehen aufgrund von genetischen Anomalien, die zu Fehlfunktionen in den biologischen Prozessen des Körpers führen (GV1_CGPT).

Im direkten Vergleich mit den Texten aus der Mitte des 20. Jhs. muss es erstaunen, welche Homogenität im sprachlichen Ausdruck sich in den Texten zeigt.

Auch die Kriegsmetaphern mussten einen deutlichen Bedeutungsverlust erfahren. Sie sind zwar nach wie vor Bestandteil des sprachlichen Ausdrucks, treten aber hinsichtlich der relativen Häufigkeit und der Plakativität der verwendeten Sprachbilder kaum noch in Erscheinung. Wenn dann begegnen sie noch in Widerstandsmetaphern. Das weist auf einen tiefgreifenden Wandel in der medizinischen Kommunikation hin, der sich durch eine kritische Würdigung der zugrundeliegenden Metaphorik auszuzeichnen scheint. So kann angenommen werden, dass infolge der Friedensbewegungen und der zunehmenden Sensibilität gegenüber den Auswirkungen von Krieg und Gewalt ein Wandel des sprachlichen Ausdrucks eingesetzt hat.

Orientierungsmetaphern gehen auf Erfahrungen mit physischer Orientierung wie „oben“ und „unten“, „innen“ und „außen“, etc., zurück und sind Grundlage für abstraktere Konzepte. Im Gegensatz zu Strukturmetaphern sind sie weit weniger offensichtlich als Bedeutungsübertragung zu erkennen und können aus dem Sprachgebrauch kaum herausgelöst werden. Der Bedeutungsverlust der Strukturmetaphern scheint dazu beizutragen, dass Orientierungsmetaphern in den heutigen Texten, für die Lesenden deutlich stärker im Vordergrund stehen. Analog zu den Textsegmenten der 1950er-Jahre findet sich in den Gegenwartstexten eine starke Differenzierung zwischen „innen“ und „außen“, hier insbesondere bezogen auf Krankheitsursachen, die entweder von außen kommen (z. B. Mikroorganismen) oder auf innere Zustände (z. B. genetische Ausstattung) zurückzuführen sind. Auch die Präpositionen „über“ / „unter“ (z. B. Unterversorgung) und „vor“ / „hinter“ folgen den bereits bekannten Mustern.

Hervorzuheben sind die Gleichgewichtsmetaphern, die vor allem – aber nicht ausschließlich – in den pflegebezogenen Texten der heutigen Lehrwerke vorzufinden sind:[9]

> Sie stört das Gleichgewicht des Organismus oder seiner Teile (GM1:20).

> Mangelernährung oder die übermäßige Zufuhr von Nährstoffen und Vitaminen sind häufig Auslöser von Erkrankungen. (GP1:62)

Gesundheit wird auch in den heutigen Texten als Gleichgewichtszustand verstanden, der sich konzeptionell durch zwei unterschiedliche Denkfiguren rekonstruieren lässt. Einerseits adressiert die Gleichgewichtsmetapher die erfolgreiche Orientierung an einer biologischen Norm, die es nicht zu unter- oder überschreiten gilt, sei es durch „übermäßige Zufuhr von Nährstoffen und Vitaminen“ (GP1:62) oder durch die „potenziell gefährliche Unregelmäßigkeiten des Herzrhythmus“ (GV2_AU). Andererseits hat der Mensch ständig dafür Sorge zu tragen, dass die inneren und äußeren potenziell schädlichen Einflüsse, die auf die Person einwirken, aktiv ausgeglichen werden. Dass

9 Eine Durchsicht mehrerer zusätzlicher Lehrbücher konnte den Eindruck erhärten, dass in pflegebezogener Literatur die Gleichgewichtsmetapaher zwei- bis dreimal häufiger genutzt wird als in der Medizin.

diese Metaphorik insbesondere in den Pflegeberufen als besonders attraktiv wahrgenommen wird, dürfte verschiedene Ursachen haben. Durch die Akademisierung und Professionalisierung der Pflegeberufe in den 1990er-Jahren stand die Pflege vor der Herausforderung, sich einen genuinen Gegenstandsbereich erschließen zu müssen. Dies gelang, indem der medizintypische Krankheitsbezug zugunsten einer Orientierung am Gesundheitsbegriff im Sinne einer gelebten Alltagsautonomie aufgegeben wurde [19]. Der Fokus pflegerischen Handelns liegt daher auf Erhalt, Förderung und Wiederherstellung von Gesundheit und Unterstützung in der Bewältigung von Krankheitsfolgen. Für diese Bestrebungen wurden Theorien und Modelle als wichtige Orientierungspunkte herangezogen, die freimütig mit der Gleichgewichtsmetapher operieren. Das Modell der Salutogenese von Antonovsky [20] sei an dieser Stelle stellvertretend genannt.

8.7 Diskussion und Kritik

Metaphern spielen eine wichtige Rolle in der Kommunikation medizinischer Erkenntnisse, da sie helfen können, komplexe Konzepte zu verstehen. In diesem Sinne ist die Verwendung von Metaphern auch in fachwissenschaftlichen Veröffentlichungen nicht per se zu kritisieren. Nichtsdestotrotz lässt sich der Trend feststellen, ausdrucksstarke Metaphern zugunsten eines nüchternen und deskriptiveren Sprachgebrauchs zu ersetzen. Interessanterweise lässt sich dieser Effekt weniger stark in der heutigen Vergleichsliteratur beobachten, die sich an Lai*innen richtet. Das könnte dafür sprechen, dass der Wandel in den Lehrwerken als Ergebnis eines reflexiven Vorgangs und wissenschaftlichen Selbstverständnisses zu verstehen ist. Wie gezeigt werden konnte, sind es vor allem raumorientierte Metaphern, die in den heutigen Texten anzutreffen sind, von denen die Gleichgewichtsmetaphern in besonderer Weise herausstechen. Eine differenzierte Metaphernkritik muss sich nun der Frage der Angemessenheit der vorgefundenen Sprachbilder stellen. An dieser Stelle soll das vor allem anhand der Frage untersucht werden, welche Aspekte des Quellbereichs betont werden und welche in den Hintergrund treten.

Hinsichtlich der raumbezogenen Metaphern, die durch „innen“ / „außen“, „vorne“ / „hinten“ etc. gekennzeichnet sind, zeigt sich ein enormer Verstärkungseffekt zugunsten einer konkreten räumlichen Verortung von Krankheiten und Faktoren, die Krankheitsentstehung begünstigen bzw. verursachen. Krankheiten kommen entweder von außen und befallen die Person oder sie sind im Inneren bereits angelegt. Auch feststehende Begriffe wie *Innere Medizin* repräsentieren diese Metaphorik. Eine weitere Variante dieser Vorstellung findet sich in der Differenzierung zwischen somatischen und psychischen Erkrankungen, die weite Teile der medizinischen Praxis strukturiert. Diese Metaphern sind gut geeignet, ein Verständnis von der grundsätzlichen Unterschiedlichkeit bestimmter Krankheitsklassen zu vermitteln. Bei näherer Betrachtung zeigt sich aber der kognitive Effekt des „entweder hier oder dort“, die gegenstandsunangemessen scheint und gleichzeitig relevante Aspekte verdeckt: Krankheitsgeschehen lassen sich in den seltensten Fällen monokausal auf den ein oder anderen Faktor reduzieren. Genetische Disposition, Krankheitserreger, individuelles Verhalten, erlernte Muster, sozialstaatliche Strukturen, Umgebungsfaktoren u. a. bilden ein Konglomerat aus sich gegenseitig bedingenden Einflussfaktoren. Einfache Orientierungsmetaphern sind zumindest in vielen Fällen nicht geeignet, den Blick für diese Komplexität zu öffnen.

Die Gleichgewichtsmetapher ist insbesondere in der Pflegefachliteratur präsent und wird dort auch herangezogen, um zentrale theoretische Positionen zu beschreiben. „Das Gleichgewicht zu verlieren" bedeutet, die bewusste Kontrolle über die horizontale Position im Raum einzubüßen. Diese konkrete leibliche Erfahrung wird auf abstrakte Krankheitsgeschehen übertragen. Betrachtet man unterschiedliche Zielbereiche, zeigt sich, dass der Abstraktionsgrad von Fall zu Fall variiert. Bei einer Mittelohrentzündung kann diese sensomotorische Fähigkeit tatsächlich verloren gehen, wird bei einer psychischen Erkrankung das „seelische Gleichgewicht" gestört, ist die Differenz zwischen Quell- und Zielerfahrung beträchtlich größer. Welches Verhältnis z. B. bei Erkrankungen des schizophrenen Formenkreises gestört wird – das der Neurotransmitter, das aus individueller Vulnerabilität und Stressoren, das von Mensch und Welt – bleibt vage und es wäre jeweils kritisch zu hinterfragen, ob nicht relevante Aspekte der Pathogenese verdeckt werden. Die Gleichgewichtsmetapher wird aber nicht nur auf Einzelkrankheiten angewendet, sondern auch auf Krankheit *an sich*. Das führt insbesondere im Kontext des bereits eingeführten Normierungsaspekts zu schwerwiegenden Implikationen. Diese zweite Variante der Gleichgewichtsmetapher legt nahe, dass Gesundheit und Krankheit als Erfüllung bzw. Abweichungen von einem definierten Normbereich oder Idealzustand beschrieben werden können. Dadurch wird eine in der Medizin beliebte Deutung von Krankheit als objektives, messbares Naturphänomen in den Vordergrund gestellt. Es verdeckt aber, dass Gesundheit und Krankheit nicht auf Fragen von Norm und Abweichung reduziert werden können, ja sogar ohne diese Denkfigur auskommen. Das biomedizinische Modell konzentriert sich stark auf die biophysikalischen und biochemischen Aspekte von Krankheiten und neigt dazu, den Menschen auf einzelne, isolierte Teile oder Systeme zu reduzieren. In dieser Sichtweise werden komplexe, mehrdimensionale Gesundheitsprobleme simplifiziert und es wird ignoriert, dass der Mensch eine biologische, psychologische und soziale Einheit bildet. Zurückkehrend zu den eingangs vorgestellten Krankheitstheorien zeigt sich, dass durch die Normierungsvariante der Gleichgewichtsmetapher normatavistische Theoriepositionen konzeptionell ausgeblendet werden. Gesundheit kann aber nicht nur als vortreffliche Erfüllung der Norm verstanden werden, wie es naturalistische Positionen nahelegen, sondern auch als der Zustand, in dem der Mensch über die körperlich-geistigen Voraussetzungen verfügt, selbst gesteckte Ziele zu erreichen [21, 22].

Und noch ein letzter Aspekt ist zur Diskussion zu stellen. Die Gleichgewichtsmetapher hat den medizinischen Diskurs seit dem antiken Griechenland geprägt. Die von Hippokrates eingeführte [23:35–41] und später durch Galen populär gemachte

[23:103–109] Humoralpathologie verfolgt die zentrale Idee, dass das Gleichgewicht oder Ungleichgewicht der vier grundlegenden Körperflüssigkeiten die Gesundheit eines Menschen bestimme. Bis ins 19. Jh. hinein konnte diese sog. *Vier-Säfte-Lehre* Gültigkeit beanspruchen und wurde erst durch die 1858 von Rudolf Virchow begründete Zellularpathologie endgültig abgelöst [23:303–307]. Sie ist aber z. B. in „alternativmedizinischen" und esoterischen Gesundheitsvorstellungen bis heute präsent.[10] Vieles spricht dafür, dass die Gleichgewichtsmetapher so stark in unserer kollektiven Wahrnehmung verankert ist, dass der metaphorische Charakter unkenntlich geworden ist und die Modellvorstellung mit einer wie auch immer gearteten Realität verwechselt wird. Eine kritische Auseinandersetzung mit Metaphern in den Gesundheitsberufen hätte an dieser Stelle anzusetzen.

Literatur

[1] Boorse C. Health as a theoretical concept. Philos Sci. 1977;44(4):542–73.

[2] Nordenfelt L. The concepts of health and illness revisited. Med Health Care Philos. 2006;10(1):5–10.

[3] Nordenfelt L. The opposition between naturalistic and holistic theories of health and disease. In: Carel H, Cooper R, editors. Health, Illness and Disease. Philosophical Essays. London: Routledge; 2016.

[4] Werner M. Der Krankheitsbegriff zwischen Naturalismus und Normativismus. In: Hucklenbroich P, Buyx A, editors. Wissenschaftstheoretische Aspekte des Krankheitsbegriffs. Münster: Mentis; 2013.

[5] Wilhelms B. Hybridism als Konzept zum Krankheitsbegriff zwischen Naturalismus und Normativismus – the best of both? In: Sell A, editor. Diskurse über Krankheit. Zum Krankheitsbegriff in Philosophie, Medizin und Psychologie. Bielefeld: Transcript; 2024.

[6] Sonntag S. Krankheit als Metapher & Aids und seine Metaphern. Frankfurt am Main: Fischer; 2003.

[7] Lakoff G, Johnson M. Leben in Metaphern. Konstruktion und Gebrauch von Sprachbildern. Göttingen: Carl-Auer; 2021.

[8] Schmitt R, Schröder J, Pflücker L. Systematische Metaphernanalyse. Eine Einführung. Wiesbaden: Springer; 2018.

[9] Gallagher S, Zahavi D. The Phenomenological Mind. 3rd ed. London: Routledge; 2021.

[10] Gallagher S. Phenomenology and embodied cognition. In: Shapiro L, editor. Routledge Handbook of Embodied Cognition. London: Routledge; 2014. p. 9–18.

[11] Schmitt R. Rezension: Lakoff, George & Mark Johnson. Leben in Metaphern. Konstruktion und Gebrauch von Sprachbildern [Internet]. [zitiert 2024 Jul 25]. Verfügbar unter: https://www.systemagazin.de/buecher/klassiker/lakoff_johnson_metaphern.php

[12] Glaser B, Strauss A. The Discovery of Grounded Theory: Strategies for Qualitative Research. Chicago: Aldine; 2012.

[13] Oertner M. ChatGPT als Recherchetool? Is ChatGPT a Useful Research Tool? Bibliotheksdienst. 2024;58(6):259–97.

[14] Briganti B. How ChatGPT works: a mini review. Eur Arch Otorhinolaryngol. 2024;281(1):1565–156.

---

10 Unter dem Label der *Traditionellen europäischen Medizin (TEM)* lassen sich zahlreiche Versuche identifizieren, humoralpathologische Konzepte im Kanon pseudomedizinischer Verfahren zu verankern. Besonders eindrücklich: [24].

[15] Brüllmann P. Ethische Schriften. In: Rapp C, Corcilius K, editors. Aristoteles-Handbuch. Leben – Werk – Wirkung. 2nd ed. Heidelberg: Metzler; 2021.
[16] Nennen H-U. Die Metapher vom Gleichgewicht. Ideale der Ordnung in der Kritik. In: Neumaier O, editor. Gerechtigkeit. Auf der Suche nach einem Gleichgewicht. Berlin: De Gruyter; 2005.
[17] Schmitt A. Über die Bedeutung der Philosophie in der Medizin der Antike. Hippokrates und Galen über die Grundlagen der Gesundheit. In: Bergdolt K, Herrmann I, editors. Was ist Gesundheit? Antworten aus den Jahrhunderten, Impulse – Villa Vigoni im Gespräch, Bd. 3. Stuttgart: Steiner; 2011.
[18] Descartes R. Die Passionen der Seele. Hamburg: Meiner; 2014.
[19] Müller K. Berufsverständnis. In: Büker C, Lademann J, Müller K, editors. Moderne Pflege heute. Beruf und Profession zeitgemäß verstehen und leben. Stuttgart: Kohlhammer; 2018.
[20] Antonovsky A. Salutogenese. Zur Entmystifizierung der Gesundheit. Tübingen: dgvt; 1997.
[21] Nordenfelt L. On the Nature of Health. An Action-Theoretic Approach. Dordrecht: Springer; 1995.
[22] Whitbeck C. Eine Theorie der Gesundheit. In: Schramme T, editor. Krankheitstheorien. Berlin: Suhrkamp; 2011.
[23] Bergdolt K. Leib und Seele. Eine Kulturgeschichte des gesunden Lebens. München: Beck; 199.
[24] Stern U. Traditionelle Europäische Medizin [Internet]. 2020 [zitiert 2024 Jul 25]. Verfügbar unter: https://www.science.de/artikel/traditionelle-europaeische-medizin

Stefan Dübel, Stefan Heuser, Hans G. Ulrich

9 Metaphern in den Wissenschaften. Ein Gespräch zwischen Biotechnologie und Ethik

1 Einleitung

Das folgende Gespräch zwischen dem Biotechnologen Stefan Dübel und den beiden Theologen und Ethikern Hans G. Ulrich und Stefan Heuser geht auf Diskussionen im Rahmen des Workshops „How Metaphors shape Biotechnology" vom 23.–24. November 2023 an der Technischen Universität Braunschweig zurück. Im Nachgang des Workshops haben wir Schlüsselthemen gesichtet und offene Fragen gesammelt, an denen entlang wir mithilfe eines webbasierten Texteditors ein kollaboratives Schreibgespräch geführt haben, das im Folgenden dokumentiert ist. Die Beiträge wurden nachträglich von den Autoren redigiert und um Abbildungen und Fußnoten ergänzt. Der sprachliche Charakter dieses Austauschs bewegt sich zwischen mündlicher und schriftlicher Kommunikation und wurde weitgehend beibehalten.

2 Ein Gespräch zwischen Biotechnologie und Ethik über Metaphern in den Wissenschaften

Stefan Heuser: In den Diskussionen, die wir auf dem Workshop „How Metaphors shape Biotechnology" geführt haben, wurde wiederholt auf die Wissenschaftskommunikation in der Corona-Pandemie Bezug genommen. In der Zeit der Pandemie und in ihrer bisherigen Aufarbeitung ließ sich eindrücklich beobachten, wie sehr die Wissenschaftssprache und deren Vermittlung von Metaphern geprägt ist – und welches Wirkungsspektrum die jeweilige Metaphorik in der Öffentlichkeit haben kann. Da war beispielweise davon die Rede, das „Virus" zu „bekämpfen", es zu „verstehen", mit ihm zu „leben" und durch „Impfstoffe", die die mRNA als „Botenstoff" und „Bauplan" zur Herstellung von „Antigenen" verwenden, das Immunsystem zu „(re)programmieren". Welche Metaphern spielen in Deiner Forschung im Feld der Biotechnologie eine wichtige Rolle? Gibt es vielleicht sogar eine für Deine biotechnologische Forschung besonders signifikante Metapher?

Stefan Dübel: Ja. Das fängt schon bei meinem Hauptarbeitsgebiet an, dem „Antikörper-Engineering" [1]. Antikörper sind Moleküle, die uns gegen Krankheiten schützen. Sie sind der zweithäufigste Eiweiß-Stoff (Protein) in unserem Blutserum, und wir haben davon buchstäblich Billionen unterschiedlicher Varianten – grob gesagt mindestens einen Antikörper gegen jeden möglichen Eindringling, den es zu bekämpfen gilt, also vor allem Krankheitserreger wie Viren, Pilze, Bakterien oder Parasiten, welche uns als Lebensraum besiedeln und uns dadurch auch schädigen können. Der Be-

https://doi.org/10.1515/9783112215685-009

griff „Antikörper“ ist gleich ein wunderbares Beispiel für eine historisch entstandene und keinesfalls exakte Metapher für Immunglobuline, mehr Details dazu erläutere ich später. Das Immunsystem, zu dem die Antikörper gehören, ist ganz generell eine Fundgrube für Metaphern. Es wird bezeichnet als ein „Waffensystem“ des Körpers, das in der Blutbahn patrouillierende Polizisten (eben die „Antikörper“) hervorbringt welche „Eindringlinge“ „bekämpfen“, „Krankheitserreger“ werden durch „Abwehrzellen“ oder sogar „Killer-Zellen“ „verfolgt“ und „zerstört“, es ist ein dauernder „Kampf“ in unserem Inneren, usw.

Stefan Heuser: Die Kampf- bzw. Kriegsmetaphorik hat die öffentliche Wissenschaftskommunikation während der Corona-Pandemie lange dominiert. Welche genaue Funktion hat die Kriegsmetaphorik für die interne Verständigung der Forschenden und in der öffentlichen Wissenschaftskommunikation? Offenbar findet die Wissenschaftssprache mit dieser Metaphorik einen leichten Anschluss an lebensweltliche Erfahrungen oder jedenfalls an Vorstellungen, die das Publikum leicht abrufen kann. Ich frage mich, wie weit diese Metaphorik den biologischen Vorgängen entspricht, die als „Immunsystem“ (selbst eine sehr implikationsreiche Metapher) der Forschung zugänglich sind bzw. welches Spektrum an immunbiologischen Phänomenen sie einfängt, welche sie nicht mit abdeckt und welche sie vielleicht sogar verdeckt? Wir nehmen die Wirklichkeit des Immunsystems – wie jede Wirklichkeit – im Medium von Sprache wahr, versuchen es zu verstehen und zu deuten und antworten entsprechend dieses Verständnisses bzw. dieser Deutungen darauf mit unseren Einstellungen, Emotionen und unserem Verhalten und Handeln, auch mit den Methoden der Forschung und mit Therapieansätzen – bis hin zum politischen Handeln. Entsprechend hat die dominante Kriegsmetaphorik die Wahrnehmung der Viren und des Immunsystems in der Pandemie vom individuellen Erleben bis hin zu politischen Maßnahmen gewiss auch mitgeprägt. Ist es aber eine kluge Betrachtung der Wirklichkeit, die uns mit den Viren angeht, sie als „Feinde“ zu sehen und den „Kampf“ gegen sie auszurufen, um die Bevölkerung für bestimmte Schutzmaßnahmen zu mobilisieren? Jedenfalls sind die gesundheitspolitischen Maßnahmen in Deutschland in der Prime Time der Pandemie einer dem „Kampf gegen das Virus“ entsprechenden Logik gefolgt. Man hatte aufgrund der politischen Rhetorik teilweise den Eindruck, sich im Ausnahmezustand zu befinden. So wurden auch soziale, kulturelle und ökonomische „Kollateralschäden“ in Kauf genommen, deren problematische Folgen uns teilweise erst jetzt, in der Zeit nach der Pandemie, vor Augen treten. Führt die Übertragung vom quasipolitischen Metaphern-Quellbereich des Krieges auf den biologischen Metaphern-Zielbereich des Immunsystems nicht dazu, „Viren“ mystisch als „Feinde“ zu überhöhen und alternative Antwortmöglichkeiten auf die von ihnen ausgehende „Bedrohung“ auszublenden? Erst langsam wurde in der öffentlichen Kommunikation die Metapher vom „Kampf gegen das Virus“ vom „Leben mit dem Virus“ abgelöst – und entsprechend haben sich auch die Politik und die soziokulturellen Praktiken des Umgangs mit dem Virus und den Mitmenschen als potentiellen Überträgern des Virus wieder verändert.

Mich würde interessieren, ob dieser Wandel in der Metaphorik auch bis hinein in die Labore stattgefunden hat – ob in der internen Kommunikation in Forschung und Lehre weiterhin – oder überhaupt – die Kriegsmetaphorik vorherrscht? Wie weit entspricht der metaphorische Quellbereich des Krieges der biologischen „Wirklichkeit" der „Anti"-körper, der Viren und den Vorgängen im Immunsystem, wie sie die Forschung beobachtet – oder leitet diese Metaphorik die Wahrnehmung in eine Richtung, die den Phänomenen nicht oder nicht vollumfänglich gerecht wird – jedenfalls bezogen auf die Komplexität des möglichen Zielbereichs?

Stefan Dübel: Die „Waffensystem/Polizisten" – Metaphorik ist aus vielen Gründen weit verbreitet, und wenn man einige der biochemischen Vorgänge dabei anschaut, versteht man auch, warum die Forschenden, welche diese Metaphern prägten, diese Wahl trafen. Eine zentrale Funktion des Immunsystems ist das physikalische Unterscheiden von „selbst" und „fremd" mithilfe biochemischer Vorgänge. Dieses Unterscheiden auf Ebene einzelner Moleküle ist ganz entscheidend für die physische Abgrenzung unseres Körpers vom Rest der Welt – und damit für eine der biologischen Antworten für die Frage, was der Mensch eigentlich ist. Biochemisch wird diese Abgrenzung durch physischen Kontakt einer zu prüfenden Struktur mit einer Immunzelle erreicht. Die „prüfende" Immunzelle hat dafür Moleküle auf ihrer Oberfläche, welche genau definierte Gegenstücke auf der anderen Struktur vorfinden müssen. Werden diese Strukturen von der prüfenden Zelle erkannt, gibt es je nach Art dieser Struktur und der sie präsentierenden Entität (also entweder fremde oder eigene Zelle) verschiedene Reaktionen, die dadurch ausgelöst werden.

Zum einen haben viele Zellen des Immunsystems „Steckbriefe von bekannten Gangstern" dabei, also Bindemoleküle, welche nicht-menschliche Strukturen direkt erkennen können. Während der Evolution unserer Spezies hat das Immunsystem zahlreiche angeborene Abwehrwege entwickelt, die uns gegen fremde Organismen schützen, welche seit Millionen von Jahren in unserer Umwelt präsent sind. So können zum Beispiel zahlreiche Bakterienarten direkt durch die Beschaffenheit ihrer Zellwand erkannt werden – ein einfaches und verlässliches Merkmal, da menschliche Zellen selbst keine Zellwand besitzen. Biochemisch gesehen geschieht diese Erkennung durch zahlreiche „Rezeptoren", also Bindemoleküle, auf der Oberfläche der Immunzellen, welche bekannte Eindringlinge in unseren Körper – typischerweise Viren, Bakterien, Pilze und Parasiten – direkt identifizieren können. Bindet also ein solcher Rezeptor auf der Oberfläche einer Immunzelle an den fremden „Eindringling", löst diese Zelle eine Alarmreaktion aus, welche weitere Elemente des Immunsystems zur Bekämpfung aktiviert, und oft kann sie die als fremd erkannten Strukturen auch direkt abtöten. Auch Antikörper repräsentieren auf molekularer Ebene so etwas wie einen Steckbrief, denn sie beinhalten eine genau zu einem Eindringling passende atomare Struktur. Sie können also einen ganz bestimmten „Gangster" inmitten Zehntausender anderer „Nicht-Gangster" effizient erkennen und ihn dann buchstäblich gefangen nehmen. Antikörper werden deshalb oft mit „Zielfahndern" verglichen, denn sie zirkulieren durch unsere Blutbahn, und können buchstäblich einen ganz bestimmten „Gangster“ auf molekularer Ebene festhalten. Biochemisch ausgedrückt: Immunglobuline erkennen hochspezifisch eine bestimmte körperfremde molekulare Struktur. Dabei binden sie nur an diese Struktur, trotz der Gegenwart von Zehntausenden anderen hochkonzentrierten biologischen Stoffen um sie herum, und können sie dadurch für andere Mechanismen des Immunsystems markieren, welche sie dann zerstören oder entsorgen können, z. B. durch Makrophagen (Fresszellen). Die Metaphorik stößt aber auch an ihre Grenzen, denn im Immunsystem werden die an den „Gangster“ gebundenen „Zielfahnder“ von den Fresszellen gleich mit verspeist.

Zum anderen können Zellen des Immunsystems aber auch „Eindringlinge“ erkennen, ohne dass sie bereits molekulare „Steckbriefe“ für sie haben. Diese Funktion ist sehr wichtig für die Bekämpfung der dauernd neu über uns Menschen herfallenden Krankheitserreger, wie kürzlich das SARS-CoV-2 Virus, dem ja unser Immunsystem im Laufe der Evolution noch nie vorher begegnet ist. Auch verändern sich Viren und Bakterien oft durch Mutationen innerhalb von Tagen und Wochen, dann nützen vorhandene molekulare „Steckbriefe“ nichts mehr zu ihrer Erkennung und Bekämpfung. Das Immunsystem löst dieses Problem dadurch, dass alle körpereigenen Zellen Moleküle auf ihrer Oberfläche präsentieren, welche sie eindeutig als körpereigen ausweisen. Mit der Polizistenmetapher ausgedrückt: sie haben einen „Personalausweis“ dabei, im Englischen oft noch treffender mit der Metapher *„living license“* bezeichnet, den sie vorzeigen müssen. Sind diese „Personalausweis“-Moleküle nicht vorhanden, so wird umgehend eine Abwehrreaktion gegen die geprüfte Struktur ausgelöst – sie ist als körperfremd erkannt und wird angegriffen und entfernt.

Einen ganz ähnlichen und gleichermaßen faszinierenden Vorgang zur Erkennung körperfremder „Eindringlinge“, nur diesmal statt auf zellulärer Ebene im Bereich der löslichen Blutfaktoren, existiert in Form des „alternativen Aktivierungswegs“ des Komplementsystems. Das Komplementsystem besteht nicht aus Zellen, sondern nur aus verschiedenen miteinander reagierenden Eiweiß-Molekülen (Proteinen), und bilden eine sogenannte Protease-Kaskade. „Proteasen“ sind Eiweiße, welche andere Eiweiße zerstören können, indem sie sie in Teile zerschneiden. Eine „Kaskade“ entsteht daraus, indem ein Protein von einem ganz bestimmten anderen Protein einen Teil abscheidet, wodurch dieses geschnittene Protein so aktiviert wird, dass es danach selbst das nächste Protein schneiden/aktivieren kann, und so weiter. Ihr vollständiger Ablauf löst sehr schnell eine lokal begrenzte Entzündungsreaktion aus, welche dadurch „Eindringlinge“ bekämpft. Nun wird diese Protease-Kaskade ständig zufällig und spontan, aber mit niedriger Häufigkeit im Blut aktiviert – in der Polizei-Metaphorik vergleichbar mit zufälligen Ausweiskontrollen in einer Fußgängerzone. Der vollständige Ablauf der Protease-Kaskade nach der spontanen Aktivierung wird aber im gesunden Gewebe ohne körperfremde Strukturen sehr schnell durch dort stets anwesende hemmend wirkende körpereigene Moleküle verhindert – wieder eine Version des Vorzeigens einer zelluären *„living license“*, welche die Proteasen inaktivieren. Nur wenn etwas diese hemmend wirkenden Moleküle nicht „vorweisen“ kann – also eine körperfremde Zelle, Virus oder Parasit – dann geht die Aktivierung weiter. Kann eine Struktur in unserem Körper nicht die richtigen „Ausweis" vorzeigen, erfolgt umgehend die Bekämpfung. Das Geniale daran ist, dass das Immunsystem dafür keinerlei Informationen über die Struktur des Eindringlings braucht, und deshalb damit auch neue Mutationen oder uns bisher fremde Krankheitserreger erkennen kann.

Weitere Beispiele für die Polizei & Gangster-Metapher: Unser Immunsystem kann unerwünschte Zellen buchstäblich durchlöchern, zum Beispiel durch das oben erwähnte Komplementsystem. Nach dessen Aktivierung sehen die Zellaußenhüllen unter dem Elektronenmikroskop tatsächlich sehr ähnlich aus wie die Bilder der Einschusslöcher in der Tür des Autos, in dem Bonnie und Clyde starben. Es gibt auch „Killer-Zellen" (heute meist Zytotoxische T Zellen genannt), welche genau das machen, was der Name suggeriert: andere Zellen gezielt abzutöten (auch unter anderem wieder durch „Perforine", welche Löcher in Zellaußenhüllen erzeugen).

Stefan Heuser: Wenn die Befunde der Biologie derart die Kampf- bzw. Kriegsmetaphorik nahelegen, wie Du es beschreibst, stellt sich aus ethischer Perspektive dennoch die Frage, was diese Metaphorik an weiteren Dimensionen der Interaktion eines Organismus mit seiner Umwelt auslässt oder sogar verdeckt. Ein Beispiel ist die systemische Innen-Außen-Metaphorik, die mit der „Polizisten"-Metapher verbunden ist. Metaphorisch gesprochen: „Polizisten" sind keine „Soldaten", weil sie nicht einfach nur alles Fremde abwehren, sondern prüfen, was innerhalb des Systems und seiner Funktionen anschlussfähig ist und was nicht. Die verschiedenen Ebenen, auf denen sie intervenieren, dienen dem Erhalt, aber auch der Weiterentwicklung des Organismus, zu dem nicht nur der komplette „Ausschluss" des „Fremden" und der „Kampf ums Überleben", sondern auch die Koexistenz sowie die Interaktion von Fremdem und Eigenem gehört, bis hin zur Mutagenese. Mir erscheint es als fragwürdig, wenn in der Pandemie die Metaphorik vom „Kampf" des Immunsystems gegen das Virus ihren bestimmten biologischen Zielbereich verlassen und direkt die politische Sprache und Imagination affiziert hat. Bestimmte politische, ökonomische, kulturell und sozial einschneidende Maßnahmen – wie beispielsweise die diversen Lockdowns mit Schul- und Kitaschließungen – erschienen so als alternativlos, schon bevor die Urteilsbildung eingesetzt hat. Der Schutz von gesundheitlich besonders gefährdeten Personen hat aus Sicht der Ethik immer Vorrang vor anderen Interessen. Umso wichtiger war und ist es, kluge Maßnahmen zum Umgang mit einem solchen neuen Virus zu ergreifen, die nicht den Ausnahmezustand auf Dauer stellen, sondern damit rechnen, dass wir uns die Welt mit dem neuen Virus in seiner konkreten Bedrohlichkeit teilen müssen.

Stefan Dübel: Ja, die Funktion des Immunsystems geht über die Kontrolle der Interaktion eines Organismus mit seiner Umgebung weit hinaus, es kann auch nach „innen" schauen. Tatsächlich beseitigt es auch unzählige Krebszellen, welche im Laufe unseres Lebens entstehen. Diese weisen in aller Regel Mutationen auf, welche sie überhaupt erst bösartig werden lassen. Auf molekularer Ebene bedeutet es, dass die Struktur eines oder mehrerer Proteine sich verändert – zu einer für den Körper bisher unbekannten Form. Mit diesem neuen molekularen Merkmal sehen sie nun für das Immunsystem „fremd“ aus und werden beseitigt. Krebs entsteht nur, wenn Mutationen der Immunabwehr „entkommen“. Zum vermehrten Auftreten von Tumoren bei älteren Menschen trägt bei, dass die Effizienz der Immunantwort mit dem Alter stetig nachlässt.

Es wird aus diesen vielen Beispielen deutlich, dass es ist gar nicht so leicht ist, für das Immunsystem eine gänzlich andere Metaphorik zu finden, welche im gleichen Maße die biochemischen Vorgänge abbildet, obwohl es natürlich gute Gründe gäbe, von der „Kriegs“ bzw. „Polizei“-Begrifflichkeit wegzukommen. Ich habe hierzu einiges versucht in meinen Vorlesungen, z. B. Metaphern aus dem Sport oder technische Analogien, aber damit ist nicht in gleicher Weise das ganze Spektrum anschaulich zu erklären. Immerhin geht es bei Immunreaktionen buchstäblich tausendfach um Leben und Tod, wenn auch im mikroskopischen Maßstab. Bei einer Infektion mit einem Krankheitserreger geht es eben nicht um „Dabeisein ist alles“, sondern um das für unser Überleben als Individuum nötige Abtöten von Bakterien oder Pilzen, aber auch Krebszellen. Viele Viren, Pilze oder Bakterien bedrohen uns ganz konkret, täglich und individuell mit dem Tode. Würden sie nicht vom Immunsystem in einem unermüdlichen und unter Verbrauch eines erheblichen Teils der mit unserer Nahrung aufgenommenen Energie (Schätzungen gehen bis 20%) neutralisiert, wären wir bald aufgefressen. Das klingt erstmal dramatisch – und das ist es auch. Was ohne diese Abwehrfunktion aus uns würde, sogar ohne dass besondere Krankheiten drohen, kann jeder selbst einfach ausprobieren, indem er einfach mal im Hochsommer (um unsere Körpertemperatur von 37°C ungefähr zu simulieren) ein Stück Fleisch (in welchem das Immunsystem ja nicht mehr intakt ist) mal ein paar Wochen ungekühlt herumliegen lässt. Der beeindruckende Unterschied zu Gewebe mit einem lebendigen Immunsystem zeigt, wie viel wir den Antikörpern, Abwehrzellen, Komplementsystem und anderen Mechanismen der Immunabwehr täglich zu verdanken haben. Alleine die hochwertigen Nährstoffe, aus welchem wir uns zusammensetzen, würden es vielen Mikroorganismen ermöglichen, sich massenhaft in uns zu vermehren, sobald dies nicht durch den dauernden Einsatz des Immunsystems verhindert wird. Dazu braucht es gar keine besonderen Krankheitserreger – wir sind einfach superlecker für Bakterien und Pilze. Unser Gehirn mag für viele von uns als das entscheidende Organ erscheinen, das uns zur „Krone der Schöpfung“ macht. Ohne das Immunsystem wäre es aber nur ein paar Tage lang ein leckerer Snack für eine blühende Gemeinschaft anderer Organismen. Wie ich finde, eine wunderschöne Metapher für das produktive Zusammenwirken von unterschiedlichsten Fähigkeiten bei gelungenem Teamwork, denn erst das Immunsystem (und natürlich der ganze Rest unserer Organe) gibt dem Gehirn die Möglichkeit, lange genug zu leben, um seine Fähigkeiten zu entwickeln und zu nutzen.

Hans Ulrich: Bei dem Gebrauch von Metaphern geht es immer auch um die Frage, wie – sinnvoller Weise – begrenzt der Beobachtungsbereich ist, den sie abdecken – hier also etwa den menschlichen Körper als ein „Immunsystem", das ankommende Angreifer, die die Fähigkeit haben „einzudringen", abzuwehren und so „Immunität" zu bewahren. Man kann sofort freilich dieses „Immunsystem" verortet wissen in weiteren ineinander liegenden oder sich überlagernden Systemen – wie eben das, was wir vage „Natur" oder auch „lebende Natur" nennen – eine Metaphernbildung mit einer eigenen signifikanten Geschichte. Von dem menschlichen Körper als Immunsystem zu sprechen, heißt ihn in seiner doch stabilen Gegebenheit „in der Natur" bestimmt zu sehen – eben so, dass er darin bewahrt bleibt. Und es muss als erstaunlich erscheinen, über wie lange Zeiträume es diesen „Menschen" doch identisch als diesen Menschen gibt. So ist dafür „gesorgt", dass dieser so erhalten bleibt. Andererseits ist ja doch die „Koexistenz" mit den Viren derart, dass sie auch die Möglichkeit haben, so „anzudocken", dass sie bleibend „eingebaut" werden. So wäre also nicht nur von einem „Immunsystem" zu sprechen, sondern zunächst überhaupt von einem „System", das – wie jedes System – der Unterscheidung von System und Umwelt entsprechend aus der Umwelt selektiert, was es wie gebrauchen kann und was nicht. Die Metapher „System" lässt sich so als „Theorie" fassen, mit der solche Vorgänge zwischen einem „Innen" und „Außen" zu erfassen sind, und zwar so, dass es immer um das zu bewahrende „Innen" geht, also darum, etwas identisch Gegebenes zu erhalten. Das gilt aber für jede gegebene „Entität", die als „System" zu beschreiben ist. So brauchen wir eine Metapher für die Koexistenz von Systemen, die sich nicht gegenseitig als „Umwelt" definieren. Eine gängige Metapher haben wir wohl nicht. Davon unterschieden sind dann „Entitäten", die nicht als Systeme derart zu beschreiben sind, sondern eine bestimmte Teilfunktion in einem System ausüben, wie auch bestimmte Viren. „Metaphern" bezeichnen ja eben bestimmte „Funktionen" – und diese sind dann in bestimmten Systemen verortet, wo sie ausgeübt werden und dann hoffentlich am richtigen Ort im richtigen System. Dies sollte nur anzeigen, dass mit dem Gebrauch von „Metaphern", die wir unserer Sprache entnehmen und die in ihrer Bedeutung dort ihren Ort und ihr Bedeutungsfeld haben, direkt die Frage verbunden ist, wo die metaphorisch erfassten Entitäten ihrerseits dann ihren genuinen Ort, in welchem Funktionszusammenhang, haben. Es geht insofern um die Erfassung und Beschreibung einer gegebenen „Ordnung" und die „Sprache" ist dafür das Paradigma. So müssen und können etwa Grammatikfehler in der Sprache korrigiert werden, wenn Verständigung funktionieren soll.

Stefan Dübel: Die zugrundliegende Sprache ist sicher ein weiterer Faktor, der die Rezeption von Metaphern in der Forschung und Wissenschaft beeinflusst. Metaphern sind oft nicht ohne eine Verzerrung der Aussage zu übersetzen. Ein Beispiel ist schon die Benennung meines eigenen Arbeitsgebietes, des „*antibody engineering*"[1]. Der englische Begriff suggeriert zurecht eine aktive Konstruktionstätigkeit, denn ein großer Teil meiner Arbeit ist es, verschiedene von der Natur entwickelte Elemente neu zusammenzusetzen und so zum Beispiel neue Medikamente zu entwickeln. Im Deutschen fehlt jedoch eine passende Übersetzung von *engineering*. Die Wörterbücher nennen uns Begriffe wie „Technik“ oder „Ingenieurwesen“, welche aber die aktiv gestaltende Tätigkeit des englischen Begriffs in keiner Weise ausdrücken. Eine passende Metapher für meine Tätigkeit in deutscher Sprache habe ich deshalb noch nicht gefunden, und nutze deshalb den englischen Begriff. Auch klingt der Titel unserer Konferenz „*How Metaphors shape Biotechnology*“ im Deutschen weniger schwungvoll. Die Frage der verwendeten Landessprache ist aber zumindest in der Biotechnologie nicht wirklich maßgeblich, da in diesem Fach alle nennenswerten Publikationen in Englisch verfasst werden.

Stefan Heuser: Was wäre denn eine für die theologische Forschung zentrale Metapher, die von ihrer Bedeutung her vergleichbar mit der „Engineering“-Metapher in der biotechnologischen Forschung wäre?

Hans Ulrich: In der Theologie ist die Metapher „Tradition“ eine der für die Forschung zentralen Metaphern, die durch nichts zu ersetzen ist. In den Geisteswissenschaften wird diese Metapher auch gebraucht, diese müssen sich aber fragen, inwiefern sie genuin ihnen zugehört – oder nicht eben aus der Theologie metaphorisch übernommen ist. In der Theologie hat die Metapher einen genuinen Ort. Sie kennzeichnet die „Weitergabe“ dessen, was inhaltlich artikuliert als Bekenntnis, Lehre, Gebot, Geschichte fassbar ist und eben so – in seinem Bestand – „weitergegeben“ oder „überliefert“ wird. Die Metapher impliziert vor allem, dass das Weitergegebene „empfangen“ ist und nicht selbst generiert. Dies ist in der Theologie insofern genuin gegeben, als das, was von „Gott“ zu erfahren ist, anders als empfangen (logischer Weise) nicht zu denken ist. Es wäre ein Widerspruch, sich „Gott“ und das, was ihn kennzeichnet, zu „denken“, selbst zu generieren, wie die Metapher vom „Gottesbild“ (das man sich macht) nahelegt. Die Metapher Tradition impliziert den Vorrang der Bewahrung, der unveränderten „Weitergabe“ im Unterschied zu fortlaufenden Transformationen oder Lernprozessen. Die Metapher „Tradition“ hat ermöglicht, – prominent in der alttestamentlichen Bibelwissenschaft – Texte in ihrer mehrschichtigen (verschiedene Traditionen einschließenden) Genese und ihrer Weitergabe als „Traditionsgeschichte“ zu rekonstruieren und so Ausrichtungen und Tendenzen (Strategien) zu identifizieren. Die Metapher ermöglicht, „Traditionen“ als Entitäten verschiedener Substanz zu identifizieren und historisch zu verorten – also damit einen „Gegenstand“ zu haben, der zu bearbeiten ist. Es wäre interessant zu sehen, was sich in der Genom-Forschung verändert, wenn sie nicht nur die Metaphern „Transkription“ und „Translation“, sondern auch „Tradition“ einsetzt. Diese Metapher wiederum würde sich auch von der Metapher „Vererbung“ unterscheiden, sofern sie auf einen eher allgemeinen Vorgang kohärenter „Reproduktion“ verweist. Freilich erfasst die Metapher „Reproduktion“ nicht die Tatsache, dass innerhalb der „Reproduktion“ und ihr entgegen zugleich „Variationen“ verschiedener Art stattfinden. In der Theologie und ihrer Geschichte ist dafür auch die Kategorie des „Neuen“ als eines absolut unableitbaren Neuen, eines

Neuen, das auch nicht gegen ein bestimmtes „Altes“ steht, in Gebrauch. Mit dieser Kategorie wie in der Rede von der „neuen Schöpfung“ ist festgehalten, dass alles Gegebene in seiner Begrenzung nicht nur auf ein ihm zugehöriges Jenseits (transzendental) zu verstehen ist, sondern daraufhin, dass ein Neues in das Gegebene einbricht, das aber gleichwohl kein absolut Anderes ist, das auch als „Fremdes“ nicht verortet werden kann. Die Frage nach diesem „Neuen“ ist ein treibendes Movens, das die Suche nach Erkenntnis als mit einer unbedingten Wachsamkeit verbunden sieht.

Stefan Heuser: Ich würde den Blick nun gerne von der Metapher des „Neuen“ zum Beitrag von Metaphern bei der Generierung neuer Erkenntnisse in der Forschung richten. Gibt es spezifisch im Feld der Biotechnologie bzw. in der Biologie exemplarische Beispiele für Metaphern, die zur Gewinnung neuer Erkenntnisse beigetragen haben?

Stefan Dübel: Ich glaube, es war der Mathematiker Poincaré, der erstmals darauf aufmerksam gemacht hat, dass der Erkenntnisprozess in den so rational erscheinenden Naturwissenschaften in oft komplett irrationale, kreative Wurzeln hat. Denn Fortschritt kommt manchmal eben nicht durch noch mehr Messen des Bekannten zustande, sondern durch eine neue Idee, etwas zu messen, an das bisher niemand vorher gedacht hatte. Die Geschichte der Entdeckung der Kohlenstoff-Ringbindung (Benzolringe) durch Kekulé geht der Erzählung nach auf einen Traum zurück, in dem er die Atome in Ringen herumwirbeln sah. Bis dahin kannte man in der Chemie nur Kohlenstoff-Atome in gestreckter Kettenform, die aber etliche Eigenschaften einiger Verbindungen nicht erklären konnten. Erst der völlig irrationale Schaffensakt des Träumens hat eine neue Metapher geliefert, die die organische Chemie revolutionierte und völlig neue Wege eröffnete, zum Beispiel bei der Medikamentenentwicklung. Ein anderes Beispiel sind die Relativitätstheorien von Albert Einstein. Der kreative Akt war, sich vorzustellen, dass die Zeit den Raum krümmt. Keine Messergebnisse oder vorhandenen Daten hatten damals darauf hingewiesen. Dieser kreative Schaffensakt der Erstellung einer neuen, revolutionären Hypothese über Vorgänge in der Natur ist nicht durch noch so langes Nachdenken oder Analysieren des gesamten bis dahin verfügbaren Wissens zu erzwingen, sondern bedarf einer neuen kreativen Hypothese, die sich oft gerade NICHT aus dem Bekannten ableiten lässt. Wenn man wissenschaftliche Hypothesen als komplexere Metaphern für das ansonsten Unbeschreibbare begreift, ist klar, dass die Formulierung dieser Art von Metaphern entscheidend ist für die darauffolgende experimentelle Strategie. Natürlich gibt es neben dem Wissensgewinn mithilfe solcher kreativen „Sprunginnovationen“ auch noch weitere Arten, wie in der Biologie Fortschritt entsteht – die Korrelationsanalyse sein hier vor allem genannt, und sogar Zufallsbefunde tragen manchmal dazu bei. Bei allen diesen Mechanismen spielen jedoch die konkreten Metaphern, mit denen individuelle Forschende über die Befunde, Rohdaten oder Beobachtungen nachdenken und die sie verwenden, um diese zu kategorisieren und katalogisieren, sicherlich auch eine Rolle. Jedes unserer naturwissenschaftlichen Experimente öffnet ja – bitte diese simplen Metaphern hier verzeihen – ein kleines „Fenster" mit einem neuen Blick auf die „ewige Wahrheit der Welt". Dabei ist es extrem wichtig, nicht zu vergessen, dass wir als Experimentatoren durch die Wahl der Parameter, die wir einsetzen und testen, bestimmen, wohin wir dieses Fenster „hinbauen". Damit definieren wir auch, auf welchen kleinen Teil der „Wahrheit" wir damit schauen. Blicken wir in die falsche Richtung – und knapp vorbei ist hier auch daneben – ist der Erkenntnisgewinn gering oder nicht vorhanden. Und jede Metapher, die für etwas neu Beobachtetes gebildet wird, definiert durch die gewählte Metapher automatisch einen assoziativen Denkrahmen, in den wir das Neue einordnen, d. h. wir definieren somit auch ein begrenztes Fenster in unserem Denken, welches damit auch die Art der Erkenntnis definiert. Dieser Einschränkung sind wir uns aber meist nicht in gleichem Maße bewusst wie bei den Grenzen des Parameter-„Fensters", das wir für ein Experiment bewusst definieren.

Die Wahl der richtigen Hypothese ist aber natürlich essentiell von einer Sprache abhängig – normalerweise den bisher in diesem Bereich der Wissenschaft benutzen Termini – und natürlich schränkt dies unser Denken ein. Da die Hypothese also in sehr vielen Fällen der experimentellen Forschung vorausgehen muss – ansonsten kann man das experimentelle „Fenster" ja gar nicht richtig beim Blick auf die Welt „positionieren", dürfte die Wahl der Begriffe, mit denen die Hypothese formuliert wurde, stark dazu beitragen, wie das Ergebnis aussieht. Es gibt auch viele Beispiele, die zeigen, dass die gewählte Metapher nützlich ist, aber bei weiteren Fortschritten in der Forschung bemerkt wird, dass die Metapher am Rande etwas „ausfranst" und teilweise nicht mehr zum Problem passt. Ein Beispiel geben die Definitionen von biologischer Art und Gattung – für Jahrhunderte eine zentrale Säule der Biologie. Die Nomenklatur zur Benennung unterschiedlicher Lebewesen wurde von Linné konzipiert, um überhaupt die belebte Welt grundsätzlich in ihrer Vielfalt systematisch wissenschaftlich erfassen zu können. Er entwarf ein System für die Klassifizierung der unterschiedlichen Arten von Lebewesen mithilfe von zwei Namen, welches auch heute noch Standard ist. Es besteht aus einem „Nachnamen", welcher die Gattung beschreibt, und einem „Vornamen" für die Art (wobei die Gattung vorne steht). *„Homo sapiens"* ist ein Beispiel. Dieser Name als Metapher für alle Menschen ist eingängig, und die Linné'sche Nomenklatur war ein riesiger Fortschritt bei der wissenschaftlichen Kartierung der Vielfalt des Lebens. Das gewählte System dieser Artnamen suggeriert aber auch eine eindeutige Zuordenbarkeit, und sogar noch aufgeteilt in 2 genau definierte Ebenen, die Gattung (= Gruppe nah verwandter Arten) und die eigentliche Art (Spezies). Die Vielfalt des Lebens, welches wir um uns herum vorfinden, ist aber nicht in solche „Schubladen" mit fest definierten Außengrenzen gegliedert, sondern ein stetig fließendes und dauernd sich verändernder Prozess. Die „Schubladen" haben im Detail also keine klar definierten Grenzen, womit die Metapher ungenau wird, i. e. an den Rändern etwas „ausfranst". Spätestens seit der Evolutionstheorie von Darwin verstehen wir auch warum. Arten können sich durch Anpassung verändern, und da dies ein kontinuierlicher Prozess ist, finden wir dabei in der Natur natürlich alle Zwischenstufen und Übergänge, zum Beispiel, wenn eine Spezies sich gerade durch Mutationen und Evolution in zwei verschiedene Arten diversifiziert. Das führt natürlich in vielen Fällen zu Problemen bei der exakten Beschreibung. Jedes Kind kann einen Esel von einem Pferd unterscheiden (nach Linné zwei verschiedene Spezies: *Equus ferus* bzw. *Equus asinus*). Welchen Artnamen nimmt man aber dann für Maultiere – die Produkte einer Romanze zwischen Pferd und Esel? Wir sind Zeuge einer Dichotomie in der Evolution, wobei beide Arten sich offensichtlich noch nicht soweit auseinanderentwickelt haben, dass gemeinsamer Nachwuchs gar nicht mehr möglich ist.

Noch verwirrender wird es bei Organismen, die Linne noch nicht kannte: Bakterien und Viren. Zwar werden auch hier oft noch Gattungen und Artnamen vergeben, aber die Veränderung von Mikroorganismen durch Anpassung an ihre Umgebung erfolgt oft so schnell, dass jede wissenschaftliche Untersuchung nur eine Momentaufnahme sein kann – schaut man die gleiche „Art" ein paar Monate später wieder an, hat sie schon viele Veränderungen in der Erbsubstanz angehäuft, und damit neue Eigenschaften, denn mit jeder Vermehrung mutiert die DNA und damit verändert sich die Art.

Das bringt uns auf die Problematik der Definition von Metaphern für wissenschaftliche Phänomene. Naturwissenschaftlich Forschenden ist natürlich bewusst, dass Hypothesen immer nur in einem bestimmten Bereich gelten, mathematisch würde man „innerhalb eines definierten Intervalls" sagen, außerhalb dessen wir einfach keine Aussage treffen können. Praktisch definiert sich dies zum Beispiel aus der „Größe des Fensters", das wir experimentell öffnen konnten, um einen Blick auf die „ewige Wahrheit der Welt" zu erhaschen. Sehr oft ergibt sich aus mehr und genaueren Messungen aber, dass die Hypothese angepasst werden muss. Damit entsteht oft auch die Notwendigkeit, Begriffe nach ihrer Einführung immer genauer – und oft eingeschränkter – zu definieren. Natürlich hat dies direkte Auswirkungen auf die metaphorischen Begrifflichkeiten der Hypothesen.

In der Biologie – wie auch in den anderen Naturwissenschaften – ist dieser Prozess unvermeidbar aufgrund der stetigen Entwicklung immer neuer Analysemethoden, die immer breitere, tiefergehende, hochauflösendere und/oder genauere Messungen erlauben. In Bezug auf den Linné'schen Artbegriff ist hier vor allem die DNA-Sequenzierung zu betrachten, also die heute selbstverständliche Fähigkeit der Molekularbiologen, die Abfolge der einzelnen „Buchstaben" der genetischen Information verschiedenster Lebewesen schnell und ohne großen Aufwand bestimmen zu können. Erfolgte zu Linnes Zeiten die Einordnung einer Tier- oder Pflanzenart in Gattungen, Familien und übergeordnete Gruppierungen weitestgehend nach äußerlich sichtbaren Merkmalen wie Körperform, Blütenstruktur, Art der Früchte, Blattformen usw., so wird heute allgemein davon ausgegangen, dass Organismen desto enger verwandt sind, je ähnlicher ihre DNA-Sequenz ist, also der Text, der durch die Abfolge der vier verschiedenen Nukleotid-„Buchstaben" des genetischen Codes in ihrer Erbsubstanz gebildet wird. Diese Einschätzung geht wiederum von der Hypothese aus, dass sich die DNA langsam, relativ stetig und mit gleichbleibender Geschwindigkeit verändert – was keinesfalls immer der

Fall ist, aber immer noch eine weit bessere Verallgemeinerung als Linnés ursprüngliche Hypothese, dass z. B. alle Bäume mit ähnlicher Blatt- Wuchs- und Blütenform auch eng verwandt sind.

Hans Ulrich: Das Beispiel zeigt, dass es bei der Wahl von Metaphern für „wissenschaftliche Phänomene" offensichtlich darauf ankommt, was sie für ein bestimmtes Erkenntnisziel leisten – wenn denn das Erkenntnisziel wirklich auch bestimmt ist – wie hier das Ziel, die Welt der Organismen in einer bestimmten Ordnung zu erfassen – hier mit der Metapher „Verwandtschaft" angezeigt. Es geht also hier nicht um irgendeine andere Ordnung – etwa die Ordnung nach Maßgabe der Verwertbarkeit für den Menschen, oder die Ordnung nach ihrer jeweiligen Bedeutung für das Ganze der organischen Welt etc. Wenn die Ordnung im Blick auf „Verwandtschaft" erfasst werden soll, wird nun die „genetische" Verwandtschaft, auch wenn diese sich verändern kann, als die gesehen, die tiefer greift und das Differente im Unterschied zum Gleichen genauer festmachen kann, als die auf sichtbare Merkmale bezogen ist (Blattform ...). Auch die Art und Geschwindigkeit von Veränderungen der verschiedenen „Verwandten" lässt sich offensichtlich mit der „genetischen" Verwandtschaft besser erfassen, die dann nicht zuletzt so zu verstehen ist, dass sie nur als dynamisch different zwischen gleichbleibend und variierend – oder auch mutierend – zu erfassen ist. Dann aber ist die kenntlich gewordene Ordnung weniger in Übereinstimmung mit der Ordnung in der Sprache und der Alltagswelt, sofern diese auf eigenen Unterscheidungsmerkmalen beruht, die zur Orientierung gebraucht werden – wie z. B. „essbar" oder „nicht essbar". Generelle Metapherntheorien haben erklärt, dass Metaphern „funktionale" Bedeutung haben – so hier Funktionen für die Feststellung verschiedener Arten von Ordnung in der Welt der Organismen.

Stefan Heuser: Eure Beispiele sind eindrückliche Belege dafür, dass sich Metaphern gut auf ihre Funktionen hin analysieren und verstehen lassen: Wir wollen etwas mit unseren Metaphern erreichen – und zugleich zeigen sie eine Funktion an, die dem jeweils Bezeichneten zukommt und die die Metapher aus ihrem Quellbereich in ihren Zielbereich „mitnimmt". Jedenfalls besteht Klärungsbedarf mit Blick auf die Frage, welche Funktionen eine Metapher erfüllt bzw. erfüllen soll. Linné beispielsweise wollte zeigen, dass die Welt der Lebewesen geordnet ist – ein Ansinnen von Ordnung und Stabilität, das sich an der Beobachtung rapider Anpassungsvorgänge bei Mikroorganismen bricht, dessen Erklärungskraft deshalb aber nicht obsolet ist, wenn man sich die gleichzeitig zu beobachtende erstaunliche Stabilität beispielsweise der DNA und die Weitergabe ihrer Buchstabenfolge an die Folgegenerationen vor Augen hält. Nur erweist sich dann die Metaphorik von „Stabilität" bzw. „Variabilität" als erklärungskräftiger als die Ordnungsmetaphorik, ohne diese komplett abzulösen. Stefan Dübels Hinweis, dass das Leben und seine Prozesse nicht in „Schubladen" eingeordnet werden können, verstehe ich als eine solche notwendige Form der Metaphernkritik, die eine doppelte Funktionalität von Metaphern in ihrem epistemischen, erkenntnisgenerierenden Gebrauch sichtbar macht:

Metaphern können – wie bei Linné – erstens die Funktion haben, etwas sichtbar zu machen, das jemand für die grundlegende Wahrheit der Wirklichkeit hält – zum Beispiel, dass die Dinge wohl geordnet sind. Sie bleiben im Horizont eines übergeordneten Sinnzusammenhangs, wie er beispielsweise von absoluten Metaphern wie dem „Kosmos“ eröffnet wird, dem einfache Metaphern dienen bzw. dessen Funktionalität sie entsprechen – und einem bestimmten prioritären „Weltbild“ verpflichtet ist. Am Beispiel von Linné lässt sich das gut sichtbar machen. Metaphern haben demnach eine Funktion, z. B., dass sie die Dinge, die sie bezeichnen, wiederum auf eine bestimmte Funktion bzw. einen bestimmten Sinn hin erschließen. Sie artikulieren dann die Funktion, die etwas hat, bzw. das „Woraufhin“ der Dinge gemäß einer Theorie, die bereits existiert und die das Erkennen leitet. Dass die Metaphernbildung bzw. der Einsatz von Metaphern von einem bestimmten Grundverständnis über die Wahrheit von Wirklichkeit geleitet wird und dabei eine Funktion bei der Erkenntnisgewinnung hat, ist ja keine besonders originelle Einsicht. Interessant ist aber, dass uns bei der Metaphernbildung offenbar der Gedanke nicht loslässt, dass das, was die Metaphern artikulieren, selbst eine Funktion bzw. einen Sinn hat bzw. irgendwie haben muss, und dass sich dieser Sinn nicht formalsprachlich, sondern nur metaphorisch ausdrücken lässt. Man könnte hier weiterfragen, inwiefern dieser Sinn von uns Menschen kommt, und wir diesen „Glauben“ an Sinn nicht gut loslassen können, weil wir uns sonst nicht in der Wirklichkeit einrichten und in ihr „zu Hause sein“ können. Für die Metaphernkritik bedeutet es aber, dass wir eine ziemlich radikale Auseinandersetzung mit unseren Vorannahmen brauchen, um wahrnehmen und sprachlich erfassen zu können, was die Forschung an Erkenntnissen über den Sinn von Wirklichkeit zutage fördern *soll*.

Metaphern können aber auch – zweitens – erfassen, was sich beobachten lässt, aber bislang rätselhaft bleibt oder mit Blick auf seinen möglichen, immer schon vorausgesetzten Sinn erklärungsbedürftig erscheint. Sie können so auch neue Erkenntnisbedarfe markieren. Metaphern führen dann potentiell in einen neuen Sinn- und Entdeckungszusammenhang hinein, z. B. die Metapher der „Evolution“.

Stefan Dübel: Genau – die Entwicklung von Linnés ersten Versuchen, darunterliegende Zusammenhänge greifbar zu machen (ohne dabei irgendetwas von Genen oder Evolution zu wissen), deutete ja schon ganz konkret auf die Abstammungslehre hin: die Grundhypothese der Struktur der Nomenklatur Linnés zeigt, dass er die fortschreitende Veränderung und Diversifizierung der verschiedenen Lebewesen instinktiv bereits erkannt hatte, denn er wählte die Metapher „Familie“ als nächste Gliederungsebene zum Zusammenfassen ähnlich aussehender Gattungen. Familienmitglieder sind nahe verwandt, stammen oft voneinander ab. Damit ebnete Linné metaphorisch bereits den Gedankenweg bis hin zur modernen DNA-Systematik und natürlich Darwins Evolutionslehre.

Interessant finde ich in diesem Zusammenhang auch die Fähigkeit unseres Gehirns, Kategorien zu bilden, ohne dafür Sprache zu benötigen. Einige davon scheinen sogar angeboren zu sein, zum Beispiel das Erkennen von einer Kategorie von Lebewesen, ohne etwas von Linné'scher Systematik zu wissen – z. B. bei der Angst vor Spinnen bei Kindern, die vorher noch nie eine solche gesehen haben. Aber damit verlassen wir die Ebene der Metaphernkritik; auch deren Definition „franst" offensichtlich hier an den Rändern etwas aus.

Stefan Heuser: Ich finde es interessant, dass Du Linnès Wahl der Metapher der Familie als „instinktiv" bezeichnest. Gewiss war es Linné bewusst, dass er aus dem lebensweltlichen Quellbereich der Metapher „Familie" einen großen Sinnüberschuss und eine mit der Sprache verbundene Grammatik – auch eine moralische Grammatik – in den biologischen Zielbereich mitnimmt. Die Funktion der Metapher ist es, Dinge mit einem bestimmten Sinn zu versehen, ohne den Linné den Gegenstand seiner Untersuchung nicht verstehen wollte oder konnte – und den er anderen nahegelegt hat. Er wollte den Dingen etwas „ansinnen". Michel Foucault hat diesen Vorgang kritisch als eine sprachliche Operation gekennzeichnet, durch die Naturdinge nomenklatorisch identifiziert und geordnet und an einen beherrschbaren Platz gestellt werden sollen.

Das bringt mich zu einer dritten Funktion von Metaphern: sie zeigen an, wie mit den Dingen in ihrer je eigenen Funktionalität und ihrem angesonnenen Sinn umgegangen werden kann. Man könnte dies eine pragmatische bzw. praxisbezogene, vielleicht sogar: moralische Funktion von Metaphern nennen, die mit deren propositionalem Gehalt verbunden ist. Metaphern legen Praktiken nahe bzw. sprechen diejenigen, die mit ihnen kommunizieren, auf bestimmte Praktiken an. Um zu Linnés Familienmetapher zurückzukommen: Mit einem als „Ordnung" verstandenen Gegenstand ist – je nach Praxiszusammenhang – anders umzugehen als mit chaotischen oder fluiden Zuständen. Das hängt daran, wie der Quellbereich der Metapher kulturell und praxeologisch kodiert ist. Dies gilt auch in dem Sinne, dass eine „Ordnung" selbst die Frage nach ihrer Funktion bzw. ihrem Sinn als Ordnung und ihrer Veränderbarkeit wachruft – während Chaos geradezu als der Mangel an Sinn bzw. Funktion erscheint und eigene Fantasien nach einem Umgang mit dem als „chaotisch" Klassifizierten freisetzt, wenn es auf einen Praxiszusammenhang trifft. Diese Funktion von Metaphern zeigt einen weiteren Grund für Metaphernkritik an: und zwar hinsichtlich des Gebrauchs von Metaphern in der öffentlichen Kommunikation und den damit verbundenen politischen und moralischen Implikationen von Metaphern sowie hinsichtlich ihres Gebrauchs in der gemeinsamen, interdisziplinären Kommunikation sowie in der Lehre und den damit verbundenen Implikationen für den Zusammenhang von Methoden und Medien unseres Erkennens.

Stefan Dübel: Eine weitere Relevanz der sorgfältigen Auswahl von Metaphern liegt in der Kommunikation wissenschaftlicher Inhalte an Patienten in der Medizin. Da Placebo-Effekte Patienten helfen können, dass tatsächlich Medikamente besser wirken, ist die Auswahl verständlicher und positiv aufzunehmender Metaphern zur Erklärung der wissenschaftlichen Hintergründe der Wirkung von Medikamenten oder Behandlungsmethoden hier sorgfältig zu treffen [2]. Und in Zukunft wird die sorgfältige

Auswahl von Metaphern noch aus einem anderen Grund wichtig: Die überwiegende Mehrheit der biologischen und biotechnologischen Ergebnisse werden in Textform publiziert. Gleichzeitig wird so viel publiziert, dass einzelne Forschende nur noch in einem sehr eng begrenzten Spezialgebiet die Chance haben, überhaupt alle neuen Ergebnisse zu verfolgen. Das behindert vor allem, neue Zusammenhänge mit etwas entfernteren Forschungsgegenständen zu erkennen – nicht ideal für das Erkennen hochvernetzter Zusammenhänge, wie sie uns die Biochemie lebendiger Systeme präsentiert. Hier wird künstliche Intelligenz in naher Zukunft die Ausbeute das Ergebnissen potenzieren, denn im Gegensatz zu bisherigen „*big data*" Computeranalysen, welche meist zahlenbasiert sind, ist die Spezialität der neuesten KI Systeme vor allem der Sprachvergleich. Die Identifikation von neuen Zusammenhängen, welche menschliche Experten übersehen hatten, aus einer Vielzahl von publizierten Studien mithilfe von Computern wurde bereits nachgewiesen [3]. Die heute verfügbaren *large language models* wie GPT sind im Gegensatz zu den bisherigen zahlenbasierten Analysen ideal geeignet, um die Riesenmengen von Texten der publizierten Forschungsergebnisse zu verarbeiten. Sie werden uns in den nächsten Jahren in bisher nicht vorstellbarer Weise helfen, zahlreiche neue Erkenntnisse zu gewinnen, deren Lösungen in der heute bereits vorhandenen enormen Sammlung an Daten bereits schlummern, deren Zusammenhänge von Menschen aber bisher nicht erkannt wurden. Damit werden sie zu einem mindestens dem Menschen gleichwertigen, wenn nicht sogar effektiveres Instrument zum Verständnis der komplexen und vernetzten Vorgänge der belebten Natur, und deshalb haben wir als Forscher heute auch eine Verantwortung, unsere Publikationen auch für diese Verarbeitung zu optimieren. Als für die Metaphernkritik relevante Frage ergibt sich daraus, ob wir deshalb besser in der Wahl unserer Metaphern versuchen sollten, diese nicht allzu oft zu wechseln, und etablierte Begriffe weiter zu verwenden, auch wenn sie nach neueren Ergebnissen etwas ungenau werden, oder ob wir Metaphern stets so genau wie möglich an neue Entwicklungen anpassen sollten, um mögliche neue Zusammenhänge nicht zu verdecken. Im ersten Fall hat die KI ein geringeres Risiko, relevante Publikationen zu übersehen, im zweiten Fall sind dagegen vielleicht detailliertere Aussagen möglich. Diese Frage kann zum Glück mithilfe der Analyse entsprechender Datensätze in Zukunft experimentell beantwortet werden.

Stefan Heuser: Gibt es in der biotechnologischen Forschung eigentlich Beispiele dafür, dass neue Erkenntnisse zur Umgestaltung von Metaphern und zur Erneuerung der Wissenschaftssprache (z. B. auch zur Ersetzung einer Metapher durch eine andere) beigetragen haben?

Stefan Dübel: Ja, sehr viele. Zum Beispiel bei TNF („Tumornekrosefaktor"), oder bei der historischen Sukzession von „Antitoxin" zu „Antikörper" und dem heute meist „Immunoglobulin" genannten Molekül. Ich habe dazu ja zuvor schon einiges ausgeführt und kann darauf gerne noch weiter eingehen.

Stefan Heuser: Bevor Du das näher ausführst, möchte ich noch Hans Ulrich fragen, ob es auch in der theologischen Forschung Beispiele für einen Wandel oder eine Substitution von einer Metapher durch eine andere gibt?

Hans Ulrich: Es kennzeichnet die Theologie in ihrer Arbeit am Reden von Gott, dass beständig Metaphern, die in Gebrauch sind, durch neue ersetzt werden – also wirklich „ersetzt“, sodass die ersetzte Metapher als definitiv unbrauchbar erscheint. Es gibt abgesehen von vielen nicht signifikant hervortretenden Ersetzungen auch bekanntermaßen höchst signifikante, die tief in die „Grammatik“ der Rede von Gott eingreifen und die im theologischen Diskurs entsprechend dramatisch in den Blick gerückt wurden. Dies hat immer auch im Vorgang der Übersetzung biblischer Texte stattgefunden. Ein hervorragendes Beispiel der neueren Theologiegeschichte ist die Ersetzung der Metapher „Zukunft“ im Sinne dessen, was sich von hier aus in ein Folgendes erstreckt, durch „Zu-kunft“ im Sinne dessen, was auf dieses hier und jetzt „zukommt“, hier und jetzt „ankommt“ – also die Ersetzung von „Zukunft“ in jenem herkömmlichen Sinn durch „Adventus“, in der Erkenntnis, dass die biblische Rede von Gott entscheidend in solcher „adventlichen“ Grammatik erfolgt. Welche Metapher die theologische Arbeit am Reden von Gott leitet, hängt weitgehend davon ab, wie die in den biblischen Texten vorgegebenen Metaphern in der Übersetzung erscheinen. Manche Ersetzungen freilich bleiben weitgehend unentschieden, so dass Unklarheit herrscht, welcher Metapher zu folgen wäre. Dies hat seinen Grund auch darin, dass die Metaphern in der Theologie nicht allein auf ihre Funktion hin zur Diskussion stehen, sondern auch auf ihre Herkunft hin, sofern sie biblische Metaphern ersetzen und es dafür mehrere Ersatzmetaphern gibt. Metaphern lassen sich nicht in eine andere Sprache „übersetzen“, sondern nur ersetzen, so die Metapher „Pistis“ (Vertrauen) durch „Glauben“. Doch der Metapher „Vertrauen“ in der Wahrheitsfindung zu folgen ist ein gänzlich anderer Vorgang, als die „Gründung“ der Wahrheit auf einen „Glauben“, der etwa als „Für-Wahr-Halten“ oder als „Glauben, dass“ verstanden wird. Gewiss ist die Diskussion darüber unabsehbar und doch ist darin eine klare Unterscheidung von Metaphern enthalten, die ganze Welten theologischer Arbeit voneinander scheidet – eine „hermeneutische Theologie“, die „Wahrheit“ im „Verstehen“ von Gegebenen gewinnt und eine Theologie, die „Wahrheit“ als (fundamental) nachweisbare Gewissheit verfolgt. Für das Zusammenwirken der Theologie mit der Naturwissenschaft ergeben sich daraus gänzlich verschiedene Konstellationen.

Stefan Heuser: In der Religionsdidaktik hat man für das Zusammenspiel der unterschiedlichen Weltzugänge von Naturwissenschaft und Theologie das Konzept des „komplementären Denkens“ entwickelt. Demnach benötigen wir – wenn wir die Welt, in der wir leben, nicht reduziert wahrnehmen wollen – beide Zugänge, können diese aber nur komplementär, nie gleichzeitig verfolgen, wenn wir keine Widersprüche erzeugen wollen. Das ist ein ganz gutes Konzept, wenn es um die Frage geht, wie sich unterschiedliche Arten der Deutung von Welt miteinander vermitteln lassen. Wenn es aber um eine gemeinsame Arbeit an einer metapherngeleiteten Erschließung von

Wirklichkeit geht, kommt man mit „Komplementarität" nicht weit. Das Modell setzt voraus, dass schon feststeht, was „Wirklichkeit" ist und dass es nur noch darauf ankommt, diese auf verschiedene Art zu deuten bzw. verschiedene Perspektiven auf die eine „Wirklichkeit" zu entwickeln. Es geht dann eigentlich nur noch darum, sich der Zulässigkeit einer arbeitsteiligen Multiperspektivität zu versichern. Ein „Zusammenwirken" von Geisteswissenschaft und Naturwissenschaft beim Verstehen von dem, was die Forschung in dem riesigen, für unsere Augen unsichtbaren Feld der Molekularbiologie antrifft und sichtbar macht, ist bei solchen Konzepten nicht im Blick. Diese „Sichtbarkeit" bzw. „Unsichtbarkeit" ist ja auch ein Problem des „Forschungsgegenstands" der Theologie: Gott. Noch dazu ist Gott nicht im naturwissenschaftlichen Sinne nachweisbar, sein Wirken ist nicht aus den wahrnehmbaren Ereignissen einfach ablesbar und auch nicht ableitbar, sondern ausschließlich im Medium der Sprache, also im Medium des Redens von Gott und zu Gott, zu erforschen. Bei der Erforschung Gottes geht es primär ums Hören, nicht ums Sehen. Mich würde an dieser Stelle interessieren, welche methodische Funktion der Metaphernbildung in der Molekularbiologie zukommt, die ja ihren Forschungsgegenstand nicht ohne technische Vermittlung mit bloßen Augen sehen kann.

Stefan Dübel: Alles, was wir Biologen im molekularbiologischen Labor von unserem Forschungsgegenstand jemals in den Händen haben, sind winzigste Mengen klarer Flüssigkeiten. Wir können niemals die Moleküle, die darin herumschwimmen und das Wunder der molekularbiologischen Wissenschaft und Gentechnologie ermöglichen, direkt sehen. Schon deshalb müssen wir ständig mit Metaphern arbeiten. Bei überraschenden neuen Ergebnissen oder Beobachtungen ergibt sich unter den Forschenden im „Labor-*Slang*" oft schnell ein Begriff, der deren Eigenheiten und Neuheit metaphorisch versucht, griffig zu kommunizieren. Die Begriffe ändern sich deshalb anfangs noch oft und vielfältig, um sie dem Fortschritt der Ergebnisse der Experimente anzupassen. Selten schaffen es die „Labor-*Slang*"-Metaphern in die später daraus hervorgehende wissenschaftliche Publikation, manchmal aber doch, weil einem einfach nichts besser Passendes einfällt. Ein Beispiel sind die „Monster-Zellen" der Gattung *Acetabularia*, an denen ich in meiner Diplomarbeit arbeitete [4], Abb. 9.1. Die zunächst fadenförmige einzellige Alge *Acetabularia* bildet zur Vermehrung wunderschön filigran geformte Schirmchen. In Laborkulturen tauchten aber manchmal unförmige Zellen auf, die nicht fadenförmig waren und auch keine Schirme bildeten. Sie sahen aus wie unregelmäßige Blobs. Wir nannten sie im Labor einfach Monster-Zellen, auch weil sie oft dicker angeschwollen waren als die feinen Strukturen der normalen Form der Alge und dabei irreguläre Pusteln und Auswüchse entwickelten. Bei der Erzählung dieser alten Geschichte ist mir wieder aufgefallen, wie schwierig die Wortwahl für die Beschreibung dieser Zellen war und ist – damals habe ich in keiner Weise an die Bedeutung der Metaphern-Wahl gedacht, heute würde ich gegen das natürlich negativ assoziierte Wort „Monster" stimmen. Dieser Labor-*Slang* Begriff hat es aber dann doch als *„amorphous monster cells"* in die wissenschaftliche Literatur geschafft.

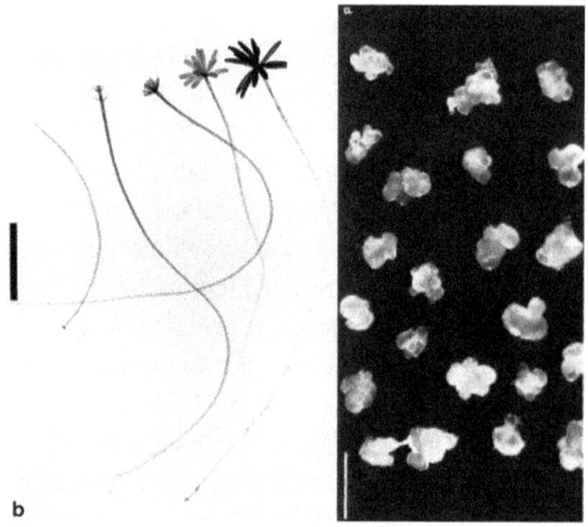

Abb. 9.1: Links: Acetabularia cliftonii in verscheidenen Wachtstumsstadien. Rechts: 3 Monate alte „Monster"-Zellen der gleichen Algenart. Maßstab: links 1 cm, rechts 1mm. Fotos: S. Dübel.

Wir konnten auch Unterschiede in der Zusammensetzung der Proteine (Eiweiße) zwischen den Monster-Zellen und den „normalen" Zellen feststellen – einer der frühesten Befunde eines neuen Wissenschaftszweiges der Biochemie, der mittlerweile als *„proteomics"* weltweit breit beforscht wird. Übrigens ist die Rede von „Eiweiß" für Proteine auch ein wunderbares Beispiel einer historischen biologischen Metapher, welche aus der Herkunft begründet wurde und eigentlich nicht wirklich mehr zum modernen Erkenntnisstand passt. Tatsächlich ist im Eiweiß eines Hühnereis weniger „Eiweiß" (also Protein) enthalten als im Eigelb. Wenn man Proteinlösungen herstellt, erscheinen diese meist gelb statt weiß – ein bekanntes Beispiel ist die gelbliche Farbe unseres Blutserums, nachdem man die roten Blutkörperchen abzentrifugiert hat – Serum ist eine hochkonzentrierte „Eiweiß"-Lösung.

Hans Ulrich: Offensichtlich machen die hier erwähnten Metaphern verbal auf etwas Sichtbares aufmerksam, wie eine Farbe (Eiweiß) oder „Monster". Was die Funktion von „Eiweiß" ist, muss anders erfasst werden – auch hier kann dann wieder eine Metapher eingesetzt werden, also „Protein" (das was von primärer Bedeutung oder Funktion ist). Die Metapher „Monster-Zellen" ist hier wohl primär des Aussehens wegen gewählt. Anders wäre es auch hier, wenn stattdessen eine bestimmte dominante Funktion dieser Zellen in einem bestimmten Organismus metaphorisch erfasst würde. Anders wiederum wäre es, wenn Metaphern aufgrund spezifischer Aufgaben des Verstehens, Erkennens und Identifizierens von „Objekten" und ihrer Bedeutung etc. gewählt werden – wie *„Homo sapiens"*. Freilich bleibt hier offen, in welcher begrenzten Reichweite die Bedeutung von Metaphern gesehen wird – hier also etwa begrenzt auf ein bestimmtes Merkmal, das den „Menschen" von anderen vergleichbaren „Gattungen" unterscheiden lässt, nicht etwa um „den Menschen" etwa seinem „Wesen" nach zu bestimmen. Diese wenigen Anmerkungen sollten deutlich machen, dass die Analyse von Metaphern sehr differenziert ausfallen wird, sofern Metaphern auf viele verschiedene Bedeutungskontexte verweisen, wie auf den einer *prima vista* Identifikation im Labor (Monster-Zellen), auf einen alltäglich-lebensweltlichen (*Homo sapiens*), oder einen theoretisch und experimentell erschlossenen funktionalen etc. Letzterer (Beispiel „Protein“) kann wohl die Forschung leiten, sofern sie eben mit dieser Metapher etwas festhält, was gilt und im Ganzen des Forschungsfeldes bis auf Weiteres gilt, d. h. bis die Metapher geändert werden müsste. Sofern Metaphern irgendwie festzustellendes Gegebenes als so oder so Sichtbares kennzeichnen – also einem gemeinsamen Sehen zugänglich machen, das zunächst von keinem weiteren Verstehen abhängig ist – entsteht in ihnen auch eine Art von „gemeinsamer Welt“. Damit ist das Problem gegeben, dass eben diese als solche auch daraufhin zu befragen ist, ob sie für die gemeinsame und verlässliche Orientierung hilfreich ist – oder eher irritierend, störend etc. Das betrifft dann etwa die Kommunikation zwischen dem Labor und der „Öffentlichkeit“. Dies freilich ist ein eigenes Kapitel, das die auch „politische“ Verantwortung der Wissenschaft und die Offenheit der öffentlichen Diskurse für die Wissenschaft betrifft.

Stefan Dübel: Nochmal zum Begriff Eiweiß: Anscheinend hatte der Begriff sich schon so weit in der naturwissenschaftlichen Literatur und darauffolgend in der allgemeinen Sprachkultur verbreitet, dass er nicht mehr so einfach ausgetauscht werden konnte. Heute benutzt man in der deutschen Fachliteratur und auch vielfach in der Umgangssprache den Begriff „Protein“, ein Kunstwort, welches anfangs für alle möglichen Substanzen verwendet wurde, da die heutigen biochemischen Unterscheidungsmethoden noch nicht bekannt waren. Auch dieses Wort kann man als Metapher verstehen, denn der niederländische Chemiker Gerhard Johan Mulder wollte damit auf die herausragende Bedeutung dieser Stoffe für das Leben hinweisen und leitete es vom Griechischen *prōteios* („erste Qualität“) ab. Da Proteine immer noch als sehr wichtig angesehen werden, bestand seitdem keine weitere Notwendigkeit mehr zur Änderung des Begriffs. Tatsächlich kannte ich als des Griechischen nicht mächtiger Proteinforscher die Etymologie des Wortes und damit die metaphorische Bedeutung vor dem Schreiben dieses Berichtes selbst bis zu meiner Recherche zum Verfassen dieses Textes nicht – was mich wahrscheinlich immun gegen Einschränkungen bei meiner Hypothesenbildung durch die Wahl der Metapher machte. Gerade bei diesem sehr allgemeinen Begriff ist aber auch die chemische Definition sehr viel eindeutiger – dann heißen Proteine „Polypeptide“, beschreibend nach der Art der chemischen Verbindung ihrer Untereinheiten, die allen gemeinsam ist. Diese Metapher bietet damit von vorneherein weniger Platz zum „Ausfransen“ an den Rändern – ganz anders als bei dem Begriff „Eiweiß“!

Stefan Heuser: Wie stark hängt die Metaphernbildung in Deinem Forschungsfeld, der Biotechnologie, vom Stand der Technik ab – und von identifizierbaren kulturellen Faktoren?

Stefan Dübel: Der Einfluss kultureller Faktoren ist eindeutig vorhanden, da die Forscher, die neue Metaphern prägen, diese nur aus den Begriffen schöpfen können, die sie kennen. Die erste Limitation ist ganz technisch ausgedrückt der Umfang ihres Wortschatzes. Weiterhin ist es naheliegend, dass kulturelle Unterschiede den assoziativen Begriffsbildungsprozess für eine Beschreibung von neuen biologischen Funktionen, Effekten oder Strukturen stark beeinflussen, genauso wie Altersunterschiede und die persönliche Geschichte, Elternhaus, Freunde, Hobbies usw. Ich vermute, dass die meisten Forscher neue Begriffe nicht im vollen Bewusstsein, dass es Metaphern sind, gezielt als solche einführen. Zumindest war es bei mir so, bis wir unser gemeinsames Projekt zur Metaphernkritik begannen. Vermutlich wird jedoch die Wortwahl unausweichlich von der Hypothese, unter der die Experimente durchgeführt wurden, beeinflusst.

Das muss aber nicht heißen, dass das immer so zu sein hat. Gerade mit Blick auf die Perzeption unserer Forschungsergebnisse in einer immer komplexer werdenden und deshalb wohl auch immer allgemein technik- und wissenschaftskritischen Welt müssen wir diesem Punkt in Zukunft sehr viel mehr Aufmerksamkeit widmen. Die Naturwissenschaftler sollten hier aus der Politik und Werbung lernen, und viel bewusster bedenken, was wir eigentlich an Inhalten transportieren wollen. Damit meine ich keinesfalls, dass „negative“ Informationen unterdrückt oder vorenthalten werden sollen, aber etwas Nachdenken über die möglichen Interpretationen eines Begriffes durch Fachfremde und Nichtwissenschaftler ist sicher hilfreich. Allerdings ist dabei der Grat zur unethischen bewussten Manipulation schmal, und die möglichen Implikationen davon können schwerwiegend sein.

Eine radikale Beschreibung der Steuerung des Denkens durch machtpolitisch diktierte Wahl von Bezeichnungen finden wir in George Orwells dystopischen Zukunftsroman „1984“, in dem ein faschistisch-kommunistisches Regime die Gedanken seiner Untertanen durch Verbot unerwünschter oder kritischer Worte und deren Ersatz durch irreführende neue Begriffe formt. Die bewusste Veränderung der Sprache wird von den Protagonisten des diktatorischen Regimes im Orwell'schen Roman somit gezielt zur Gedankenkontrolle genutzt. Wir kennen milde Versionen dieser Methode auch aus eigener Erfahrung, aus durchaus erfolgreich umgesetzten Beispielen unserer aktuellen Sprachwelt. So wurde aus „weggeworfenem Müll“ die Metapher „entsorgter Wertstoff“. All diese nicht-naturwissenschaftlichen Beispiele von problematischen Begriffsbildungen illustrieren ein Grundrisiko jeder Metaphernbildung. Bewusst und bösartig angewendet wie bei Orwell'scher *Newspeak* ist der Versuch zur Gehirnwäsche meist einfach zu erkennen. Die dagegen in aller Regel unschuldig-unbewusste Wahl von Metaphern in der Naturwissenschaft kann sich dennoch nicht vor der Wahrheit verstecken, dass alleine durch das Nutzen einer bestimmten Metapher für neue wissenschaftliche Vorgänge oder Strukturen deren Urheber automatisch den Blick in Richtung der eigenen Ausgangshypothese fokussiert, welche der Anlass zu der Entdeckung war. Das ist gar nicht vermeidbar, jedoch wird uns hoffentlich alleine ein stärkeres Bewusstmachen der Bedeutung der wichtigen Rolle der Metaphern bei unserer Arbeit helfen, über deren Einschränkungen bewusst hinaussehen zu können – sowohl wenn wir Metaphern für unsere Forschungsergebnisse neu kreieren, als auch um sie bei der Rezeption der Arbeit anderer besser kreativ transzendieren zu können.

Stefan Heuser: Provozieren denn bestimmte Gegenstände Deiner Forschung die Bildung von Metaphern – und wenn ja, wie bzw. womit?

Stefan Dübel: Hierzu gibt es sicher viel Literatur aus dem nicht-naturwissenschaftlichen Bereich, der auch auf diesen Spezialfall anwendbar ist – denn ein Forscher schöpft neue Metaphern ja auch nur aus der Sprache seiner Lebenswirklichkeit. So werden Kriegs- und Polizei-Metaphern beim Erklären des Immunsystems angewendet, Maschinenanalogien für unseren Bewegungsapparat oder Computeranalogien für das Verstehen unserer Hirnfunktionen. Mir kommen dagegen keine Beispiele in den Sinn, bei dem Gegenstände aus unserer Forschung die Bildung von Metaphern direkt inspiriert haben. Ich vermute, wir vermeiden sie unbewusst, da wir ahnen, dass sie keine allgemeine Verständlichkeit haben, weil sie dann oft bereits Forschenden geringfügig außerhalb unseres eigenen Spezialgebiets schon nicht mehr verständlich sein könnten.

Ein Sonderfall in den Naturwissenschaften sind vielleicht die in früherer Zeit viel populäreren Begriffe, die aus griechischen und lateinischen Silben und Stämmen zusammengesetzt wurden; das Beispiel *„Homo sapiens“* hatten wir ja bereits erwähnt. Dabei werden dann zur Zeit der Entdeckung besonders wichtig scheinende Faktoren oder Eigenschaften ausgewählt, um in der Metapher transportiert zu werden. Selbstgefällig gaben sich hier sich die Forscher den Namen „verständiger, vernünftiger, kluger, weiser, einsichtsvoller Mensch“ in Latein. Heute ist Englisch die Wissenschaftssprache, und englische Metaphern dominieren. Ein Beispiel, wie der Fortschritt der Forschung einmal vergebene Metaphern irreführend macht, ist TNFα, der *„Tumor necrosis factor (alpha)“*. Anfangs gab es mehrere Namen für TNF, einige Forscher nannten ihn Kachektin (engl. *cachectin*), abgeleitet aus dem medizinischen Begriff *„cachexia“* für einen schlechten allgemeinen Gesundheitszustand – ein erstmal wenig aussagekräftiger Name, der den geringen Verständnisstand der damaligen Zeit widerspiegelt. Aber auch der heute dominante Begriff *tumor necrosis factor* beschreibt nur einen sehr kleinen Teil der Funktionalität dieses zentralen Schalters in der Regulation der Immunantwort, und dies ungenau. Denn TNF kann, wie wir heute wissen, Tumore gar nicht selbst angreifen und töten, wie es der Name suggeriert. Heute wissen wir, dass er einer von mehreren wichtigen Signalstoffen ist, der die Reaktion der Immunzellen gegen Tumore verstärkt, damit diese dann Tumore abtöten können. Heute nutzt man Medikamente, welche TNF neutralisieren können, wie zum Beispiel den gentechnologisch hergestellten Antikörper Adalimumab, sehr erfolgreich zur Behandlung von weit verbreiteten Autoimmunerkrankungen wie Rheuma.

Stefan Heuser: Gibt es in der Biotechnologie oder allgemein in der Biologie Metaphern, die eine bestimmte Art des Umgangs mit dem, was sie bezeichnen, nahelegen?

Stefan Dübel: Vielleicht dazu ein Beispiel aus meiner Doktorarbeit: ich beschäftigte mich mit der Funktion eines kleinen Eiweiss-Bruchstücks (eines „Peptids“) bei der Ausbildung der Körperformen des Süßwasser-Polyps *Hydra*. Meine Doktormutter hatte die Hypothese aufgestellt, dass dieses Peptid die Ausbildung des Kopfes mit dem Mund und den Tentakeln stimuliert, und es deshalb „Kopfaktivator“ genannt. Natürlich suchte das ganze Labor mit Experimenten im Bereich der Ausbildung von Zellen im Bereich von Mund und Tentakeln nach der Wirkung des Peptids. Mir gelang es nicht, eine entsprechende Wirkung auf die von mir untersuchten Epithelgewebe nachzuweisen, aber ich investierte mehr als ein Jahr in die erfolglose Suche – sicher auch getrieben von der suggestiven Macht des Begriffes. Eine skurrile Anekdote war die Lizenzanfrage eines Shampoo-Herstellers, ob sie den „Kopfaktivator“ für ihre Produkte verwenden dürften – nicht etwa, weil sie glaubten, dass das Peptid auch beim Menschen den Haarwuchs tatsächlich fördern würde, sondern nur weil sie den Namen passend fanden und dann auf wissenschaftliche Studien hinweisen konnten.

Hans Ulrich: Man kann fragen, ob nicht jede Metapher eben per se einen bestimmten Umgang – ihre Funktion – nahelegt, der auch nahegelegt bleibt, wenn die Metapher und die damit angezeigte Funktion nicht übereinstimmen, weil neue Erkenntnisse dazukommen oder die Metapher nicht gezielt auf die Funktion hin gewählt worden ist. So ist die Metapher „genetischer Code“ gewählt worden, um eine Funktion wie „Codierung“ zu markieren, die per se nahelegt, ihn so zu „entziffern“ (auf eine andere Schrift umzuschreiben), dass man selbst entsprechende Vorgänge codieren kann.

Stefan Heuser: Der „genetische Code“ besteht sogar aus zwei Metaphern, insofern mit „genetisch“ die „Genese“, also das spezifische, mit einer bestimmten Zeit des Werdens versehene Entstehen jenes informationellen Systems von Regeln (des „Codes“) bezeichnet wird. Mit Blick auf die von der Code-Metapher nahegelegte Um- oder Neu-Codierung wäre jedenfalls der Faktor „Zeit“ im Blick zu behalten. Der Zeitraffer durch manuelle, nicht „genetische“, sondern „technische“ Veränderungen scheint doch einer der Gründe für das öffentliche Unbehagen gegenüber gentechnischen Interventionen zu sein. So stellt sich neben der Frage, welche Funktion Metaphern haben und welche sie anzeigen, auch die Frage, welchen Beitrag Metaphern in der Wissenschaftskommunikation zur öffentlichen Akzeptanz von biotechnologischer Forschung leisten?

Stefan Dübel: Einen erheblichen, da jede Metapher nicht nur aufgrund ihres eigentlichen verbalen Informationsgehaltes aufgenommen wird, sondern auch stets aufgrund ihres stets unvermeidbaren assoziativen Wirkmechanismus Emotionen auslöst. Diese können und werden bei unterschiedlichen Menschen natürlich unterschiedlich ausfallen, und dieser Anteil der Metapher ist es, dem die Wissenschaftler große Aufmerksamkeit widmen sollten, bevor sie eine neue Wortschöpfung in die Freiheit der Welt entlassen. Wählen wir hier weise, dann kann die Metapher Menschen inspirieren und für die Wissenschaft interessieren. Aber die Entwicklung des Sprachgebrauchs ist auch immer etwas chaotisch, sodass langfristige Vorhersagen über die Bedeutung schwierig sind. Ein Beispiel: die Benennung der Boeing B29, die 1945 die erste Atombombe auf Hiroshima abwarf, mit dem Namen „Enola Gay“ störte damals niemanden, es war einfach ein Frauenname und „gay“ bedeutete „heiter und fröhlich“. Bereits 1980 wurde ein von diesem Flugzeug inspiriertes Anti-Kriegslied der britischen Band Orchestral Manoeuvres in the Dark (OMD) mit dem Titel „Enola Gay“ kritisiert und seine Rundfunkausstrahlung blockiert, da der Name (völlig falsch) als Anspielung auf Homosexualität verstanden wurde. Heute haben wir eine noch sehr viel schnellere Veränderung der Umgangssprache durch die neuen Medien, oft können nur wenige Jahre auseinander liegende Jahrgänge von Jugendlichen gegenseitig ihre Chats nicht mehr verstehen. Das Problem der richtigen Wortwahl wird dadurch nicht erleichtert. Dies ist aber natürlich nicht nur ein Problem spezifisch für die Naturwissenschaft.

Stefan Heuser: Gibt es in der Biotechnologie Metaphern, die intrinsisch mit Bewertungen verbunden sind bzw. bestimmte Bewertungen nahelegen?

Stefan Dübel: Ich würde sagen, jede, wobei diese aber persönlich unterschiedlich ausfallen, denn sie schöpfen sich ja stets assoziativ aus den Erfahrungen in dem Moment, in dem jemand diese Metapher liest oder hört. Da wir aktuell in einer Gesellschaft leben, in der sich viele Menschen durch immer weitergehenden Verzicht auf qualitätskontrollierte Informationsquellen immer mehr in verschiedenen Informationsblasen isolieren, wird in Zukunft die assoziative Rezeption von Metaphern immer divergenter ausfallen. Dies macht die bewusste Gestaltung durch Wissenschaftler nicht einfacher.

Stefan Heuser: Kannst Du uns bitte auch Beispiele für Metaphern nennen, die sich als dysfunktional in der Forschung erwiesen haben?

Stefan Dübel: Das Beispiel TNF (s. o.) zeigt, dass die Wissenschaftler selbst mit schlechtsitzenden Analogien und Namenswahlen oft recht gut umgehen können. Das wird dann oft noch vereinfacht durch die Nutzung einer Abkürzung, hier: TNF, die erstmal nichts mehr aus sich heraus suggeriert.

Es gibt aber auch andere Fälle. Ein aktuelles Beispiel einer sich nach vielen Jahrzehnten problemloser Nutzung aufgrund neuer Erkenntnisse dysfunktional entwickelnden Metapher im Bereich meiner eigenen Forschung ist der Begriff „Monoklonale Antikörper“. Hier wurden die Effekte auf die Perzeption neuer Erkenntnisse durch eine bestehende Metapher offensichtlich. Der Wortteil „Klon“ bezeichnet biologisch eine Vielzahl identischer Zellen, wie sie für die Produktion ausreichender Mengen eines Antikörpers notwendig sind, welche aber alle aus einer einzigen Ursprungszelle stammen. Im Immunsystem erzeugt jede einzelne antikörperproduzierende Zelle (B-Zelle) jeweils nur einen einzigen, ganz bestimmten Antikörper. Die Vielfalt von Milliarden unterschiedlicher Antikörper, welche wir benötigen, um die vielen verschiedenen „Eindringlinge“ zu bekämpfen, wird in unserem Körper dadurch erzeugt, dass es ebenso viele unterschiedliche Klone von B-Zellen in unserem Körper gibt.

„Monoklonale Antikörper“ werden nun im Reagenzglas künstlich durch Fusion einer B-Zelle mit einer Krebszelle erzeugt, wobei letztere der antikörperproduzierenden B-Zelle das unlimitierte Wachstum eines Tumors „beibringt“. Durch diesen Trick können die entstehenden Zellen unbegrenzt wachsen und somit ausreichende Mengen des gewünschten Antikörpers produzieren. Die aus solchen „Hybridom-Zellen“ gewonnenen monoklonalen Antikörper wurden nach ihrer Nobelpreis-gewürdigten Entdeckung 1975 schnell zum der „Gold-Standard“ für beste Qualität beim Nachweis einzelner Eiweiße in unzähligen Experimenten. Der Grund dafür war, dass bis dahin als Quelle von Antikörpern ausschließlich Blutseren zur Verfügung standen, die aber immer „polyklonal“ waren, also immer ein Gemisch von verschiedenen Antikörpern enthielten, welche aus vielen verschiedenen B-Zellen stammen. Diese polyklonalen Antikörper-Gemische waren aufgrund ihrer Herstellung aus Blut niemals genau in ihrer Zusammensetzung bekannt. Es war zwar nachweisbar, dass sie eine gewisse Menge von Antikörpern mit der gewünschten Reaktivität enthielten – sonst wären sie ja als Nachweisreagens für Experimente nutzlos – jedoch enthielten sie immer noch viele andere unbekannte Antikörper, dessen Spezifität anders und unbekannt war. Schließlich stammten sie aus dem Blut eines Tieres, welches zwar mit dem gewünschten Antigen geimpft wurde und deshalb dagegen durchaus die gewünschten spezifischen Antikörper erzeugte, aber zusätzlich dazu auch noch jede Menge andere Antikörper enthielt (geschätzter Anteil 95–99%) welche mit anderen „Eindringlingen“ reagierten, welche das Spendertier sonst noch infiziert hatte. Dies führte verständlicherweise oft zu Problemen mit falsch-positiven Resultaten, Nebenreaktionen oder starker Hintergrundfärbung. Bei den monoklonalen Antikörpern dagegen verringerte die Herkunft aus einer einzigen B-Zelle, welche ja bekanntermaßen in unserem Körper nur einen einzigen Antikörper produzieren kann, das Risiko, falsche Resultate zu erhalten, erheblich. Die Metapher „monoklonal“ suggerierte also den Forschern, dass darin im Gegensatz zu den polyklonalen Antikörpern stets nur ein Antikörper mit einer einzigen Spezifität („monospezifisch“) enthalten war, dass monoklonale Antikörper stets nur ein einziges Eiweiss erkannten. Das sollte sich aber als falsch erweisen.

In den frühen 1990er Jahren begann ich, die Gene aus solchen monoklonalen Hybridom-Zellen zu isolieren und auszulesen (d. h. ihre DNA zu „sequenzieren“), um sie dann biotechnologisch im Reagenzglas herstellen zu können. Dabei fand ich mehrfach in einem einzigen monoklonalen Hybridom-Zell-Klon unterschiedliche abgelesene Antikörper-Gene, welche somit auch die Produktion mehrerer verschiedener Antiköper ermöglichten. Eine einzige Hybridom-Zelle konnte offensichtlich mehrere unterschiedliche Antikörper herstellen, obwohl dieser Klon aus einer einzigen B-Zelle hervorgegangen war. Wie war dies zu erklären? Zum einen hatten die krebsartig wuchernden Hybridom-Zellen durch die für ihre Herstellung nötige Fusion einer antikörperproduzierenden B-Zelle und einer Tumorzelle sowieso schon vier verschiedene Genkopien für Antikörper zur Auswahl, denn jeder der beiden Zellen brachte ja jeweils ein mütterliches und ein väterliches Antikörper-Gen mit. Zudem fand man vielfach eine unnatürliche Chromosomenzahl, oft viel mehr als in den natürlichen B-Zellen. Ganz offensichtlich blieben bei der Zellfusion zur Herstellung der Hybridomzellen die jeweiligen Eigenschaften der zwei Ausgangszellen nicht komplett erhalten. Wir vermuten, dass die künstlichen Wachstumsbedingungen im Reagenzglas ohne jegliche Kontrolle durch das restliche Immunsystem dazu führt, dass in der künstlichen Umgebung oftmals mehr als eines dieser Gene „angeschaltet" und damit abgelesen und so für die Antikörperherstellung genutzt wird. Dazu kam noch, dass Zellen während der massenhaften Vermehrung zur Herstellung der Antikörper auch mutieren und damit zusätzliche Versionen der Gene erzeugen. Dadurch kann auch ein einziger Zell-Klon mehrere unterschiedliche Antikörper produzieren, und diese können wie bei den polyklonalen Antikörpern dann auch unerwünschte Nebenreaktionen erzeugen. Diese Beobachtung versuchte ich viele Jahre erfolglos zu publizieren – niemand wollte wahrnehmen, dass „monoklonal" eben nicht immer mit „monospezifisch" gleichzusetzen war. Erst eine große multizentrische Studie, welche 185 verschiedene Hybridom-Zelllinien zur Produktion von monoklonalen Antikörpern aus 7 verschiedenen Labors in fünf verschiedenen Ländern auf Ebene der Gensequenzen analysierte, konnte die Gutachter überzeugen [5]. Die Studie wurde danach aber dennoch trotz der großen Zahl dokumentierter Beispiele, dass „monoklonal" eben nicht immer auch „monospezifisch" bedeutete, in der Folge stark angegriffen und kritisiert, besonders von Herstellern und Nutzern monoklonaler Antikörper, welche wohl ihre eigene Forschung diskreditiert sahen. Ich halte es für sehr wahrscheinlich, dass hier die für Jahrzehnte als Qualitätslabel etablierte Metapher „monoklonal" die Perzeption neuer Erkenntnisse, welche ihre implizite Interpretation als „monospezifisch" relativierte, behinderte.

Stefan Heuser: Das ist ein sehr eindrückliches Beispiel dafür, dass und inwiefern Metaphern eine bestimmte Funktion ihres Objektbereichs indizieren – und dabei die Wahrnehmung auch fehlleiten können. Die Metapher „monoklonal" hat offenbar ihre Funktionsbestimmung aus dem Kontext des Immunsystems in den Bereich der im Labor erfolgten Fusion von B-Zellen und Tumorzellen zu Hybridom-Zellen transferiert. Das ist an sich schon ein interessanter Vorgang. Als Laie wäre ich bei der Verschmelzung von B-Zellen mit Tumorzellen vermutlich aus ganz anderen Gründen als der Biotechnologe misstrauisch geworden, und zwar wegen der bedrohlich klingenden Metapher „Tumor". Auch die Metapher „Klon" oder „Klonierung" kann beim Laien ein aus Science-Fiction-Filmen und dystopischen Szenarien genährtes Unbehagen auslösen, während ein „Klon" in der Biologie eine ganz neutrale Bezeichnung ist. Das hat in der Wissenschaftskommunikation gegenüber Laien gewiss einiges an Miss- und Unverständnis, auch an Ängsten hervorgerufen. Was sind denn für Dich als Biotechnologe vorrangige Beispiele für dysfunktionale Metaphern in der öffentlichen Wissenschaftskommunikation?

Stefan Dübel: In der öffentlichen Wissenschaftskommunikation ist offensichtlich der Begriff „Gentechnologie" dysfunktional. Der Begriff ist außerhalb der Fachwelt zum

Angstwort worden, obwohl er natürlich rein deskriptiv gemeint war. Vielleicht liegt es schon ein klein wenig in der Begriffswahl begründet – schließlich suggeriert „Technik“ eine handwerkliche Zugänglichkeit der uns definierenden Erbsubstanz, und damit einen Weg, um im wörtlichen Sinne im Innersten unserer biologischen Wesenheit eine Zange oder einen Schweißbrenner anzusetzen. Skurrilerweise wird aber gerade dieser Aspekt – also die heute bereits konkret existierenden Möglichkeiten der Veränderung der Spezies Mensch im biologischen Sinne, und damit die weit offenstehende Tür zur gesteuerten physischen „Verbesserung“ von Menschen – in der öffentlichen Diskussion um Gentechnologie fast völlig ignoriert, obwohl sie die derzeit meiner Ansicht nach die eigentliche Gefahr dieser Technologie ausmacht. Dagegen werden in den sozialen Medien postulierte Gefahren in anderen Bereichen, z. B. bei Lebensmitteln, heiß diskutiert und immer wieder ohne Belege kolportiert, welche mittlerweile durch jahrzehntelange Forschungen und Erfahrungen ausgeschlossen wurden – schließlich essen Milliarden von Menschen seit mehr als 25 Jahren gentechnisch veränderte Lebensmittel, ohne dass ein einziger dadurch erkrankt oder verstorben ist. Dieses Missverhältnis ist für Fachleute sehr schwer nachzuvollziehen, hat meiner Meinung aber nichts direkt mit der Wortwahl zu tun, sondern mit anderen komplexen Vorgängen, vom Versagen des kritischen Journalismus, fragwürdige Marktstrategien von Unternehmen bis zu finanziellen Interessen von Interessensverbänden, die an geschürten Ängsten gut verdienen. Aber das ist ein Thema für einen anderen Tag, denn es füllt leicht ein eigenes Buch.

Stefan Heuser: Der Metaphernwechsel von der „Vererbung“ zur „Genetik“, wie ihn William Bateson vorgenommen hat, ist folgenreich. Mit dem altgriechischen Wort γεννάω (zeugen, hervorbringen) ruft diese Metapher eine ganze Welt unterschiedlicher Referenzen hervor, nicht zuletzt biblische und theologische Referenzen. Da ist zum Beispiel das Buch vom Ursprung „Genesis“ mit seiner Urgeschichte (Gen 1–11) oder die Theologie der „Genealogien“ bzw. „Geschlechterfolgen („Toledot“, hebr.: תּוֹלְדֹת), auch die Theologie des Stammbaums Jesu (Mt 1,1–18; Lk 3,23–28). Aber das wäre auch ein Thema für einen anderen Tag. Können denn aus Deiner Sicht Metaphern bei der Identifikation neuer Probleme, Themen und (gemeinsamer) Ziele der Forschung helfen? Wenn ja, wie?

Stefan Dübel: Sie haben eine Schlüsselfunktion, denn sie ermöglichen überhaupt erst die Kommunikation über ansonsten praktisch nicht breit vermittelbare Forschungsinhalte und -ergebnisse. Ohne Metaphern – auch wenn wir wissen, dass sie nie „die Wirklichkeit“ exakt beschreiben, können wir in vielen Fächern neue Ergebnisse nicht verständlich transportieren. In der Physik und einigen anderen Fächern hilft hier sicherlich die Mathematik, aber diese „Sprache“ ist dem größten Teil der Menschen nicht ausreichend geläufig, um die hochkomplexen Fortschritte moderner Forschungen zu verstehen. Ein Beispiel für die Probleme mit umgangssprachlichen Metaphern in der Physik ist die „Verschränkung“ von Teilchen bei Quantenvorgängen: als Laie deutet man den Begriff automatisch so, dass „verschränkte“ Teilchen auch über riesige Entfernungen noch irgendwie in Verbindung stehen oder mit einander kommunizieren, was aber nicht der Fall ist. Wenn Sie ein Brötchen in eine obere und untere Hälfte schneiden, diese dann in zwei undurchsichtige Schachteln verpacken und in verschiedene Regionen der Welt verschicken, weiß derjenige, der eines der Pakete aufmacht, im gleichen Moment auch, welche Hälfte in dem anderen Paket weit entfernt ist, es kann nämlich nur die andere sein – dazu muss keine Information mit Überlichtgeschwindigkeit übermittelt werden. Hier scheint die gewählte Metapher eindeutig eher Verwirrung verbreitet zu haben. In diesem speziellen Fall ist diese Verwirrung aber auch meist bei Fachfremden entstanden, während die Physiker durch das Verständnis der dahinterstehenden mathematischen Modelle kaum betroffen sind. In der Biologie hilft dagegen die Mathematik in den meisten Fällen aber nicht, die Gegenstände unserer Forschung zu veranschaulichen. Dabei hilft eher vernetztes, ganzheitliches Denken, während die Mathematik in der Biologie meist nur Werkzeug zur Quantifizierung, Modellierung, oder statistischer Einschätzung von Signifikanzen ist. Dadurch spielen Metaphern aus umgangssprachlichen Begriffen in den Biowissenschaften wahrscheinlich eine wesentlich wichtigere Rolle als in der Physik.

Gut gewählte Metaphern können Andere inspirieren und auf neue Gedanken bringen. Damit spielen hier Metaphern eine zentrale Rolle als Auslöser der oben schon beschriebenen irrationalen und kreativen Findung neuer Hypothesen für wirkliche wissenschaftliche Fortschritte. Da Assoziationen eine der Quellen für Kreativität sind, und Metaphern bei verschiedenen Menschen unterschiedliche Assoziationen auslösen, ist ihre inspirierende Rolle beim Fortschritt der naturwissenschaftlichen Forschung hoch wahrscheinlich.

Hans Ulrich: Rückblickend kann man genau dies feststellen, dass Metaphern geholfen haben, neue Ziele und Probleme der Forschung zu identifizieren. Das Beispiel „genetischer Code" ist dafür besonders evident. Metaphern erfassen etwas, das als „gegeben" erscheint (etwa durch das Mikroskop sichtbar gemacht), das dann durch die Metapher auf weitere Erforschung hin festgehalten und – wenn die Metapher entsprechend passt – in bestimmter Weise ausgerichtet wird. Die Diskussion über „Transposons", die zur Zeit im Gang ist, hat wohl eine entsprechende Bedeutung. Für manche anderen Beobachtungen fehlen dann womöglich entsprechende Metaphern – wie für die Beobachtung der noch nicht geklärten so weitgehenden Übereinstimmung von *„patches"* zwischen den verschiedensten Organismen, oder auch andere Beobachtungen. Die Gewinnung einer entsprechenden Metapher könnte die Forschung in bestimmter Weise leiten. Stefan Dübel verweist auf diesen Sachverhalt („you never walk alone"). Was wäre eine dies aufnehmende und die Forschung provozierende Metapher?

Stefan Heuser: Mir fällt nur eine Metapher ein, die den Diskurs in der Bioethik stark geprägt hat, aber mittlerweile nur noch wenig Erschließungskraft besitzt: Donna Haraway hat zur Beschreibung des grundlegenden ökologischen Eingebundenseins des Menschen die Metapher „Entanglement" vorgeschlagen. Der Bedeutungsgehalt dieser

Metapher hat sich allerdings in den Geisteswissenschaften mittlerweile ins Allgemeine verflüchtigt. Die Aussage, dass alles mit allem verbunden ist, verdeckt eher die konkreten Zusammenhänge, wie sie uns mit übereinstimmenden DNA-Sequenzen bei verschiedenen Organismen möglicherweise vor Augen treten. Und die aus der Informatik übernommene Metapher „Patch“ (Flicken) lenkt die Phantasie in Richtung von Softwareupdates, die der Verringerung von Sicherheitsrisiken bzw. der Optimierung von Programmen dienen. Gut möglich, dass der Quellbereich dieser Metapher den Blick auf das zu beschreibende Phänomen und die Richtung, in die zu forschen wäre, vorgibt. Vielleicht wäre es nicht falsch, wenn die noch zu suchende Metapher, die das Phänomen ähnlicher DNA-Sequenzen bei verschiedenen Lebewesen erfassen soll, einen starken Lebensweltbezug aufweist. Vor dem Hintergrund von Edmund Husserls Diagnose aus seiner „Krisis“-Schrift [6] könnten sich vor allem Metaphern, die in der menschlichen Lebenswelt verwurzelt sind (z. B. Lesen, Schreiben, Verstehen), gut zur Identifizierung von Forschungsthemen und -zielen der Lebenswissenschaften eignen – auch mit Blick auf eine mögliche gemeinsame Forschung mit den Geisteswissenschaften. Husserl meinte, dass sich die Wissenschaften von der Lebenswelt der Menschen zu weit herausgelöst haben, so dass sie nicht mehr hinreichend mit den Erfahrungen, Sinn- und Lebensfragen der Menschen verbunden sind. Zugleich geht er aber auch davon aus, dass die Wissenschaften und das Wissen, das sie hervorbringen, weiterhin in lebensweltlichen Praktiken und Sinnzusammenhängen verwurzelt sind. Die Entzifferung des Genoms beispielsweise ist noch immer durch alle technischen Prozeduren hindurch mit der Praxis des Lesens und ihrer Metaphorik verbunden (z. B. die Gene als „Wörter“ einer „Sprache des Lebens“; das Genom als Text, die Nukleinbasen als „Buchstaben“) – bis dahin, dass „Eingriffe“ in das Genom sehr erfolgreich als textliche Veränderungen konzipiert werden. Die Vermutung ist, dass wir uns aus dem Horizont dieser Metaphorik nicht so leicht lösen können, weil sie in unserer Lebenswelt wurzelt und so den unhinterfragten Horizont von Selbstverständlichkeiten darstellt. Neue Themen, Theorien und Methoden der Forschung würden dann darauf beruhen, dass unser Horizont gewissermaßen durch neue Metaphern aufgebrochen wird. Diese müssten aber vermutlich selbst wiederum aus der Lebenswelt stammen.

Hans Ulrich: „Lebenswelt“ meint hier „menschliche“ Lebenswelt – und das impliziert die Frage, für wen diese „lesbare Welt“, für wen dieses Welt-Buch zum Lesen – und Verstehen – geschrieben ist. Hier kann der Gedanke verfolgt werden, dass das „Buch der Natur“ an den Menschen gerichtet ist, damit er es liest – und er dazu auch bestimmt ist (in der Logik von Heideggers Verständnis des menschlichen „Daseins“). Die Metapher „Buch der Natur“ erscheint in dieser Logik aber nicht ohne Anleihe an das „Buch der Bücher“ (der Bibel), das per se an den Menschen gerichtet ist, der darin lesen soll oder auch gerne darin liest – studiert, „Tag und Nacht“, wie es in Psalm 1 heißt. Wer fragt „Wozu Mensch überhaupt?“ (Nietzsche), kann darin – vielleicht einzig darin – eine Antwort finden, die nicht ins Leere läuft, weil die beiden Bücher (noch immer) eben da sind und darauf „warten“ gelesen zu werden. Damit ist auch eine mögliche Antwort auf eine weitere Frage gegeben: „Gibt es Metaphern, die ein tieferes Verständnis der *conditio humana*" eröffnen? Dies ist auch im Blick auf Blumenbergs „Lesbarkeit der Welt" festzuhalten (siehe dazu u.), sofern Blumenbergs ganzes Werk in die Logik der „Selbstbehauptung" (im Unterschied zu „Selbstbestimmung") einmündet.

Stefan Dübel: Der lateinische Artname „*Homo sapiens*" für unsere Spezies, bedeutet, wie schon erwähnt, „verständiger, vernünftiger, kluger, weiser, einsichtsvoller Mensch". Schaut man sich aktuell die Welt an, scheint dieser Name oft wie blanker Hohn. Aber wir machen ja hier kein Menschheits-*bashing* – positiv ist zu notieren, dass jeder von uns viele verständige, vernünftige und weise Menschen kennt. Und solange dies so ist, ist unsere Spezies nicht verloren.

Stefan Heuser: Blumenbergs Metapher von der „Lesbarkeit der Welt" ist sozusagen die „Geschäftsgrundlage" der Naturwissenschaft, die versucht, die „Welt" zu „lesen" und damit rechnet, dass sie auch lesbar ist; lesbar von uns und für uns zugänglich. Blumenberg geht davon aus, dass die Wissenschaft der Grundidee folgt, dass die Welt („Kosmos") für den „Logos" (Vernunft, Denken, Sprachfähigkeit, Wort) lesbar ist; allerdings entzieht sich der Kosmos aufgrund seiner Komplexität der vollständigen Begreifbarkeit durch den Logos. Entsprechend ist die Technik, mit der wir die Welt erforschen, mit Metaphern verbunden, z. B. auch die Labortechnologien. Mit technischer Hilfe und mithilfe von Metaphern macht die Biotechnologie etwas sichtbar bzw. lesbar, was sonst für uns unsichtbar ist, d. h. sie folgt irgendwie noch immer der Vorstellung, dass die Welt (Kosmos) lesbar ist und sich uns zu lesen gibt. Diese Leitvorstellung ist in der Metapher der Lesbarkeit der Welt ausgedrückt. Ich denke da an Stefan Dübels Hinweis auf die „klaren Flüssigkeiten" im Labor, deren Inhalte wir nicht direkt, sondern nur im Medium von Technik „sehen" können. Das Sichtbarmachen können Metaphern leisten, sie sind Techniken des Erkennens und Verstehens, und sie sind intrinsisch mit Technologien verbunden, die wir zum „Lesen" der Welt entwickeln und verwenden. Das ist gar nicht so banal, wie es sich auf den ersten Blick vielleicht anhört, denn offenbar folgen wir in der Wissenschaft noch immer einer ganz alten Idee: dass die Welt (Kosmos = eine absolute Metapher) von uns im Medium von Sprache (Logos) und Technik wirklich wie ein Text gelesen und erkannt werden kann, weil sie logische, informative Strukturen (auch so eine Metapher: „Information") enthält und sich von uns erkennen lässt. Insofern ist es nicht einerlei, welche Metaphern wir verwenden, weil wir auch metaphorisch danebenliegen können. Und zugleich führt die Metapher von der „Lesbarkeit" der „Welt" (wie Metaphern generell) auch ganz viel „Unbegriffliches" mit, das sich dem begrifflichen Erfassen entzieht, aber die Suche nach Erkenntnis immer neu triggert. Die Kritik an der Vorstellung, dass der Kosmos Strukturen und Ordnungen aufweist, die dem Logos zugänglich und nicht etwa durch das menschliche Sinn- und Herrschaftsbedürfnis in die Welt hineingelesen sind, findet sich bei vielen Denkerinnen und Denkern, z. B. bei Nietzsche. Sie zieht sich auch durch unser Gespräch, genauso wie gleichzeitig das Erstaunen über die Lesbarkeit der unermesslich komplexen Welt, die sich der Molekularbiologie auftut.

Stefan Dübel: Die ganze Naturwissenschaft basiert doch auf der Idee, dass es nicht nur Chaos und Zufall gibt, sondern unter allem, was wir erfahren, Strukturen liegen, die die Welt ordnen. Um diese Strukturen zu erkennen braucht es keinen Philosophen oder Biologen, das kann auch ein Hund, Vogel oder Tintenfisch. Die Versuche Pawlows zum später nach ihm benannten Reflex zeigten uns, wie diese Art des Lernens neuer Erfahrungen ohne jeden gezielten Willensakt, quasi automatisch funktioniert – das Pawlow'sche Lernen durch Konditionierung ist im Prinzip eine unbewusst ablaufende Korrelationsanalyse, wobei letztere ja auch eine der Kernmethoden der naturwissenschaftlichen Hypothesenbildung darstellt. Im Hirn von Pawlows Hunden entstand so von selbst die Hypothese: „Wenn's klingelt, gibt es gleich etwas zu futtern". Der biologische Nutzen, in Form eines Überlebensvorteils, besteht darin, dass dieses zwangsweise in das Nervensystem eingebaute, ständige „Lesen der Welt" für die Spezies eine bessere Vorhersehbarkeit zukünftiger Ereignisse und damit eine bessere Reaktion darauf ermöglicht. Wir können also gar nicht anders, als die Welt laufend zu lesen – zweifellos eine der wertvollsten während der Evolution entwickelten Fähigkeit größerer Gehirne.

Als Naturwissenschaftler versuchen wir dementsprechend, Regeln zu formulieren, die nicht nur das Erfahrene beschreiben, sondern erst dann validiert sind, wenn diese Erfahrungen auch in Zukunft immer diesen Regeln folgen. Die Wahl der Hypothese und der sie beschreibenden Metapher stammt dabei naturgemäß aus unserer kulturellen Einbettung und dem Wissensstand der Zeit. Ein Beispiel: Die Wikinger stellten sich vor, dass schwere Gewitter entstehen, wenn Thor (oder Donar) wütend ist. Dann ging man besser nicht vor die Tür, denn man konnte von den Blitzen, den Thor in seiner Rage auf den Boden schleuderte, erschlagen werden und sterben. Dies war erst einmal ausreichend, um Leben zu retten, und erfüllte so die Kriterien einer hilfreichen wissenschaftlichen Hypothese, denn sie sagte den Effekt des möglichen Todes durch Blitzschlag korrekt auch für die Zukunft voraus. Heute haben wir mehr Daten zur Verfügung und daraus eine andere Hypothese (die Elektrizitätslehre) abgeleitet, welche den gleichen Zweck für unsere Spezies erfüllt: Menschen davor abzuhalten, sich bei Gewitter in Gefahr zu begeben. Es ist deshalb sehr naheliegend, dass der Drang, die Welt zu lesen, eine entscheidende Rolle bei der Entstehung der Spezies *Homo sapiens* spielte – denn Neugier ist eine der stärksten Triebkräfte beim evolutionären Erfolg in der Evolution mehrzelliger Lebewesen mit umfangreicheren Nervensystemen.

Man merkt am vorigen Satz deutlich meinen Eiertanz um die Wahl der korrekten Begriffe an – ich versuchte dabei, explizit die Verwendung der verbreiteten Metapher „höhere Lebewesen" zu vermeiden. Warum dies? Weil die Wertung „höher" extrem stark von der Definition der Kriterien abhängt. Warum sollten Säugetiere „höher" stehen als zum Beispiel Tardigraden (Bärtierchen), die fast unzerstörbar sind, Bäume, die mehr als 1500 Jahre alt sind oder Hydrozoen, die bei ausreichender Futterversorgung sogar unsterblich sind? Geht man nach Zahlen oder den eroberten Lebensräumen, sind Insekten viel erfolgreicher als wir. Die absolute Spitze bei den zahlenmäßig häufigsten Lebewesen halten mit uneinholbarem Vorsprung die Mikroorganismen. Und von diesen gehören wieder zahlreiche zu unserer eigenen Person, denn jeder von uns läuft mit wesentlich mehr Zellen herum, die keine menschliche Erbsubstanz enthalten, als solchen mit den Genen unserer Eltern. In diesen Mikroorganismen wiederum sitzen Bakteriophagen, also Viren, welche speziell bestimmte Bakterien befallen können. Davon gibt es üblicherweise mehrere pro Bakterienspezies, Phagen sind also die diversesten Lebensformen in unserem Körper – und auch in der ganzen Welt, denn Phagen gibt es überall, wo Bakterien leben. Auch in unserem eigenen Genom findet man eingebaute Viren, in den verschiedensten Stadien der Integration: einige haben offensichtlich in der Evolution dazu beigetragen, unseren Ahnen biochemisch neue Fähigkeiten zu geben und sind nun fester Bestandteil unseres vererbbaren Genoms, andere sind tatsächlich noch Pathogene, z. B. die ubiquitären Herpesviren, die im Großteil der Bevölkerung vorkommen. Aber wie so oft in der Biologie: alle Übergänge dazwischen werden auch beobachtet. Offensichtlich sind Viren und Reste von Virusgenomen in unserer eigenen DNA wichtige Faktoren, die die Veränderung unserer Erbsubstanz bei der Anpassung an neue Lebensbedingungen sprunghaft beschleunigen können, und damit zum Erfolg unserer Spezies bei der Evolution beitragen. Dafür Feind- oder Freund-Metaphern zu finden ist genauso schwierig, wie die Definition, ob Viren belebt sind oder nicht – schließlich haben Viren keinen Stoffwechsel, sondern müssen immer ein anderes Lebewesen zur Vermehrung nutzen, weshalb ist zumindest umgekehrt die Metapher „Computervirus“ schon recht passend ist. Zusammengefasst: *„You never walk alone“* lehren uns die Mikrobiologen. Der Mensch kann also auch als wandelndes Ökosystem begriffen werden. Hier warten viele noch nicht definierte Metaphern auf ihre Verwendung zur Vermittlung dieser komplexen Befunde.

Damit wird auch der Begriff „Mensch“ zu einer Metapher, die hinterfragt werden kann, denn im Gegensatz zur Einschätzung der meisten Menschen ist seine exakte physikalische Grenze heutzutage biologisch gar nicht mehr genau zu definieren. Zum gesunden Überleben brauchen wir sehr vielfältige bakterielle Bewohner unserer Haut, Schleimhäute und im Verdauungssystem. Ein Beispiel: Werden mütterliche Mikroben nicht durch natürliche Geburt im Durchgang durch den Geburtskanal rabiat auf das Neugeborene übertragen, entstehen ihm dadurch Nachteile bei der Entwicklung der Abwehrkräfte gegen Krankheiten – dies weiß man aus Vergleichen von Kindern, die natürlich oder per Kaiserschnitt geboren wurden. Was natürlich die Frage nach der physischen Definition der Grenzen der eigenen Person aufwirft – zählt man die unzähligen Bakterien, die wir zum Überleben brauchen, nun dazu? Ist das schon „die Umwelt“, auch wenn es tief in unserem Innern ist? Ohne sie würden wir kaum überleben. Aber auch hier ist nichts nur schwarz oder weiss: Auf der anderen Seite würden uns viele dieser „harmlosen“ Bakterien auch sofort auffressen, würden sie nicht durch vielfältige Vorgänge, natürlich auch mithilfe des Immunsystems, daran gehindert. Es ist ein Gleichgewicht, oder besser ausgedrückt, ein Fließgleichgewicht, und Krankheiten sind oft einfach eine Störung dieses Fließgleichgewichts.

Ein Beispiel: Bakterien der Spezies *Clostridioides difficile* im Darm produzieren Toxine, welche zu schweren Erkrankungen führen können. Normalerweise werden sie aber überwachsen von für uns harmlosen Bakterienspezies, meist als „Mitesser" („Kommensalen") bezeichnet, welche besser an unser Inneres angepasst sind und sich deshalb schneller vermehren. Nach Gabe bestimmter Antibiotika zur Behandlung anderer Krankheitserreger werden diese harmlosen Bakterien jedoch oft auch mit beseitigt. Dadurch hat nun *Clostridioides difficile* genügend Raum und Nahrung, um sich stark zu vermehren, was uns krank macht. Eine der derzeit untersuchten Methoden zur Behandlung besteht darin, den Betroffenen ein gesundes Mikrobiom mit den normalen Kommensalen zurück zu verpflanzen. Gar nicht harmlos wären die gleichen Kommensalen jedoch gegenüber dem oben erwähnten Stück Fleisch im Sommer, sie würden dieses in kurzer Zeit zerlegen. Dieses Beispiel illustriert, dass jede Metapher über die Rolle von bestimmten Bakterien – oder auch des Mikrobioms als Ganzen – schwierig passend zu finden ist – eine einfache funktionale Schubladen-Definition aufgrund ihrer Rolle für uns als Individuum ist kaum korrekt zu erfassen.

All dies zeigt, dass die Metapher Mensch zumindest bei der Beschreibung unseres Körpers als eine physische Entität am Rande auch hier etwas „ausfranst", und zwar sowohl räumlich in der atomaren Zusammensetzung wie zeitlich. Sind die oben beschriebenen kommensalen Bakterien noch als einzelne Lebewesen isolierbar und können im Reagenzglas unabhängig von uns wachsen, ist es bei den Viren anders. Eine interessante Frage bist, ob die in unser Genom integrierten (und damit gegebenenfalls auch vererbbaren) Viren zu unserer Spezies gehören und damit unserer Person, oder ob sie noch eine eigene Lebensform sind? Die Wahl von Metaphern in der Biologie ist durch die Ubiquität derart unscharfer Grenzen immer problematisch, und kann ihr deshalb auch niemals völlig gerecht werden. Dazu kommt der zeitliche Faktor. Heraklit hatte mit seinem πάντα ῥεῖ (Alles fliesst) schon eine wirklich gute Intuition, die hinter allem Leben liegende biochemischen Funktionen vorherzuahnen: die Fließgleichgewichte. Für Biologen ist es selbstverständlich, alles Lebendige als Fließgleichgewicht zu verstehen, in dem ständig Stoffaustausch und Umwandlung ablaufen, und durch das alle Atome im Verlauf unseres Lebens ausgetauscht werden – das Schiff des Theseus lässt grüßen. Wir blicken auf das sich vierdimensional stetig ändernde Netzwerk aus biochemischen Fließgleichgewichten, welche den Menschen bilden, und konnten dennoch schon das bisherige Wissen darüber, obwohl noch sehr vereinfacht und lückenhaft, immerhin bereits vielfältig nutzen. Es ermöglichte zum Beispiel die Überwindung zahlreicher früher tödlicher Erkrankungen durch gezielte Entwicklung von Medikamenten. Die Lesbarkeit der Welt zeigt sich auch hier als wertvoll für das Überleben der Spezies Mensch.

In direktem Zusammenhang mit der Metapher Mensch steht auch der biologische Begriff „Keimbahn", einer faszinierenden Metapher, die in ihrer Bedeutung desto schwerer zu fassen ist, je genauer man diese definieren möchte. Elemente der Keimbahn sind diejenigen Zellen eines mehrzelligen Organismus, aus denen die Nachkommen entstehen, also Samen und Eizellen, sowie die Zellen, aus denen sie gebildet werden. Bei einzelligen Organismen, die sich typischerweise durch Teilung wie Bakterien oder auch Knospung (z. B. Hefepilze) vermehren, ist „Keimbahn“ der gesamte Organismus, eine Unterscheidung in solches Gewebe, welches in Nachkommen fortbesteht, und solches, welches das nicht kann, ist hier unnötig. Bei ihnen wird aber am einfachsten deutlich, weshalb der Begriff „Keimbahn“ meist mit „Unsterblichkeit“ assoziiert wird, denn eine sich teilende Bakterienzelle „stirbt“ dabei ja nicht, sondern lebt in den Nachkommen direkt weiter. Die Sterblichkeit entwickelte sich in der Evolution wohl erst später, insbesondere bei Mehrzellern. Es gibt bei ihnen wie bei den Einzellern immer Zellen, welche direkt in den Nachkommen weiterwachsen (Ei-/Samenzellen = Keimbahnzellen), diese wurden aber nun in definierten zeitlichen Intervallen durch eine wachsende Zahl von anderen Zellen umhüllt und begleitet, welche das nicht konnten – nur dieser Teil des Organismus wurde sterblich. So lebt ein Teil eines Menschen, jeweils in Form einer Zelle der Mutter und des Vaters, buchstäblich in Nachkommen weiter. Beide Zellen vereinigen sich und bilden gemeinsam alle Zellen des Kindes, das Leben erlischt ohne äußere Gründe niemals in diesem Prozess. Die Metapher „Keimbahn“ suggeriert dementsprechend, dass es eine übergeordnete Funktionalität gibt, eine „Bahn“, der das Leben folgt und dabei immer wieder „keimt“, also sich erneuert. Sie deutet so einen unendlichen, kontinuierlichen Pfad an, dem Teile von uns folgen – die Assoziation von einem „unsterblichen“ Teil jedes Menschen liegt nahe. Auf molekularbiologischer Ebene denkt man sofort an die Erbsubstanz DNA, denn die uns von unseren Eltern in den Keimzellen mitgegebene Erbsubstanz (DNA) reichen wir weiter an unsere Nachkommen, und diese wiederum an ihre Kinder. Es passt zu der gewählten Metapher, dass hier anscheinend die Unsterblichkeit der DNA gewährleistet wird, weil die Keimzellen ihr eine klare theoretisch unendliche „Bahn“ in die Zukunft zu geben. Bei genauerem Hinsehen franst aber auch diese Metapher deutlich aus. Was ist hier tatsächlich „unsterblich“? Die einzelnen Moleküle sind es jedenfalls nicht, denn DNA wird in den Zellen kontinuierlich dupliziert und dabei aus stets neuen Baumaterialien aus unserer Nahrung neu zusammengesetzt – es wird also nichts Materielles im eigentlichen Sinn erhalten, genau wie beim Schiff des Theseus. Die Information scheint aber dabei erhalten zu werden – ist also sie das unsterbliche Element der Keimbahn? Kann auch nicht sein, denn unserer Art konnte sich überhaupt nur entwickeln, weil die DNA kontinuierlich verändert (mutiert) wurde, und auch die Existenz von zwei verschiedenen Geschlechtern hat in der Natur ja genau die Aufgabe, DNA mit anderer DNA zu vermischen und so zu verändern. Aber was gibt die Keimbahn dann kontinuierlich als „unsterblich“ weiter? Am besten hilft bei der Antwort darauf wahrscheinlich das oben schon erwähnte Konzept des „Fließgleichgewichts“. Eine einfache Metapher für das Fließgleichgewicht ist der Wasserfall: er behält die gleiche Form, sofern genügend Wasser nachfließt, besteht aber immer aus anderen Wassermolekülen.

Hochaktuell relevant für das Verständnis des Begriffs „Mensch“ und seiner Definition besonders in der direkten Zukunft ist die „Keimbahn“ aber dadurch, dass sie heute bereits gezielte körperliche „Verbesserungen“ der Menschheit ermöglicht. Keimbahnzellen sind per Nomenklatur der Biologie „totipotent“ – eine etwas unglücklich gewählte Metapher, denn sie suggeriert Allmacht. Gemeint ist dagegen lediglich, dass „totipotente Zellen“ sich zu jedem Zelltyp entwickeln können, welchen wir in unserem Körper benötigen, also Muskelzellen, Nervenzellen, Hautzellen und so weiter, aber auch neue Keimzellen. Diese „Totipotenz“ sorgt dafür, dass genetisch veränderte Keimzellen im Gegensatz zu den vielen heute klinisch verwendeten somatischen (d. h. nur für das direkt behandelte Individuum wirkenden) Gentherapien den genetischen Eingriff an die Nachkommen weitergegeben. Damit wird das Gen-Repertoire der Menschheit also permanent verändert.

Eine viel zu wenig beachtete zentrale ethische Frage, die die heute bereits vorhandenen Möglichkeiten der Molekularbiologie aufwirft, ist die nach den Grenzen der gezielten Veränderung von Menschen. Wollen wir hier alles was wir können? Ganz klar: Nein! Die ganz große Mehrheit der Biologen und Biotechnologen ist sich der Gefahren bewusst, wie schon die Geschichte der Entstehung der Gentechnologie illustriert, bei der wir unsere Forschung bereits starken Selbstbeschränkungen unterworfen hatten, bevor die Gesellschaft außerhalb unserer Fachkonferenzen deren Konsequenzen überhaupt wahrgenommen hatte [7]. Auch zur aktuellen Frage der genetischen Menschenzüchtung hat die Gemeinschaft der Forscher längst eindeutig ablehnend Stellung genommen [8]. Begehrlichkeiten von anderen Seiten, um gezielte Menschenzüchtung durch Genmanipulation an Keimbahnzellen zu erreichen, können jedoch leicht erahnt werden. Leider wird ein breiter und konstruktiver, für die Zukunft der Spezies *Homo sapiens* essentieller und meiner Ansicht nach längst überfälliger Diskurs darüber zumindest in Deutschland durch die oben beschriebene Dysfunktionalität der Metapher „Gentechnologie“ in der öffentlichen Wahrnehmung verhindert.

Stefan Heuser: Mich beschäftigt die Frage, was die Metapher von den „Übergängen“ als Kennzeichen der Biologie und die Metapher der (fehlenden) „Grenze“ zwischen einem individuellen Organismus z. B. eines Menschen und anderen Organismen wie z. B. Bakterien für unser Verständnis der conditio humana, also für unser Selbstverständnis bedeutet. Deine Beschreibung der vielen Übergänge und Symbiosen geht mit der Metapher des Fließgleichgewichts einher. Das ist sicherlich ganz heilsam gegenüber einem Selbstverständnis, das uns Menschen als eine Art „Krone“ der Schöpfung aus allen biologischen Vorgängen heraushebt oder das – wie Du Deine Überlegungen einleitest – auf eine hierarchische Kategorisierung des Organischen in höhere und niedere Lebewesen abzielt. Eine Bevorzugung der eigenen Spezies wäre dann einfach nur „Speziesismus“, wie Peter Singer das genannt hat – und ein Beharren auf der individuellen Vorzugswürdigkeit wäre einfach nur Egoismus. Man könnte angesichts der Welt, die diese Metaphorik eröffnet, aber auch darüber staunen, was und wer alles dazu beiträgt, dass menschliches Leben bzw. Leben überhaupt erhalten bleibt –

und dass die Lebewesen nie nur auf Kosten anderer existieren. Die Organismen leben ja sogar nicht nur voneinander und miteinander, sondern sie „dienen" einander auch. Ein solches Narrativ wäre dann ebenfalls ein Übergang, allerdings einer von der Beschreibung bloßen Lebens und Überlebens zu einer Lebensgeschichte, also eines Übergangs vom „Bios" zur „Zoe", zu einem Leben, das wir Menschen wirklich „leben" und nicht nur „fristen". Wenn im Zusammenhang mit dem Selbstverständnis des Menschen von einem „Übergang" bzw. „Übergängen" die Rede ist, schwingt aber zugleich auch Nietzsches furchtbares Wort aus dem Zarathustra mit, dass alles, was er am Menschen lieben kann, ein Übergang ist. Und im Anschluss an Nietzsche machen sich transhumanistische Phantasien an der Metapher „Mensch" fest. Da taucht im Windschatten unserer Rede vom Menschen als mehrdimensionales Fließgleichgewicht auf einmal Nietzsches „Übermensch" auf, vielleicht weil uns auch angesichts einer so schönen Metapher die Frage nicht loslässt: Wozu das ganze, wozu eigentlich „Mensch"? Hans Ulrich hat diese Frage in seinem Beitrag zu diesem Tagungsband aufgegriffen. Ich will damit nur sagen, dass die Frage, mit welchen Metaphern wir im Feld biologischer Entdeckungen von uns selbst als „Menschen" reden, vor dem Hintergrund des Menschen, der sich selbst zum „Problem" geworden ist, nicht nur wichtig, sondern auch potentiell abgründig ist. Das ist in unserem Gespräch ja immer wieder deutlich geworden. Zum Ende unseres Gesprächs daher die Frage: Was folgt für Dich, Stefan und für Dich, Hans, aus der Auseinandersetzung mit diesen Fragen für die Verwendung, Kritik und Transformation von Metaphern in der Wissenschaftssprache?

Stefan Dübel: Wir Forscher sollten lernen, viel bewusster mit dem metaphorischen Charakter der von uns verwendeten Begriffe umzugehen, da alle Assoziationen, die die gewählte Metapher erzeugen, später Auswirkungen auf unsere Wissenschaft haben kann. Natürlich kann man nicht in die Zukunft sehen und welche Verschiebung der Begriffsbedeutungen sich hier ergeben könnten, dennoch sollten wir als Naturwissenschaftler lieber mal ein paar Minuten länger über die von uns vorgeschlagenen neuen Begriffe für unsere neuesten Forschungsergebnisse nachdenken, bevor wir sie publizieren.

Hans Ulrich: Weitergehend könnte man die Suche nach Metaphern selbst zu einer gezielten wissenschaftlichen Aufgabe in den verschiedenen Forschungsbereichen machen und so die Metaphernbildung gezielt für weiteren Erkenntnisgewinn einsetzen, etwa indem man verschiedene ausprobiert.

Stefan Heuser: Dann lasst uns als Ausblick noch die Frage beantworten, an welcher Metapher Ihr beide gerne interdisziplinär weiterarbeiten würdet?

Stefan Dübel: Natürlich „Antikörper", dem Alltagsbegriff für Immunglobuline [1]. Antikörper bezeichnen in der Immunologie eine Gruppe von Proteinen, welche ganz allgemein damit befasst sind, uns gegen Krankheiten zu schützen. Das machen sie wie oben schon kurz angesprochen dadurch, dass sie alle möglichen molekularen Strukturen erkennen können, die nicht zu uns gehören – womit im biochemischen Sinn gemeint ist, dass deren Aufbau nicht in unserer eigenen Erbsubstanz festgelegt ist. Mit anderen Worten, die helfen uns, „selbst" von „fremd" zu unterscheiden. Damit können sie Krankheitserreger, die uns besiedeln, erkennen, und abwehren. Zu diesem Zweck läuft jeder Mensch buchstäblich mit Milliarden unterschiedlicher Antikörpermoleküle herum, welche ständig durch unsere Blutbahn und unsere Gewebe patrouillieren. Aufgrund ihrer molekularen Struktur können sie aus dem ganzen Gemisch verschiedener Stoffe, die unseren Organismus bilden, gezielt einen einzigen herausfinden, der nicht zu uns gehört, und sich dann fest an ihn koppeln („binden"). Sie markieren so Eindringlinge und ermöglichen ihre Entsorgung.

Entdeckt wurden Antikörper von Emil v. Behring 1890 als Bestandteile im Blutserum, welche die tödlichen Giftstoffe neutralisieren konnten, die Tetanus- und Diphtheriebakterien produzierten. Dementsprechend nannte v. Behring sie zuerst pragmatisch „Antitoxine", also „Gegengifte". Er bekam den ersten Medizin-Nobelpreis für eine völlig neue, auf dieser Erkenntnis basierende Medikamentenart: den „Antiseren", welche in den folgenden Jahrzehnten unzähligen an Diphtherie erkrankten Kindern das Leben retteten.

Später lernten wir, dass Antikörper nicht nur Toxine neutralisieren, sondern eine große Zahl individueller Antikörperversionen auch an unzählige andere Eiweißstoffe binden können. Damit verbreiterte sich die Metapher zum heutigen „Antikörper" – eben einem Gegenstück zu einem bestimmten anderen Biomolekül. Der Begriff wurde aufgrund der als ersten beobachteten Funktion geprägt, und das geschah in einer Zeit, in dem das Wissen um unterschiedliche Moleküle und ihre Struktur noch extrem rudimentär war. Jeder assoziiert mit dem Wortbildungselement „Anti-" etwas diametral Entgegengesetztes, eine Negierung. Heute ist der genaue atomare Aufbau zahlreicher Antikörper bekannt. Immunglobuline verfügen über zwei „Greifarme" (vgl. Abbildung unten), welche den physischen Kontakt zur „fremden" Substanz vermitteln, und sie somit buchstäblich festhalten.

Biochemisch nennt man dies eine „hochaffine Bindung". Ein weiterer Teil des Antikörpers bindet aber nicht an das fremde „Antigen", sondern hat eine ganz andere Funktionspalette. Er stimuliert die Immunantwort und ruft sozusagen Hilfe herbei, nachdem er den „Eindringling" festgehalten hat. Eine Beobachtung in Bezug auf unser Thema, wie Metaphern die Erkenntnisgewinnung beeinflussen könnten, ist, dass diese „aktivierenden" Funktionen der Antikörper erst 50–80 Jahre nach ihrer ursprünglichen Entdeckung untersucht und beschrieben wurden (Abb. 9.2). Die Hypothese ist retrospektiv sicher nicht mehr verifizierbar, aber es wäre doch denkbar, dass die meisten Forscher, die damals mit Antikörpern arbeiteten, die im Wort suggerierte Assoziation des „gegen etwas sein" unbewusst gedanklich bevorzugten bei ihren experimentellen Fragestellungen. Damit ist der Gedanke, dass Antikörper „für" statt „gegen" etwas funktionierten, beim Ausdenken neuer Versuche einfach weniger naheliegend. Jedenfalls wurden die ersten aktivierenden Funktionen von Immunglobulinen erst mehr als 50 Jahre nach ihrer Antitoxin-Wirkung entdeckt, und die neueste dieser Funktionen sogar erst nach 1970, also 80 Jahre nach den Arbeiten

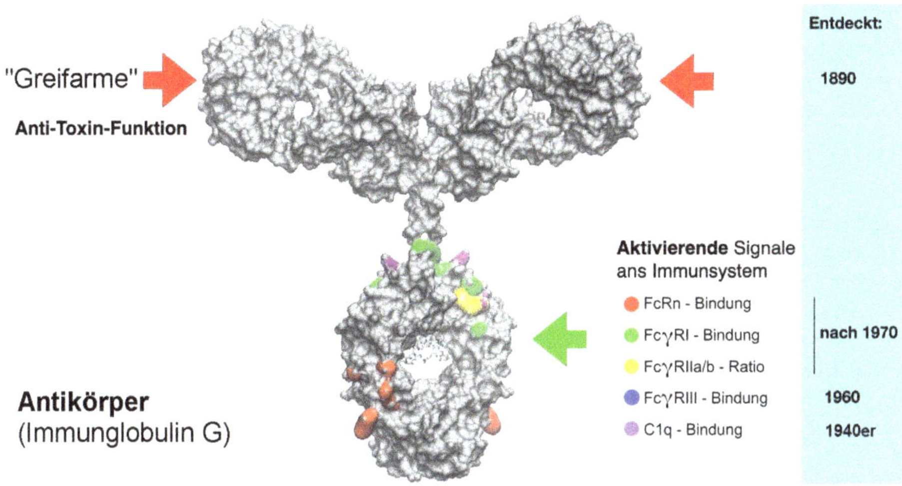

Abb. 9.2: Atomare Struktur eines Antikörpermoleküls (IgG). Die roten Pfeile deuten auf den Bereich des Moleküls, welche die Zielstrukturen binden können, also die „Anti-“ Funktionen vermitteln. Der grüne Pfeil deutet auf die Molekülregion, welche die aktivierenden Funktionen vermittelt, wobei die jeweiligen Kontaktstellen zu verschiedenen Aktivierungsmechanismen farbig markiert sind. Der blaue Balken gibt die Jahre der Erstbeschreibung der entsprechenden Funktionen an (Grafik: S. Dübel).

v. Behrings. Hat hier die durch den Wortbestandteil „Anti-“ dominierte Metapher die Aufklärung der vielen aktivierenden Funktionen verzögert? Die Frage, ob solche Effekte tatsächlich aufzufinden sind wäre sicherlich mal einen Blick wert.

Hans Ulrich: Die Arbeit an Metaphern wird in den Geisteswissenschaften oft auch als Arbeit an „Begriffen“ in begriffsgeschichtlichen Untersuchungen geleistet, sofern „Begriffe“ nicht ausdrücklich in ihrem metaphorischen Charakter gesehen werden – wie z. B. der Begriff „Gedächtnis“ der das, was „Erinnerung“ – wiederum eine Metapher – signifikant bestimmen kann, wie umgekehrt „Erinnerung“ für das, was als „Gedächtnis“ festgehalten werden soll. An solchen Metaphern gilt es, beständig zu arbeiten, das heißt kritisch daran, wo und wie sie gebraucht werden, was sie leisten und – vor allem auch – nicht leisten. So schließt beispielsweise das, was aus dem biblischen Hebräisch als „Gedenken“ übersetzt wird, sowohl die Bedeutung der Bewahrung von etwas Vergangenem ein wie auch zugleich die Bewahrung für Zukünftiges, sodass „Bewahrung“ ohnehin die bessere Übersetzung wäre. Die Metapher „Bewahrung des Lebens“ enthält beides. Damit trägt die Metapher eine Bedeutung mit sich, die biologisch Gegebenes auch „zeitlich“ versteht etc. Die Verschränkung von „Lebendigem“ mit „Zeit“ ist ein immer gegebenes mitlaufendes Problem der Beschreibung und Erfassung biologischer Gegebenheiten und Vorgänge. Wenn von „Nachhaltigkeit“ gesprochen wird, so wird damit eine gänzlich unbestimmte Zeitdimension mitgesetzt, was die Metapher nutzlos macht – es müsste immer ein bestimmter Zeitindex hinzugefügt werden.

Stefan Heuser: Es würde mich freuen, wenn wir die Arbeit an diesen Metaphern an anderer Stelle weiterführen könnten. Vielen Dank Euch beiden für dieses Gespräch!

Literatur

Einen allgemeinen Überblick über Antikörper und die modernen Methoden zu ihrer Herstellung gibt das Lehrbuch:

[1] Dübel S, Breitling F, Frenzel A, Jostock T, Marschall A, Schirrmann T, Hust M. Rekombinante Antikörper. Heidelberg. Springer Verlag, 2019.

Einzelnachweise:

[2] Pinheiro A P M, Pocock R H, Dixon M D et al. Using metaphors to explain molecular testing to cancer patients. Oncologist 22, 2017: 445–9.

[3] Tshitoyan V, Dagdelen J, Weston L. et al. Unsupervised word embeddings capture latent knowledge from materials science literature. Nature 571, 2019: 95–98.

[4] Dübel S, Neuhaus G, Berger S, Schweiger H. Characterization of haploid Acetabularia cells. *Eur. J. Cell. Biol. 38*, 1985: 328–334.

[5] Bradbury A R M, Trinklein N D, Thie H, Wilkinson I C, Tandon A K, Anderson S, Bladen C L, Jones S, Force Aldred S, Bestagno M, Burrone O, Maynard J, Ferrara F, Trimmer J S, Görnemann J, Glanville J, Wolf P, Frenzel A, Wong J, Yu X, Eng H-Y, Lane D, Lefranc M-P, Clark M, Dübel S. When monoclonal antibodies are not monospecific: hybridomas frequently express additional functional variable regions. mAbs, 10, 2018: 539–546 doi.org/10.1080/19420862.2018.1445456.

[6] Husserl E. Die Krisis der europäischen Wissenschaften und die transzendentale Phänomenologie. Eine Einleitung in die phänomenologische Philosophie. 2. Aufl. Husserliana 4. Den Haag: Martinus Nijhoff, 1976.

[7] Berg P, Singer M F. The recombinant DNA controversy: twenty years later. Proc. Natl. Acad. Sci. USA. 92, 1995: 9011–9013.

[8] Max-Planck-Gesellschaft. Stellungnahme zu den wissenschaftlichen und translationalen Auswirkungen der Genom-Editierung und daraus resultierenden ethischen, rechtlichen und gesellschaftlichen Fragen (2019), https://www.mpg.de/13501764/positionspapier-genom-editierung-mpg-de.pdf (download 27.12.2024).

Bruno Gransche, Arne Manzeschke, Stefan Heuser

10 Anthropomorphisierungen. Ein Gespräch über Metapherntechnik und Technikmetaphern

Stefan Heuser: Auf dem Workshop im vergangenen Jahr in Braunschweig hat Bruno entlang des Titels „Die Reize von Metapherntechnik und Technikmetaphern“ eine „Kritik des Übertragens als Kultivierungsaufgabe“ entfaltet. Arne hat über „Metaphern und Anthropomorphisierungen im KI-Diskurs“ gesprochen. Mit Blick auf die zunehmende Digitalisierung der Biotechnologien bzw. die Verschränkung lebenswissenschaftlicher Forschung mit KI-basierten Informationstechnologien finde ich die beiden Vortragsthemen in ihrem Zusammenklang sehr reizvoll. Könnt Ihr unseren Leser:innen bitte zum Auftakt unseres Gesprächs kurz schildern, was Euch zu Eurer jeweiligen Themenwahl bewogen hat und was für Euch in Euren Vorträgen die wichtigsten Aspekte bzw. Fragestellungen sind?

Bruno Gransche: Metaphern sind faszinierend, nicht nur im Alltag, sondern auch philosophisch und wissenschaftlich. Das Spannende daran ist, dass Metaphern nicht nur eine Art des Redens sind, sondern Grundmerkmale des Denkens ausdrücken. Wir können, wenn wir uns Metaphern anschauen, besser verstehen, wie wir denken und wie wir vor allem Neues fassen.

Das macht Metaphern relevant im Umgang mit Neuem. Das ist vor allem in der Wissenschaft so, wo neue unbekannte Phänomene untersucht werden oder manchmal auch alte Phänomene neu verstanden werden müssen. Das ist etwa in der Innovationsforschung interessant, generell in Forschung und Entwicklung, wo Neues entsteht und beurteilt und bewertet werden muss, ob es besser als Altes ist, also als Innovation gelten kann.

Das ist aber auch immer da relevant, wo wir etwas Neuem begegnen. Das kann alt sein, aber wenn es für uns neu ist, wir es also nicht kennen, dann versuchen wir es in Begriffen oder mit Konzepten von Bekanntem, von Vertrautem zu kombinieren und zu verstehen. Das heißt, Metaphern helfen uns, Unbekanntes in vertrauten Termini, in vertrauten Kategorien zu sehen.

Das ist ein Riesenvorteil, denn es macht die unbekannte Welt, die voll von Neuem und präzedenzlosen Phänomenen ist, die uns begegnen, ein Stück vertrauter, wenn wir Neues in Begriffen oder in Bedeutungsräumen von Vertrautem und Bekanntem sehen. So können wir Neues als eine andere Art von Vertrautem auffassen und haben zunächst mal eine Orientierung, was wir davon halten sollen und wie wir damit umgehen könnten. Das ist eine hervorragende Strategie, um spontan mit Neuem umgehen zu können. Ein Computervirus ist also wie ein Grippevirus, nur nicht in biologischen Systemen, sondern in technischen; die Infektiosität, Schadhaftigkeit

https://doi.org/10.1515/9783112215685-010

und prinzipielle Coping-Strategien wie Immunantworten (Anti-Virus-Programme) ähneln sich genug, um zunächst das eine (ein IT-Programm) als das andere (organische Strukturen) sehen zu können. Wo aber die Metapher hinkt, die Ähnlichkeit also genau endet und damit das Als-Vertrautes-Verstehen in ein In-spezifischer-Neuheit-Missverstehen wird, ist eine zentrale Frage, die eine nähere Beschäftigung mit Metaphern sowie den jeweiligen Bedeutungsdomänen erfordert.

Das zeigt: Wir müssen zunächst und zumeist auf solche Strategien zurückgreifen. Aber sie haben auch ihre Probleme da, wo das Neue gerade darin besteht oder gerade darin uns herausfordert, dass es sich unterscheidet von der Art der Bedeutung, Konzepte und Begriffe, mit denen wir metaphorisch auf sie zugreifen. Wenn also für eine Handlungsorientierung, für eine richtige Reaktion, ein richtiger Umgang mit einem neuen Phänomen gerade das entscheidend ist, was uns daran nicht vertraut ist, dann kann es passieren, dass wir mit Metaphern ungeeignete, potenziell gefährliche Handlungsorientierungen erzeugen.

Arne Manzeschke: Von der Anthropologie herkommend interessiert es mich, wie wir Menschen uns als Menschen jeweils verstehen. Dieses „Verstehen als" ist noch mal etwas anderes als die vermutlich landläufigere Frage, wer und was der Mensch „ist". Sich in bestimmter Weise als Mensch(en) verstehen, hängt einmal von der Welt ab, die die Menschen umgibt. Sie ist – in unseren Breiten – in sehr bestimmender Weise eine von Menschen gemachte Welt: Häuser, Straßen, Trambahnen auf Schienen und mit Oberleitungen, Flughäfen, Kanäle, Schiffe, Computer, Smartphones, smart homes, smart cities, Röntgenapparate und Operationssäle, Funkmasten, Satelliten ... Man kann sagen: Wir werden zu bestimmten Menschen durch die Welt(en), die wir uns schaffen und in denen wir dann leben. Und auf der Grundlage dieser Lebenswelt verändern wir die Welt weiter – und damit auch uns selbst. Der Mensch der Renaissance hat sich anders verstanden als ein Mensch zu Beginn der 20. Jahrhunderts und der wieder anders als einer in unserer Zeit.

Um uns zu verstehen, brauchen wir zum anderen eine Sprache, die uns hilft, dieses Verstehen in Worte zu fassen und uns in dieser von uns geschaffenen Welt zu orientieren, zu wissen, woran wir sind und welche Lebensmöglichkeiten damit verbunden sind. Wir benutzen Sprache jedoch nicht nur, um Bestehendes zu benennen, sondern auch um Neues hervorzubringen und es dann zu benennen. Wie aber erschließt man sich das Neue, von dem man noch gar keinen Begriff hat? Hier kommen Vergleiche, Analogien, Metaphern ins Spiel. Sie ermöglichen einen sprachlichen Umweg, weil die direkte begriffliche Benennung des Neuen noch gar nicht möglich ist. Stattdessen wird über ein Drittes, Bekanntes mit Formulierungen wie „so ähnlich wie ..." sprachlich verwiesen. Blumenberg hat das so formuliert: „Aber etwas als etwas zu begreifen, unterscheidet sich radikal von dem Verfahren, etwas durch etwas anderes zu begreifen. Der metaphorische Umweg, von dem thematischen Gegenstand weg auf einen anderen zu blicken, der vorgreifend als aufschlußreich vermutet wird, nimmt das Gegebene als das Fremde, das Andere als das vertrauter und handlicher

Verfügbare." [1, S. 116] Damit die Metapher aber als solche funktioniert, bedarf es eines gemeinsamen Sprachhorizontes, vor dem die miteinander Sprechenden sich verständigen. Auf die Erschließung von Neuem durch sprachliche Metaphern hat Bruno ja hingewiesen. Die Sprache erschließt uns nicht nur die Welt um uns herum, sondern sie ermöglicht es auch, dass wir uns selbst neu bzw. anders verstehen.

Stefan Heuser: Deine Ausführungen zum gemeinsamen Sprachhorizont finde ich interessant und würde gerne nachhaken: Was genau ist damit gemeint? Geht es um das Sprechen einer gemeinsamen natürlichen Sprache, um Übersetzung einer natürlichen Sprache in eine andere oder um eine gemeinsame Fachsprache? Geht es um die Fähigkeit, bestimmte Sprachspiele so zu spielen, dass die Beteiligten im Gebrauch der Wörter und über deren Bedeutungen übereinstimmen? Beim Stichwort „Horizont" denke ich auch an Gadamers „Wahrheit und Methode" und an seine Metapher vom „Verschmelzen" der Horizonte. In deiner Rede vom „Sprachhorizont" scheint es ja eher um die Rolle von Metaphern bei der Erweiterung von Horizonten zu gehen, um neues Verstehen bzw. Neuverstehen. Auf unserem gemeinsamen Workshop war diese epistemische Funktion von Metaphern ein wichtiges und wiederkehrendes Thema. Mithilfe von Metaphern können wir unsere Horizonte des Verstehens von Wirklichkeit kreativ überschreiten und zugleich versuchen, im Horizont dessen zu bleiben, was wir bereits sprachlich fassen können. Da stellt sich die Frage, worin die sprachliche und epistemische Horizonterweiterung dann jeweils genau besteht, worauf – auf welche Aspekte von Wirklichkeit – die jeweiligen Metaphern die Aufmerksamkeit lenken. Diese Funktion von Metaphern ist ja vielfältig reflektiert worden, auch mit Blick auf die Frage, welche Rolle wissenschaftliche Methoden dabei spielen – und wie es überhaupt zu Veränderungen in der Metaphorik kommt. Deine Überlegungen scheinen mir aber vor dem Hintergrund von Gadamers Überlegungen über das Verhältnis von Wahrheit und Methode noch in eine weitere Richtung zu weisen, nämlich in jene Richtung, in der es um den Beitrag von Metaphern zu den methodischen Anforderungen beim interdisziplinären Zusammenwirken von Lebenswissenschaften und Geisteswissenschaften geht. Was auf methodisch gesicherte Weise als „Wahrheit" von Wirklichkeit gewonnen werden kann, braucht demnach einen Verständigungsprozess, für den „wir" im Dialog der Wissenschaften kreativ an Metaphern arbeiten müssen. Dabei ginge es aber weniger um die Übersetzung aus einer methodisch gesicherten Domäne exakter Aussagen der Wissenschaft in die notorisch unscharfe Domäne der Alltagssprache, sondern darum, dass sich hermeneutische Fragen an jedem Punkt im Prozess des Verstehens von Wirklichkeit stellen, auch dort, wo es – wie in den Naturwissenschaften – scheinbar nur um das Erklären von Gesetzmäßigkeiten geht. Man könnte vor dem Hintergrund der Metaphorologie Blumenbergs dabei auch fragen, inwiefern Metaphern nicht nur dazu beitragen, uns die Wirklichkeit nahezubringen, sondern auch, sie auf Distanz zu halten und als beherrschbar erscheinen zu lassen – inwiefern sie also auch die Funktion haben, mit dem wissenschaftlichen Wissen über die Wirklichkeit zurechtzukommen. Freilich stellt sich dann die kritische

Frage, was uns davor bewahren kann, dass wir uns die Bedeutung von Wirklichkeit bis tief hinein in unsere naturwissenschaftlichen Beobachtungen metaphorisch so zurechtlegen, wie wir das gerne wollen bzw. wie es unseren Herrschaftsinteressen entspricht. Die kritische Metaphernanalyse, der es um den Aufweis von ideologischen Elementen des Gebrauchs von Metaphern in Diskursen geht, greift hier möglicherweise nicht weit genug, jedenfalls insofern sie nicht die Frage berührt, in welchem existentiellen „Horizont" unsere Metaphernbildung angesiedelt ist – die Frage, die bei Blumenberg immer mitschwingt. Bei den Lebenswissenschaften stellt sich diese Frage nach der Sprache, die wir für das Leben finden, mit besonderer Dringlichkeit, weil uns mit den Lebensprozessen immer schon eine „Sprache" entgegenkommt und es nicht ausgemacht ist, was wir da „hören" und wie wir darauf „antworten".

Arne Manzeschke: Betrachten wir ‚die Sprache' etwas genauer, so können wir verschiedene Ebenen ausmachen: Wir nutzen Begriffe, die sehr genau (vielleicht sogar abschließend, also definierend) beschreiben, was der Begriff bezeichnet. Ein Kreis ist eine Ansammlung von Punkten, die alle gleich weit entfernt sind von einem gemeinsamen Mittelpunkt. Ein Tisch ist eine waagrechte Fläche, auf der verschiedene Tätigkeiten ausgeübt werden können (z. B. essen, nähen, schreiben ...), und die von einer Anzahl von ‚Beinen' getragen wird. Auch wenn Tische sehr verschieden aussehen können und sehr verschiedenen Aktivitäten dienen können, so ist es für uns Menschen nicht schwer, Tische als solche zu erkennen.

Auf einer zweiten Ebene nutzen wir Metaphern, um uns Gegenstände oder Sachverhalte zu verdeutlichen, ohne sie vereindeutigen zu können oder zu wollen. So ist z. B. die Luftschraube eine Metapher, mit der man sich die Funktion des Antriebs von Luftfahrzeugen verdeutlichen konnte: Der Propeller schraubt sich durch die Luft und treibt so das Fahrzeug voran. Heute wird dieses Wort kaum noch verwendet, es ist vom Propeller abgelöst worden – Metaphern haben ihre Zeit. Dass bei Flugzeugen der Propeller (= Luftschraube) vorn für den Auftrieb und bei Schiffen (also auch bei Luftschiffen wie dem Zeppelin) der Propeller hinten für den Vortrieb angebracht ist, ist insofern bemerkenswert, als das Treibende der Luftschraube verschiedene Antriebsorte erlaubt.

Das Beispiel zeigt also auch, dass Metaphern nur vor einem bestimmten Horizont ‚funktionieren' und da ist ihre Leistung enorm, sie orientieren, wo Begriffe oder Definitionen (noch) nicht existieren. Ändert sich der Horizont, weil z. B. die technische Entwicklung über gewisse Artefakte oder Verfahren hinweggegangen ist, so sinken diese Metaphern gleichsam ab. Sie verschwinden nicht vollständig, aber ihre Orientierungskraft schwindet, was allerdings die Gefahr des Missbrauchs nicht ausschließt, weshalb der Umgang mit Metaphern immer auch ein kritischer sein muss.

Auf einer dritten Ebene nutzen wir absolute Metaphern, bei denen die metaphorische Dimension gar nicht gleich in den Blick kommt. Die absolute Metapher ist dem Symbol sehr ähnlich und findet sich in Worten wie „Sehen" (für Blumenberg die absolute Metapher par excellence) oder „Welt" oder „Leben". Anders als bei transitorischen Metaphern ist bei diesen nicht zu erwarten, dass sie irgendwann einmal absinken oder gar in Begriffe überführt werden können. Man könnte auch fragen, ob nicht der Terminus „Intelligenz“ so eine absolute Metapher darstellt. Damit komme ich auf das Thema meines Vortrags zu sprechen. Künstliche Intelligenz ist eine Technologie, die unsere Welt in einer rasanten Geschwindigkeit in sehr, sehr vielen Lebensbereichen verändert und vor komplexe Herausforderungen stellt in Bezug auf die Gestaltung dieser Welt (die klassische moralische Frage: Was sollen wir tun?) und in Bezug auf unser Selbstverständnis als Menschen (Wer können und wer wollen wir sein?). Manchmal wird in diesem Zusammenhang von der vierten großen Kränkung der Menschheit gesprochen:

1 Kopernikus hat die Welt der Menschen dezentriert; sie ist nicht das Zentrum des Universums, sondern ein sehr kleiner Planet eher am Rande.
2 Darwin hat gezeigt, dass die Menschen einer Evolution unterliegen wie alle anderen Arten auch; er ist also (naturwissenschaftlich betrachtet) keine herausgehobene Sonderschöpfung.
3 Freud hat mit seiner Psychoanalyse darauf hingewiesen, dass Menschen nicht nur bewusste und selbstbestimmte Wesen sind, sondern auch von einem Unbewussten getrieben werden – „der Mensch ist nicht Herr im Haus“.
4 Künstliche Intelligenz wirft die Frage auf, ob Denken, Lernen oder auch Emotionen tatsächlich genuine Fähigkeiten von höher entwickelten Lebewesen sind – oder ob diese Fähigkeiten nicht auch durch entsprechend „intelligente“ Maschinen geleistet werden können.

Damit sind sehr weitreichende und tief gehende Fragen für uns Menschen, für unser Verhältnis zur Welt und zu uns selbst verbunden. Sie lassen sich als „Kränkungen“ begreifen, weil sie eine Sonderstellung des Menschen auf allen denkbaren Ebenen infrage stellen: planetarisch, biologisch, psychisch und nun auch intellektuell. Dass wir die Dinge so beschreiben, betrachten und bewerten, hat mit Sprache zu tun.

Die Rede von der Kränkung der Menschheit lässt sich im Grunde als eine Metapher verstehen: Ein Vorgang in dieser Welt wirkt sich verletzend, schwächend auf alle Menschen aus, und es stellt sich die Frage, wie die Menschen sich schützen, therapieren und wieder gesunden können.

Der Gebrauch von Metaphern findet aber nicht nur auf der Ebene der Gesamtbetrachtung und -bewertung („Das ist eine Kränkung.“) statt, sondern ebenso auf der Ebene der einzelnen Phänomene, wenn z. B. die Arbeit von Menschen in der Filmindustrie nun durch KI ersetzt werden kann.

Der Begriff „Künstliche Intelligenz“ oszilliert zwischen einer sprachlichen Unterscheidung über *genus proximum* (Intelligenz) und *differentia specifica* (künstlich) und einem metaphorischen Gebrauch (Was die Maschinen da leisten, ist so ähnlich wie der lösungsorientierte Denkvorgang bei (intelligenten) Menschen).

Die Metapher müsste uns nun – wenn es gut geht – Eigenschaften aus dem Quellbereich (menschliche Intelligenz) für den Zielbereich (künstliche Intelligenz) erschließen. Wir haben dieses formale Moment sehr ausführlich diskutiert [2].

Stefan Heuser: Ausgehend von diesen Gedanken würde ich gerne einmal zwischendurch fragen, woran wir Menschen uns denn orientieren, wenn wir uns mithilfe von Metaphern „neu" verstehen wollen. Es könnte ja ohnehin sein, dass wir mit unseren Metaphern für uns selbst danebenliegen und uns damit zugleich auch über die „Welt" um uns herum irren. Ein Beispiel hierfür wäre die Metapher vom Menschen als „Krone der Schöpfung", mit der wir an einem Mythos über uns selbst und gleichzeitig über unser Verhältnis zur „Welt" und am Umgang mit ihr weiterstricken. Das Wort „Mensch" selbst ist ja schon eine absolute Metapher, bei der mehr mitschwingt, als wir begrifflich fassen können und die sich auch nicht auflösen lässt. Heißt „neu" verstehen demgegenüber einfach, die Selbstbeschreibungen zu entmythologisieren? Dann bleibt vielleicht der Ausweg über die begriffliche Sprache und die empirisch gestützten, im engeren Sinne „anthropologischen" Aussagen über den Menschen. Aber auch diese bleiben im Horizont von Metaphorik, zum Beispiel der Metapher vom „Leben" oder der Metapher von der „Natur". Wir bleiben in den bekannten Bahnen der Selbsterkenntnis, verstehen uns aber nicht „neu", oder? Was würde es demgegenüber bedeuten, dass wir uns „neu" verstehen und nicht nur im Rahmen des immer gleichen Kreisens um uns selbst?

Dann würde ich in diesem Zusammenhang gerne noch die Frage nach der Funktion stellen, die eine Metapher aus ihrem Quellbereich übernimmt und auf ihren Zielbereich überträgt, und der Art und Weise, wie wir uns in unserer Wahrnehmung und in unserem Handeln auf diese Funktion beziehen. Wir können uns ja schon in der Wahl der Metapher täuschen, und erst recht in der Funktion, die sie dem Gegenstandsbereich nahelegt. Im vorherigen Schreibgespräch hat der Biotechnologe Stefan Dübel auf ein analoges Problem beim Gebrauch bewährter Metaphern in einem neuen Kontext hingewiesen. Er berichtet, dass sogenannte Hybridom-Zellen zur Herstellung von Antikörpern verwendet werden, also künstlich hergestellte Zelllinien, die aus der Fusion einer antikörperproduzierenden B-Zelle mit einer Tumorzelle entstehen, sich im Labor dauerhaft vermehren können und zur Produktion großer Mengen von Antikörpern nutzen lassen. Diese „monoklonalen" Antikörper werden in der Forschung und auch in der Therapie eingesetzt. Allerdings hat die Metapher „monoklonal" suggeriert, dass diese Hybridom-Zellen wie im Immunsystem nur „monospezifische" Antikörper produzieren, die es auf ein einziges Zielmolekül abgesehen haben. Bei der Herstellung von Hybridom-Zellen können allerdings mehrere unterschiedliche Antikörper-Gene gleichzeitig aktiv bleiben, sodass ein einzelner Hybridom-Klon verschiedene Antikörper produziert. Die beim Laborprodukt einfach weiterverwendete Metapher „monoklonal" hat den Blick der Forschung für diesen Effekt allerdings verdeckt, so dass sich bestimmte Beobachtungen aus Experimenten nicht erklären ließen. Diese Metapher hat sich demnach als dysfunktional erwiesen, d. h. sie hat eine falsche Eindeutigkeit mit Blick auf die Funktion ihres Gegenstandsbereich nahegelegt und dessen weitere Erforschung mindestens verzögert.

Bruno Gransche: Das Interessante ist, dass Metaphern nicht nur etwas aussagen, sondern sie geben uns auch etwas zu denken. Sie lehren uns, *etwas als etwas anderes zu sehen*. Zum Beispiel die Metapher des DNA-Codes: Informationen sind geschrieben wie in einem Buch, nur in einem anderen Medium, mit anderen Buchstaben und Substanzen als Papier. Diese Metapher legt nahe, DNA als ein Buch zu sehen, in dem ein Text steht, der jedoch verschlüsselt ist und spezielle Kenntnisse zur Entschlüsselung erfordert, wie entsprechende Labortechniken und theoretische Hintergründe der Genetik. Metaphern schlagen vor, etwas in Bedeutungsaspekten von etwas Bekanntem zu sehen. Das griechische Wort „Metapher" bedeutet „Übertragen", also das Übertragen von Bedeutung von einem bekannten Bereich – der Quelldomäne – auf einen unbekannten Bereich – der Zieldomäne. Metaphern helfen, Ereignisse für unser Verständnis zu strukturieren, ermöglichen neue Perspektiven und das Hinterfragen von Selbstverständlichkeiten. Jedoch verändern sich beide Domänen, wenn sie metaphorisch gekoppelt werden. Dabei ist stets eine Kombination aus Simulation (etwas zeigen, was nicht ist) und Dissimulation (etwas nicht zeigen, was ist) im Spiel. Indem – formal gesprochen – ein X für ein Y zu verstehen gegeben wird, wird es zugleich erschwert das X als Nicht-Y zu sehen. Es ist schwierig konkrete Gegenkonzepte paarweise zu fassen, aber das Nahelegen einer Zieldomänen-Sichtweise in Hinsicht einer Quelldomäne erschwert Verstehensperspektiven, die mit der gewählten Quelldomäne inkompatibel sind. Wenn etwa gewisse DNA-Abschnitte (und die Rede war sogar von 98%) als Müll bezeichnet werden (Junk-DNA), dann sind Konzepte wie wegwerfen, loswerden, mitschleppen, verunreinigt, entrümpeln kompatibler mit einer solchen Metapher als funktional, wertvoll, nützlich, hüten, pflegen oder schützen. Nicht weil das letztere Set irgendwie weniger mit DNA semantisch kompatibel wäre, sondern weniger mit Müll. Unsere Quelldomänen-Wahl schickt anziehende und abstoßende Wellen durch unser gesamtes semantisches Territorium und kann nicht ohne solche *push-pull* oder *veil-reveal* Dynamiken verstanden werden. Diese Dynamik verläuft – und das macht es eben schwierig und erforschens- und explikationsbedürftig – meist unbemerkt, darum aber umso wirkmächtiger, da es sozusagen den kritischen Zensor einer bewussten Entscheidung der Frage ‚Will ich das so sehen oder nicht?' umgeht. Metaphern sind nicht nur stilistische Mittel der Sprache, sondern auch grundlegende Werkzeuge unseres Denkens, in denen Weltbilder, Technikbilder und Menschenbilder Eingang finden. Durch die Analyse von Metaphern können implizite Weltbilder, Menschenbilder und Technikbilder expliziert werden. Eine Konsequenz daraus ist, dass Metaphern nicht in Klartext aufgelöst werden können. Die Grundstrukturen des Denkens, die in Metaphern ausgedrückt werden, müssen als komplexes Geflecht betrachtet werden.

Arne Manzeschke: Die spannende Frage, die sich aus Brunos Überlegungen ergibt, ist folgende: Welche Flexibilität und Ungenauigkeit müssen wir in der Sprache zulassen, um sich durch die Unschärfe von Metaphern neue Felder (oder bekannte Felder anders) zu erschließen? Zugleich bedarf es aber auch einer gewissen Präzision, Schärfe und Eindeutigkeit in der Sprache, damit wir uns tatsächlich gemeinsam verständigen können. Gehen wir dieser Frage weiter nach, dann stellen wir schnell fest, dass es Felder/Bereiche/Domänen (alle drei selbst Metaphern) gibt, in denen mit sehr scharf umrissenen Begriffen gearbeitet wird, insofern diese z. B. über Normen gefasst werden (ISO, DIN, Gesetze und Verordnungen u. a.). In anderen Feldern/Bereichen/Domänen braucht es im Gegenteil gerade Unschärfe und Flexibilität in der Begriffsverwendung, um bestimmte Prozesse in Gang zu setzen (z. B. Imaginations- und Kreationsprozesse). Genau genommen erfordern auch Gesetze eine Auslegung; sofern sie das Soziale, also Lebendige regeln, kann hier nicht mit logisch eindeutigen Deduktionen gearbeitet werden, sondern allenfalls mit Subsumptionen oder Induktionen. Metaphorik erfordert Hermeneutik.

Nehmen wir das Beispiel des monoklonalen Antikörpers: Hier hat das „mono" wohl auf eine falsche Fährte geführt. Die weitergehende Frage, die ich als Laie auf diesem Feld stellen möchte, lautet: Ist das überhaupt eine echte Metapher und mit welcher Absicht wurde sie gewählt? Inwiefern erschließt der Begriff „monoklonaler Antikörper" Eigenschaften des Hybridoms? Ist der Herstellungsprozess wie ein Klonieren zu verstehen oder ist die „dauerhafte Vermehrung" der Zellen ein echtes Klonieren? Wo ist hier die metaphorische Unschärfe und wo ist ihr Informationsgehalt, der für die Zieldomäne einen Erkenntnisgewinn verspricht – und außerdem: für wen? Gerade dieses Beispiel zeigt m. E., dass Metaphern ihren Adressatenkreis haben, über den hinaus sie womöglich nichtssagend bleiben.

Bruno Gransche: Die Frage ‚für wen?' bzw. des Adressatenkreises finde ich sehr wichtig an dieser Stelle. Oft wird von Metaphern – oder auch von Begriffen und Konzepten – geredet wie von feststehenden Bedeutungskonstellationen, aber ähnlich wie Ironie verstehen nicht immer alle das Gemeinte und nie alle ausschließlich und vollständig das Gemeinte. Das liegt viel an Kontextvarianz, aber v. a. meines Erachtens daran, dass Individuen selbst bei großen historisch-kulturellen Überschneidungen nie zwei deckungsgleiche Sets an Bedeutungen haben, die ihre Quelldomäne ausmacht. Bei allen Schwierigkeiten zu verstehen, welche Bedeutungsaspekte der Quelle auf das Ziel übertragen werden sollen, bestimmt vorrangig das Set der in der Quelle allererst vorhandenen Elemente, worüber überhaupt entschieden werden kann. Wir haben es also immer mit einer unsicheren und letztlich unkontrollierbaren Kommunikation zu tun, die dennoch hochproduktiv ist. Jeder versteht Metaphern, aber alle ein bisschen oder völlig anders. Dennoch gibt es dominante oder weit verbreitete Metaphernkomplexe, die qua Üblichkeit über viele individuelle Differenzen und Nuancen hinweg funktionieren. Historisch zeigt sich, dass der jeweilige Stand der Wissenschaft ein Set von Metaphern hervorbringt, das z. B. auf Menschen oder andere Organismen übertragen wird. So gab es pneumatische Metaphern für das Herz als Pumpe und den Blutkreislauf. Mit der Elektrifizierung kamen Metaphern wie das Gehirn als Schaltzentrale und die Nerven als Leitungen hinzu. Mit der Computerisierung entstanden IT-technische Metaphern wie „etwas nicht auf dem Schirm haben“ oder „die Festplatte formatieren“. Der Prozess des Metaphorisierens lässt sich als eine Art Dialektik des Umetikettierens beschreiben, nämlich so wie ein Etikett aus einem etablierten Kontext auf ein neues Phänomen übertragen wird. Zum Beispiel „du tickst doch nicht richtig“ überträgt die mechanistische Metapher (einer mechanischen Uhr) auf die menschliche Psyche. Dies verändert sowohl die Quelldomäne als auch die Zieldomäne. Die menschliche Psyche wird in Kategorien einer Feinmechanik gesehen, und die Mechanik erhält geistige Bedeutungseinheiten (wie primitives Gehirn, was v. a. beim Sprung zur Digitaltechnik offenkundig wird).

Bei der künstlichen Intelligenz z. B. wird der Intelligenzbegriff von Menschen auf IT-Systeme übertragen, was eine anthropomorphe Technikvorstellung anregt. Gleichzeitig wird die Intelligenzvorstellung bei Menschen technizistischer gefasst. Die Dialektik des Umetikettierens zeigt, dass Metaphern die Zielbedeutung in der Quellbedeutung *aufheben*: Auf Hegel geht eine dreifache Hinsicht dieses *Aufhebens* zurück. Das ist etwas, was nur im Deutschen so wirklich gelingt, aber man kann das Aufheben als dreifachen Bedeutungshinweis nehmen. Man kann dann etwa sagen, dass durch die Übertragung einer Metapher die Quellbedeutung in der Zielbedeutung *aufgehoben* ist. Die drei Hinsichten sind dann folgende:

1) Aufheben meint einerseits *negieren*; dadurch, dass die Bedeutung einer Hinsicht in der Zieldomäne eine andere ist als in der Quelldomäne, ist sozusagen die Fassung der Quelldomäne negiert. Sie ist nicht mehr das, was sie einmal war. Intelligenz von IT-Systemen negiert die Intelligenzvorstellung von Menschen, wenn sie übertragen wurde. Man würde sagen, künstliche Intelligenz ist eben *nicht* menschliche Intelligenz. Dieses *„ist nicht“* negiert hier die Bedeutung. Also ist die Bedeutung, die einmal in der Quelldomäne gegolten hat, in der Zieldomäne aufgehoben, so wie ein Tempolimit, das bislang gegolten hat, ab einem entsprechenden Schild nicht mehr gilt.
2) Eine zweite Hinsicht des Aufhebens ist die des *Aufbewahrens*, des Konservierens. Dadurch dass eben die Bedeutung in der Zieldomäne aus der Quelldomäne kommt, bezieht sie ihre Bedeutungsgeschichte, ihre Ursprünge und ihre Anfangsbedeutung – ihre Bedeutungstradition – noch aus der Quelldomäne, die dann in der Zieldomäne mit diesem Label noch vorhanden sind und aufgehoben werden, insofern sie nicht gänzlich in der anderen Bedeutung negiert wurden. Die Herkunft des Konzepts aus der Quelldomäne wird in der Zieldomäne aufgehoben und aufbewahrt. Im Gegensatz dazu stünde, wenn man einfach ein neues Konzept einführen würde und das Alte obsolet werden ließe, dann würde das Alte verschwinden und wäre im Sprachgebrauch negiert und eben nirgends aufbewahrt. In einer Metapher bleibt es jedoch in der Zieldomäne trotz Negation noch aufbewahrt und vorhanden. So ist die Geschwindigkeitsbegrenzung von 30 km/h im „Tempo 30 aufgehoben“ Schild sowohl negiert (sie gilt nicht mehr, ist 5-fach durchgestrichen) als auch aufbewahrt (die Zahl steht noch auf dem Schild, wenn

auch ausgegraut und durchgestrichen). An einem 30-Aufgehoben Schild kann man eben erkennen, dass davor 30 km/h gegolten hat.

3) Eine *dritte* Bedeutungsebene von Aufheben wäre das *Hinaufheben auf ein höheres Niveau*, auf eine andere Bedeutungskomplexität. In der Verwendung des Konzepts in der Zieldomäne sind beide Bedeutungsgesamtheiten aus Quelldomäne und Zieldomäne kombiniert. Über das Wechselverhältnis von Negation und Konservierung bildet sich auf Zielebene eine neue Bedeutungsebene, die sowohl Bedeutungsaspekte auf Quellebene z. B. im Fall von ‚Virus' organischer Strukturen wie Nukleinsäuren und Proteinhüllen, Wirtszellen-basierte Replikation, Wirtsspezifität etc. mit spezifischen Bedeutungen auf der Zielebene, z. B. im Fall von ‚Computervirus' Befall von Dateien und Webseiten, Datenklau mit Erpressungspotenzial (Ransomware) etc. kombiniert.

Viren *als* Computerviren gefasst beinhaltet also ein neues Bedeutungsspektrum, das sich sowohl aus der Quelldomäne als auch der Zieldomäne speist und gleichzeitig durch die Negation bestimmter Aspekte der Quelldomäne gekennzeichnet ist. Welche Aspekte in dieser Metapher zum Tragen kommen, zeigt sich daran, welche Erwartungen durch den Sprachgebrauch angeregt werden.

Jede Metapher hat eine „wache" Übertragung und eine „vergessene" Geschichte sowie ein übliches Set an Erwartungen, das sie hervorruft. Dieses historische Bewusstsein ist wichtig, um den grundlegenden Charakter von Begriffen und Konzepten zu verstehen. Die Dialektik des Umetikettierens beschreibt die Übertragung von Konzepten über verschiedene Domänen hinweg, ohne dass es eine wahre, eindeutige und in wörtliche Rede überführbare Bedeutung gäbe. Es gibt immer nur Standardverwendungen oder Üblichkeiten, die im Wandel sind.

Arne Manzeschke: Der ganze Vorgang des Metaphorisierens ist anthropologisch betrachtet auch der Tatsache geschuldet, dass wir eben nicht immer eine theoretisch abgesicherte Evidenz für die Phänomene haben, mit denen wir umgehen müssen. Hätten wir diese Evidenz, diese sicheren Beweise, dann bräuchten wir nicht „drumherum zu reden". Das aber leistet die Metapher; sie entspricht unserem Wirklichkeitsbezug. Der ist „indirekt, umständlich, verzögert, selektiv und vor allem ‚metaphorisch'", wie es Blumenberg pointiert formuliert hat [1, S. 115]. Wir müssen darüber reden, wir versuchen, den anderen von unserer Sicht der Dinge zu überzeugen, manchmal auch ihn zu ‚überreden', weil es im Alltag (und sei es auch ein komplexer biotechnologischer Alltag) in den seltensten Fällen ausreicht, logisch eindeutig zu demonstrieren, was der Fall ist. Blumenberg hat in dem von mir genannten Artikel von 1971 aufgezeigt, dass wir bei aller naturwissenschaftlichen, technischen Orientierung auf die Rhetorik als Mittel der Erkenntnis und der Handlungsorientierung nicht verzichten können. Allerdings liefert die Rhetorik keine zweifelsfreien, gesetzmäßig ableitbaren Ergebnisse, sondern sie eröffnet einen Raum zur Verständigung. Sie ist ein Mittel, um kommunikativ Ergebnisse zu erzielen, die aber immer mit dem Risiko verbunden sind, eine Scheinevidenz zu produzieren bzw. eine mögliche Erkenntnis zu verfehlen. Das bedeutet also auch, dass die metaphorische Kommunikation fehl gehen könnte. Und zwar in dreierlei Hinsicht. Einmal, dass wir die Metapher falsch verstehen und sie für das Eigentliche ansehen. Zweitens, dass wir mit der Metapher das Gemeinte nicht treffen. Drittens, dass die Metapher eigentlich rhetorisch anderen Zwecken dient und uns deshalb in die Irre leitet. Bezogen auf den monoklonalen Antikörper lässt sich – rückblickend – vielleicht auch konstatieren, dass das metaphorische Angebot nicht angenommen worden ist, sondern – aus welchen Gründen auch immer – der Begriff allzu wörtlich genommen wurde und damit der Raum für Entdeckungen und Verständigung vorschnell verengt worden ist.

Stefan Heuser: Domenico Schneider hat in seinem Beitrag zu unserer Tagung darauf hingewiesen, wie stark die Verwendung technischer Geräte und Medien in den Naturwissenschaften die dafür verwendete Sprache mitbestimmen, so dass eine spezielle „Forscher"-Sprache entsteht. Die technischen Instrumente wirken sich auf die zugehörige Metaphorik aus. Er weist auf die doppelte Gefahr hin, dass hier Wunschvorstellungen die Ergebnisse der Forschung und Missverständnisse deren Rezeption in der Öffentlichkeit beeinflussen. Wie schätzt Du bzw. wie schätzt Ihr den Zusammenhang von Technopraxis, Theorie- und Metaphernbildung in der Biotechnologie ein und was bedeutet dies für die Wissenschaftskommunikation?

Arne Manzeschke: Der Begriff des *Genome Editing*, des Genom-Editierens ist m. E. ein schönes Beispiel. Der Laie kennt den Begriff des Editierens aus den Textverarbeitungsprogrammen am Computer. Der lateinische Begriff selbst hat seinen Sitz im Leben des Buchdruckens und -herausgebens (lat. *edere* von *e-dare* = aus-geben). Genome Editing wäre dann also so etwas wie a) ein Schreiben und Ändern von genetischem Text und b) die Herausgabe dieses neuen Textes, gleichsam die Freisetzung einer selbst erstellten genetischen Sequenz in den Genpool der Lebewesen. Während das Ändern von Text bzw. genetischer Information in seiner Ähnlichkeit noch leicht nachvollziehbar sein mag, so ist die „Herausgabe" dieses erstellten bzw. geänderten „genetischen Textes" ein Bild, das in seinen realen Konsequenzen sehr viel schwerer nachvollziehbar ist. Was sprachlich so leicht daher kommt, ist in seinen individuellen und gesellschaftlichen Konsequenzen unter Umständen sehr gravierend. Um das aber tatsächlich abschätzen, beraten und entscheiden zu können, bräuchte es Zeit, die bei der technischen Beschleunigung (das Genome Editing ist im Vergleich zur ‚natürlichen Züchtung' sehr viel zielgerichteter und schneller!) immer weniger vorhanden ist. Hier tut sich eine zeitliche Schere auf zwischen Technik und Ethik, die sich womöglich nicht mehr wird schließen lassen. Technik liefert einen Zeitgewinn gegenüber nicht-technischen oder technisch vorgängigen Verfahren; dieser Zeitgewinn bedeutet auf der Reflexionsebene dessen, was technisch getan wird und nun zu verstehen wäre, einen immer größeren Zeitverzug, der faktisch nicht mehr eingeholt werden kann. Oder wie es Hans Blumenberg gesagt hat: „Die Handlung verkümmert zur Reaktion, je direkter der Weg von der Theorie zur Praxis ist, der gesucht wird" [1, S. 123 f.]. Ein geeignetes Gegenmittel wäre ein „institutionalisiertes Atemholen" [1,

S. 122], das rhetorisch, also über eine sprachliche Verständigung geleistet werden könnte – aber häufig als umwegig, unnötig retardierend und ökonomisch kontraproduktiv abgewiesen wird.

Mit Bezug auf das Phänomen der künstlichen Intelligenz haben wir einmal Vorstellungsweisen gesammelt und sortiert. Das haben wir dann nicht nur auf der rein sprachlichen Ebene getan, sondern auch auf der Ebene von Bildern, die ja ebenfalls eine Ebene der Darstellung und Verständigung bilden [3]. Zwei Punkte, die uns bei dieser Arbeit sehr wichtig geworden sind, möchte ich zunächst hervorheben. Erstens hat sich noch einmal bestätigt, was in diesem Gespräch schon mehrfach Thema war: Wir Menschen können gar nicht anders, als uns auch über Um- und (scheinbare) Abwege zu verständigen (das zeigt auch die Verwendung von Metaphern in diesem Satz). Bei der Verständigung über den ontologischen Status einer KI (Was ist das eigentlich?) können wir aus mehreren Gründen nicht auf sprachliche Unschärfen verzichten. Zum einen ist das Phänomen KI nicht nur ein technisches Ding, das in seiner Konstruktion bzw. Funktion abschließend beschrieben werden könnte. Zum anderen ist seine technologische (Weiter-)Entwicklung so rasant, dass wir zwar jeweils über einen bestimmten *state of the art* sprechen, jedoch nichts Abschließendes hierzu sagen können. Das erinnert an ein Diktum Friedrich Nietzsches aus der Genealogie der Moral, wo er gesagt hat: „definirbar ist nur Das, was keine Geschichte hat". Die KI aber hat eine Geschichte, nicht nur eine Technikgeschichte, in der man die jeweiligen kalkulatorischen Möglichkeiten und Leistungen ablesen kann, sondern eine Geschichte, die mit den menschlichen Erwartungen/Befürchtungen, mit unterschiedlichen Konzepten von Intelligenz verbunden ist [4, 5].

Bruno Gransche: Hier möchte ich ganz kurz ergänzen, was mich v. a. Paul Ricœur über Geschichte und damit dieses schöne Zitat von Nietzsche anders verstehen gelehrt hat: Wir verstehen alltagssprachlich Geschichte meist als das Vergangene; „Geschichte haben" meint aber v. a. in ein Geschehen eingelassen zu sein, in ein Werden und in Änderungsprozesse, also keineswegs nur abgeschlossene Geschichte, sondern in ein andauerndes Geschehen. Das hat auch mit Narrationen zu tun; was Geschichte hat, ist *in Geschichten verstrickt* – so nennt es Wilhelm Schapp – und Geschichte, die sich noch laufend entfaltet und von ihren Akteuren geändert werden kann, die kann auch nicht ‚definiert' werden, denn: Was kein *Ende* (*finis*) hat, das kann auch nicht *vom Ende her* (*de fine*) auf eine Bedeutung *festgestellt oder festgelegt* (*definiert*) werden. Daher nennt Nietzsche in *Jenseits von Gut und Böse* den Menschen auch „das *noch nicht festgestellte Tier*". Leben, Werden, andauernde Geschichten, reflektiert, verstanden und kommuniziert in lebendigen Metaphern, haben (noch) kein Ende und keine Grenzen und damit eben auch keine *De-Finitionen*. Das zeigt auch sprachlich und Nietzsche flankierend nochmal schön, wie sehr wir Lebendigen auf Uneindeutigkeiten und flexible Grenzen angewiesen sind und wie sehr sich eigentlich das Ansinnen einer *zu Ende bringenden*, also *de-finitorischen* Festlegung mit den Herausforderungen der im stetigen Wandel Begriffenen beißt. Aber zurück zur Geschichtlichkeit und also Wandlungsdynamik von KI.

Arne Manzeschke: Der Aspekt der Geschichtlichkeit von KI erhält noch eine besondere Wendung darin, dass die Geschichte der KI nicht nur als *genitivus objectivus* gelesen werden kann, sondern auch als *genitivus subjectivus*: In dem Maße, in dem sie Texte und Bilder generiert, also selbst das Arsenal unserer kommunikativen Möglichkeiten erweitert und bestimmt – und wir zunehmend nicht unterscheiden können, was die Quellen unserer Verständigungsgrundlagen sind –, macht die KI selbst Geschichte.

Der zweite Punkt, den ich gerne hervorheben möchte, ist der, dass das metaphorische Potenzial von KI überaus mächtig ist. Unser Sammeln und Sortieren von Vorstellungsweisen von KI hat eine große Fülle von Bildern, Vergleichen, Analogien und Metaphern zutage gefördert, die gezeigt haben, dass sich das Phänomen KI enorm reaktiv zeigt, d. h. sie verbindet sich mit sehr vielen verschiedenen, teils auch gegensätzlichen Elementen. Was uns beim Systematisieren dieser Verbindungen verwundert hat, ist die Tatsache, dass trotz dieser enormen Reaktionsfreudigkeit die Aussagengehalte über KI nicht unbedingt zugenommen haben. Mit anderen Worten: Die große Menge der Bilder und Sprachspiele informieren nicht wirklich und ermöglichen nicht wirklich ein besseres Verständnis des Phänomens.

Stefan Heuser: Deine Überlegungen zur Metaphorik der KI unterstreichen für mich die Notwendigkeit einer Metaphernkritik, die sich nicht nur mit Bezug auf Herrschafts- und Ideologiekritik stellt, sondern auch mit Blick auf die Erkennbarkeit der Phänomene bzw. des besonderen Phänomens. Die Suche nach Metaphern bleibt eingespannt in den Versuch, der Welt eine Ordnung abzugewinnen und sie erhält von dieser unabschließbaren Aufgabe ihre Dynamik. Die Suche nach wirklichkeitsgemäßen Metaphern, die unsere Wahrnehmung leiten und unser Handeln orientieren, kann also – da können wir wieder Blumenberg als Referenz nennen – nicht darauf zurückgreifen, dass sich für uns wie bei Heidegger so etwas wie der „Sinn" des Seins „entbirgt". Zugleich aber stellt sich die Frage, wie wir die metaphorische Erschließung der Wirklichkeit an eine kritische Überprüfung der Wirklichkeitsgemäßheit unserer Metaphern koppeln. Lässt sich identifizieren bzw. kategorisieren, welcher Art die Bezugspunkte, Aspekte, Widerstände, Differenzen usw. von „Wirklichkeit" sind, die unsere Metaphernbildung nicht nur in Gang halten, sondern vielleicht sogar anleiten bzw. orientieren können?

Bruno Gransche: Metaphorisierungen übertragen Bedeutungsaspekte von einem bekannten vertrauten Bereich, auch als Quelldomäne oder Source Domain bezeichnet, auf einen weniger vertrauten Bereich, der in Hinsicht der Quelldomäne verstanden werden soll oder zu sehen angeregt wird. Dieser eher unvertraute Bereich, die Konzepte, über die mittels der Metapher etwas gesagt werden soll, kann man entsprechend als Zieldomäne oder Target Domain bezeichnen – wie z. B. Johnson und Lakoff das in „Metaphors we live by“ tun. In der Metapherntheorie werden die beiden manchmal auch als Vehikel und Tenor (auch selbst wieder Metaphern) bezeichnet. Dabei ist die Quelldomäne das Vehikel, mittels dessen etwas zu verstehen gegeben wird, und die Zieldomäne der Tenor, das Konzept, das Thema, um das es geht, über das etwas ausgesagt werden soll. Es ist nicht nur so, dass wir beispielsweise Technik mit menschlichen Begriffen verstehen oder in menschlichen Bedeutungshinsichten metaphorisieren, also zum Beispiel von einem Roboter als einem Gefährten oder Companion reden und damit anregen, den Roboter als eine Art von Agenten zu sehen in einer Rolle, wie wir menschliche Gefährten sehen mit Implikationen wie Freundschaft, Beistand, Vertrautheit, wechselseitiges Interesse aneinander, geteilte Werte und Ziele etc. Das große Problem an den Bedeutungsübertragungen der Metaphorisierungen ist, dass fraglich ist, welche Bedeutungsaspekte der Quelldomäne sinnvollerweise auf die Zieldomäne übertragen werden können, in welcher Hinsicht also der Tenor mittels eines Vehikels anders gesehen werden soll und kann. So gibt es als naturförmige Technikvorstellung die Metapher von KI als Welle [6].

Damit kann zu verstehen gegeben werden, dass es sich um eine Bewegung mit großem Momentum handelt und nicht um etwa ein Werkzeug wie ein Schraubenzieher, den man weglegen und konkret kontrollieren kann. Entsprechend suggeriert die Welle-Metapher auch eine gewisse Eigendynamik oder Naturförmigkeit, eine Unkontrollierbarkeit und tendenziell auch die Dramatik von Überleben und Nicht-Überleben, wenn man von einer Welle erfasst wird; dann die Fremdbestimmtheit desjenigen, der von einer Welle mitgerissen wird, und so weiter. Dies alles sind Aspekte, die in der Rede von KI als Welle intendiert sein können. Es kann aber auch lediglich das zyklische Auftreten und Verschwinden von Interesse und Aufmerksamkeit an KI – ebenfalls physiomorph als KI-Sommer und KI-Winter metaphorisiert – gemeint sein, wie Wellen am Strand kontinuierlich kommen und gehen. Nicht gemeint sind allerdings andere Aspekte, die auch in der Quelldomäne der Welle enthalten sind. Beispielsweise möchte keiner, der sagt, KI sei eine Welle, damit sagen, dass wir KI als salzig oder flüssig oder mondphasenabhängig oder von Poseidon regiert verstehen sollten. Alles das ist jedoch auch im semantischen Raum der Welle inkludiert.

Die Frage ist nun, wie wir die sinnvoll übertragbaren Aspekte von den Aspekten unterscheiden, die in der Source Domain zurückgelassen werden müssen, weil sie sonst unsinnige Übertragungen wie salzige KI ergäben. Dazu brauchen wir einen gewissen kulturellen Kontext, einen Verstehenshorizont, eine Mindestinformiertheit über die Zieldomäne, die es uns ermöglicht, die Übertragungshinsicht, die im Metaphorisieren sprachlich selten explizit markiert wird, zu dechiffrieren und zu verstehen. Und dieses Verstehen ist kultur- und geschichtsabhängig, individuell vom eigenen Horizont und Bildungsstand und so weiter, also vom Deutungshorizont, der historisch kulturell geprägt ist. Schließlich bestehen massive interkulturelle Differenzen der Aspekte, die in einer jeweiligen Quelldomäne verbunden sind. So hat zum Beispiel die Kuh in Westeuropa sicher eine andere semantische Konnotation als beispielsweise in Indien, wo sie auch religiös konnotiert ist, während sie in Westeuropa eher als Nutzvieh instrumenteller gesehen wird. Das Übertragungsgeschehen oder das Set von Quelldomänen und Zieldomänen muss zur Erhellung der Übertragungsdynamik und Verstehenspotenziale in einer komplexen Matrix betrachtet werden, da sich nicht nur anthropomorphe Technikkonzepte, sondern auch biomorphe Technikkonzepte oder technomorphe Tierkonzepte und so weiter miteinander verschränken. Je nach Vehikel, je nach Quellkonzept der Metaphorisierung, sind andere Bedeutungsebenen und Aspekte im Spiel, die üblicherweise übertragen werden und die es zu dechiffrieren gilt.

Ein Vorschlag wäre etwa von einem Set an Zielkonzepten, oder Themen auszugehen. Wir haben dies an anderer Stelle als Matrix der Metaphorisierungen vorgeschlagen (die Matrix kann eingesehen werden unter: https://www.brunogransche.de/publikationen#PosterundGrafiken). Dieses Set könnte auch völlig anders zugeschnitten werden. Wir nehmen in der Matrix eine exemplarische Auswahl, um das Prinzip klarzumachen. Die Matrix muss allerdings weiter ausdifferenziert werden und kann und sollte in seiner Vielfalt verschieden entwickelt werden. Die Idee ist denkbar einfach: Wir tragen auf der einen Seite, der Y-Achse, Vehikel und die Quelldomänen ab und auf der anderen Seite, der X-Achse, dieselben Konzepte als Tenor-Set (also die Zieldomänen) und versuchen dann zu ergründen, was in den Schnittstellen beispielsweise phytomorphe, also pflanzenförmige Technikkonzepte sind und so weiter. So könnte man unterscheiden in Zieldomänensicht: Natur, Technik, Leben, Pflanzen, Tiere, Menschen, vielleicht unterteilt noch in Männer und Frauen (oder spezifischer Kinder etc. je nach Untersuchungsinteresse), dann so etwas wie Heroen oder Halbgötter und schließlich Gottheiten. Je nach Weltsicht wäre das dann wieder ein Kreis, der sich zur Natur schließt oder dieser entsprechend entgegengesetzt ist. Hier sieht man bereits, dass diese Tenor-Konzepte kategorial nicht auf einer Ebene liegen, sondern teils Über- und Unterkonzepte darstellen. Insofern soll hier auch keine kategorial exklusive Ontologie abgebildet werden, sondern exemplarische Hinsichten unseres Metaphorisierens verdeutlicht werden. Klar ist, dass Pflanzen, Tiere und Menschen dem Bereich des Lebendigen angehören, also Leben eine Überkategorie ist und dass all dies inklusive der Technik den Bereich der Natur umfasst. Schließlich ist selbst KI aus Erde gemacht, nämlich aus seltenen Erden und so weiter. Das heißt, diese Kategorien sind nicht exklusiv. Interessant ist ja gerade, was die geläufigen Metaphern über unsere Natur- und Menschenvorstellungen aussagen, insofern bildet die Matrix Fokushinsichten ab und häufig lassen sich konkrete Metaphorisierungen in mehrere Felder einordnen, bzw. an einer Metaphorisierung Hinsichten aus mehreren Bereichen der Matrix kombiniert und in aufschlussreicher Wechselwirkung herausheben. Dieselben Einheiten – Natur, Technik, Leben, Pflanzen, Tiere, Menschen, Heroen, Gottheiten – lassen sich nun auch auf Vehikelebene als Quelldomäne einsetzen, womit dann gewisse Vorstellungen als naturförmig, technikförmig, pflanzenförmig, menschenförmig oder -gestaltig und so weiter angeregt werden. Und entsprechend wären diese Vehikeleinheiten dann naturförmig oder physiomorph, technikförmig oder technomorph, lebensförmig oder biomorph, pflanzenförmig / phytomorph, tierförmig / zoomorph, menschenförmig / anthropomorph, männerförmig / andromorph, frauenförmig / gynomorph, heroenförmig / heromorph oder halbgottförmig / hemitheomorph und schließlich gottheitenförmig bzw. theomorph.

In einer Anordnung, wo die Quelldomänen die Y-Förmigkeit, die Y-Gestaltigkeit, die Y-Artigkeit der Vorstellung in den Zeilen abgetragen werden und die Zieldomänen, die Konzepte, über die etwas ausgesagt, etwas zu verstehen gegeben werden soll, dazu in Spalten angeordnet werden, entsteht eine Matrix, die jede Quelldomäne mit jeder Zieldomäne kombiniert (Link zur Matrix s. o.). Klarerweise ist in der entstehenden Diagonalen der Felder die redundante Selbstreflexivität zu berücksichtigen, da naturförmige Naturkonzepte oder technomorphe Technikkonzepte pleonastisch sind. Dann ergeben sich in den weiteren Matrixfeldern zum Beispiel physiomorphe Technikkonzepte oder technomorphe Pflanzenkonzepte, phytomorphe Menschenkonzepte, andromorphe Tierkonzepte oder theomorphe Menschenkonzepte, theomorphe Technikkonzepte usw.

Stefan Heuser: Diese metaphorologische Matrix finde ich sehr inspirierend und aussagekräftig – und zugleich fällt mir vor dem Hintergrund unserer Auseinandersetzung mit Blumenberg auf, dass Eure Matrix ausdrücklich bis hinein in die Welt des Mythos reicht. Die Funktion des Mythos ist es nach Blumenberg, Distanz zu einer den Menschen bedrängenden Wirklichkeit, zum „Absolutismus der Wirklichkeit" zu etablieren [7]. Dies geschieht dadurch, dass die namenlosen Dinge der uns Menschen ängstigenden Wirklichkeit im Mythos konkrete Namen erhalten und menschliche Eigenschaften zugeschrieben bekommen, so dass sie weniger bedrohlich erscheinen. Anthropomorphisierung ist demnach ein zentraler Bestandteil der Wirkweise des Mythos. Eure Matrix macht eine sehr differenzierte Spannbreite von Übertragungsphänomenen sichtbar. Kannst Du bzw. könnt Ihr für die Anwendung Eurer Matrix bitte ein paar Beispiele geben? Mich würde dabei vor allem interessieren, ob mit bestimmten Kombinationen von Quell- und Zieldomänen auch bestimmte Kategorien von Funktionen verbunden sind, die die Metaphern anzeigen.

Bruno Gransche: Fokussieren wir uns hier beispielhaft auf Natur, Technik und Leben. Physiomorphe Technikkonzepte wären etwa fließende Architektur oder Häuser sprießen wie Pilze aus dem Boden. Physiomorphe Lebenskonzepte wären der Fluss des Lebens oder der Lebensabend. (IT-Namensüblichkeiten wie Motherboard, BIOS, Master/Slave, Memory etc. stellen ein ganz eigenes Feld dar, das es lohnen würde, auf Vorstellungsorientierungen hin zu untersuchen.) Am anderen Ende des Spektrums hätten wir physiomorphe, also naturförmig gedachte oder zu verstehen gegebene Gottheiten, wie etwa die Assoziation von Donner und Blitz mit Zeus und Thor oder das Verständnis, dass diese Gottheiten ihren Ausdruck in diesen Naturgewalten finden. Vulkanausbrüche als Naturereignisse werden dem Wüten des Typhon unter dem Berg zugeschrieben oder generell Erdbeben als Ausdruck von Emotionalität, meistens Zorn des Poseidons, mit dem Epitheton "Erderschütterer" verbunden.

Das sind naturförmige Gottheitskonzepte oder Verschränkungen von Naturphänomen und -implikationen mit theomorphen Hinsichten.

Bei der fließenden Architektur oder dem Fluss des Lebens und dem Lebensabend haben wir die unbelebte Natur als Quelldomäne, als Vehikel. Wir können aber auch konkret biomorphe Hinsichten analysieren, wobei die lebendige Natur oder das Leben als Bedeutungsquelle fungiert. So haben wir zum Beispiel Metaphern wie "Felsen trotzen der Brandung", wobei das Trotzen als etwas, das mit einer Motivation oder einer Weigerung zu weichen verbunden wird, Teil von lebendigen Entitäten ist, und auf Felsen, also unbelebte Natur, übertragen wird. Oder die Metaphern wie atmende, klagende, heulende Winde oder der Atem des Zephyr oder Aiolos bezeichnen Hinsichten, die Spezifika lebender Wesen, nämlich z. B. Atem, auf unbelebte Natur übertragen und damit eine biomorphe Naturmetaphorisierung darstellen. Die „Zephyr Ventile" als medizintechnische Eingriffe bei bestimmten Lungenproblemen und Atemschwierigkeiten schlagen hier direkt die Brücke von mythisch basierten animistischen biomorphen Naturmetaphern zu physio- und biomorph orientierten Technikvorstellungen. Biomorphizität haben wir auch bei Technikhinsichten, die angeregt werden durch Metaphern wie evolutionäre Algorithmen oder selbstheilende Lacke oder Beton, wobei Vorstellungen wie evolutionäre Entwicklung, Mutation, Selektion, Variation usw. auf Algorithmen oder Geräte-Sukzessionen übertragen werden, wie die Evolution des Smartphones, oder Heilungseffekte, die Merkmale von Lebewesen sind, auf technische Fähigkeiten übertragen werden. Insofern die Wissenschaft mitsamt der Technik Elemente des griechischen techné-Begriffs sind, lassen sich verschiedene phytomorphe Vorstellungen der Wissensorganisation hier anführen: einerseits hierarchische *Baum*strukturen (Stammbaum, Entscheidungsbäume, Datenstrukturen, Organisationsbaumdiagramme, biologische Systematiken mit Art, Gattung, Familie etc.) und andererseits vernetzte *Rhizom*strukturen (Verlinkungsstrukturen zwischen Webseiten, Wikipedia, sozialen Netzwerken oder das Internet) [8]. Die Entitäten, also die Zieldomänen, die ohnehin unter den Bereich des Lebens fallen, sind wiederum als biomorph zu sehen und haben meist eine Nähe zur Selbstreflexivität und damit zum Pleonasmus. Biomorphe Pflanzenkonzepte oder biomorphe Menschenkonzepte sind insofern möglicherweise weniger instruktiv, als dass Quell- und Zielbereich nicht weit genug auseinanderliegen, um metaphorisch einen „Anders-sehen"-Mehrwert einer neuen Hinsicht zu geben. Grob gesprochen: es mag auch biomorphe Tierkonzepte und biomorphe Menschenkonzepte geben, die vor allem das Lebendigsein oder Teil des Bereichs des Lebens zu sein betonen, aber sie tragen nicht wirklich eine zieldomänenfremde Bedeutungshinsicht bei, sondern fokussieren oder explizieren eine implizite Verbindung von Quelle und Ziel.

Entsprechend der Matrix lassen sich, wenn es physiomorphe und biomorphe Technikkonzepte gibt, Ziel- und Quelldomäne tauschen und man kann von technomorphen Natur- und technomorphen Lebensvorstellungen sprechen. Eine technomorphe Naturvorstellung wäre etwa der Wald als Tempel oder die Himmelsmechanik und Weltenuhr. Das regt an, ein Naturphänomen in technischen Hinsichten unter technischen Konzepten zu verstehen, etwa naturwüchsige Konstellationen wie einen Wald und eine Konstellation von Bäumen über eine Formähnlichkeit zwischen Baum und Säule, die typisch für antike Tempelarchitekturen ist, einen Vergleich zu ziehen und dann anzuregen, dass Funktionalitäten, die im Tempel, qua Architektur und kultureller Institutionen relevant sind, sich in die Natur und den Wald übertragen lassen, also etwa Momente des Gebetes, der meditativen Einkehr, der Spiritualität usw. Ein Aspekt der theomorphen Naturvorstellung oder eine Hinsicht auf Wald als etwas Heiliges findet sich in der germanischen Mythologie, bis heute vermutlich eine Wurzel des speziellen Verhältnisses der Deutschen zum Wald. Ein theomorphes Pflanzenkonzept, also ein unter der Hinsicht von Göttlichem zu verstehendes Naturphänomen wie Pflanzen, in diesem Fall ein Baum, wäre der Weltenbaum Yggdrasil in der nordischen Mythologie, der die verschiedenen nordisch-mythologischen Welten (Asgard, Midgard usw.) miteinander vereint und an dessen Quelle Odin seine Fähigkeit, die Zukunft zu sehen, gegen eines seiner Augen eingetauscht haben soll, laut Mythos. Yggdrasil, ein Baum, ist hier also von nicht zu unterschätzender Zentralität im narrativen Reservoir nordischer Erzählungen.

Technomorphe Lebenskonzepte wären etwa der bereits erwähnte Code des Lebens für die DNA. Hier wird eine technische Zeichenform, nämlich der Code, auf das Leben metaphorisch übertragen – Arne hat auf das Editieren und Genome Editing schon verwiesen. Entsprechend ist die Rede von genetischen Programmen, aber auch andere Beispiele sind instruktiv wie ölfressende Bakterien als technisiertes Mittel und Biofakt (Fusion zwischen *Bios* und *Arte*-Fakt) gegen Ölverschmutzung oder die fadenwebenden Moiren, die Schicksalsvorstellung der griechischen Mythologie, dass die drei Moiren, die Schicksalsgottheiten, die Geschicke und das Schicksal aller Lebewesen in Form von Fäden, den Lebensfäden, miteinander verweben. Hier ist auch das Fadenspinnen und Zurechtkürzen, das Musterweben, eine technizistische, eine technomorphe Lebensvorstellung, aber auch eine technomorphe Gottheitsvorstellung. Eine Weberin zu sein, also die Funktion, einen technischen Webvorgang vollziehen zu können, zumal mit Lebensfäden, stellt dann wiederum eine Gottheitsvorstellung dar (paradigmatisch dafür auch Athene).

Entsprechend gibt es weitere Einträge in der Zeile der technomorphen Metaphorisierungen. Wir hatten technomorphe Natur- und Lebensvorstellungen, technomorphe Tiervorstellungen, zum Beispiel in der Kreuzung oder der Zucht, wie also mit technischen Mitteln neue Arten, neue Rassen usw. erzeugt werden, dann Vorstellungen der Biofakte, etwa Klonen, das Schaf Dolly oder der Affe ANDi, der mit einem Quallen-Gen gespliced wurde, oder auch funktionale Metaphorisierungen, technomorphe Tiervorstellungen wie der Hund als Alarmanlage oder die Brieftaube als Kommunikationsmittel usw. Technomorphe Menschenvorstellungen wären etwa der Cyborg, häufig männlich konnotiert, aber von Donna Haraway besonders auch auf Frauen übertragen. Dann die Kreatur, überhaupt das Kreaturkonzept: Der Mensch als geschaffen durch Gott ist in diesem Falle ein poietisch, also durch herstellende Maßnahmen erzeugtes und eben nicht evolutionär entstandenes Phänomen in der Hinsicht und damit korrelieren Menschen als Kreaturen, also gemachte, geschaffene, poietisch erzeugte Wesen und entsprechende technomorphe Gottheitsvorstellungen als Intelligent Design, Schöpfer oder Demiurg.

Stefan Heuser: In der Theologie hat es sich eingebürgert, die Rede vom Menschen als Geschöpf und vom Menschen als Produkt von Evolution als komplementäre Redeweisen zu betrachten. Dazu gehört, dass man „Kreatur" nicht kausal, sondern relational versteht, um sich von kreationistischen Vorstellungen wie dem „Intelligent Design" abzugrenzen. Dass Gott Menschen „erschafft", wird in der hebräischen Sprache durch das Verb „bara" ausgedrückt, z. B. in der Urgeschichte in Gen 1,27. Da ist das Verb ein terminus technicus für die Art und Weise, wie Gott Dinge schafft, d. h. es wird exklusiv für Gott verwendet. Aber um noch einmal in Richtung von Blumenberg zu denken, der Technik in ihrer Funktion für die menschliche Selbstbehauptung angesichts einer bedrohlichen Wirklichkeit in den Blick nimmt: Lassen sich mit Eurer Matrix auch technomorphe Vorstellungen vom Menschen analysieren, bei denen „Technik" reflexiv wird, d. h. sich in ihrer Funktion auf den Menschen selbst richtet?

Bruno Gransche: Wir haben technomorphe Menschenkonzepte etwa in der Industrie, wenn man sich „Modern Times" von Chaplin vergegenwärtigt, wie sehr Menschen da als technische Teile – als Rädchen – in Produktionsprozessen gefasst und eingespannt wurden in entsprechend dehumanisierenden Fabrikarbeitskontexten. In der Medizin finden sich technomorphe Menschenkonzepte, überhaupt anthropologische Vorstellungen, nämlich vom Herz als Pumpe oder dem Blutkreislaufsystem entsprechend als Pumpsystem, dann die Sehnen im Sinne von Seilzügen bis hin zu später elektrischen Vorstellungen, die Nerven als Leitungen und Leiterbahnen, die Synapsen als Schnittstellen usw. Die Sinne als Sensoren, das alles sind technomorphe Menschenvorstellungen oder auch auf Organismen bezogene Tiervorstellungen und Pflanzenvorstellungen. Schließlich die Idee des Enhancements, dass man mit technischen Eingriffen die Essenz dessen, was Menschen ausmacht, verändern könnte, bis hin zur Vorstellung post- und transhumanistischer Gestaltbarkeit und technischer Transformierbarkeit des Menschen. Schließlich wären technomorphe spezifische Frauenkonzepte etwa die technizistische Reduktion auf die Fortpflanzungsfunktion in der Vorstellung der Gebärmaschine. Technomorphe Heroen oder Halbgötter finden wir in Vorstellungen des „Neomythos", etwa bei Superhelden wie Batman oder Iron Man. Batman, im Gegensatz zu Außerirdischen wie Superman, ist ein ‚normaler' Mensch, der rein durch Training, Disziplin, Intelligenz und v. a. *Technik* Superheldenstatus erreicht. Freud schlug vor, dass der Mensch mit seinen technischen Hilfsmitteln zu einem „Prothesengott" würde. Hier würde die technomorphe Menschvorstellung in eine technomorphe Gott- oder Halbgöttervorstellung umschlagen. Entsprechend gibt es Figuren, die über technische Aufrüstung mythologisch in den Übermenschen- oder Superhuman-Status, also den Status eines Heroen einzuordnen wären. Beispiele sind Dädalus, das menschliche Äquivalent des Technik-Gottes Hephaestus, und Dädalus' Sohn Ikarus, der Prothesenflügler. Der Aufstieg von Ikarus durch die überragende

Technik seines Vaters zu einer Art Übermensch oder Heros, der dann mit technischer Hilfe auch fliegen kann, ist bekanntlich mit einer kritischen Mahnung der Hybris und des Falls verbunden. Ein weiteres Beispiel ist die Idee von Menschen, die mittels eines göttlichen Zusatzes, nämlich dem Technikgeschenk des prometheischen Feuers, aufgerüstet werden. Prometheus hebt die Menschen mittels dieses Feuers über den Tierstatus hinaus, wobei das Feuer *techné*, allgemein Technik, Wissenschaft und Methode symbolisiert.

Technomorphe Gottheitsvorstellungen finden wir häufig in der Science-Fiction. Die Matrix (Filme mit Keanu Reeves) oder Skynet aus den Filmen um Terminator sind Beispiele für omnipräsente und schier omnipotente technische Systeme, die gegen die Menschheit kämpfen. Ideen wie Intelligent Design oder der Schöpfergott sind insofern technisch, als sie ein Produkt schaffen und herstellen können. Zu diesen Produkten, diesen Kreationen, gehören dann auch Menschen, Tiere, Pflanzen und so weiter. Prometheus ist in gewisser Hinsicht eine technomorphe Gottheitsvorstellung, denn er hat in demiurgischer Hinsicht die Menschen aus Lehm und Asche hergestellt. In gewissen Varianten des Mythos tat er dies sogar aus der Asche von zwei durch Zeus verbrannten Giganten, die zuvor den Lieblingssohn von Zeus, Zagreus, verstümmelt und verspeist hatten. Die Asche enthielt laut Mythos sowohl die Asche von Giganten als auch von Gottheiten. Das ist das Ausgangsmaterial, aus dem der technizistische Schöpfer-Titan Prometheus, die Menschen geschaffen haben soll. Diese tragen entsprechend Teile der Mutter Gaia (Erde, Lehm), Teile der Giganten (Asche) und des olympisch Göttlichen (Asche) in sich, was erklären sollte, warum Menschen zwischen gut (hier Zagreus) und böse (hier die von Hera geschickten Giganten) changieren können.

Arne Manzeschke: 1748 erscheint *L'homme machine* von Julien Offray De La Mettrie, in dem er die – damals noch als Gotteslästerung gelesene – These vertritt, der Mensch sei nichts anderes als eine Maschine; für all sein Dasein und Tun gebe es eine materialistische Erklärung, auf Vorstellungen, wie Seele, Geist oder freier Wille könne/solle man verzichten. Das ist die seinerzeit wohl radikalste Formulierung eines Maschinen-Menschen – metaphorologisch gesprochen wirkt hier ein technisches Denkmodell auf das Selbstverständnis des Menschen unmittelbar zurück. Seitdem sind immer wieder Positionen vertreten worden, die in monistischer Weise das Materielle am Menschen betonen und dualistische Positionen (eine komplementäre Wechselwirkung von Materie und Geist) entschieden zurückweisen. Verfolgt man diese Kontroverse genauer, so stößt man auf sozialwissenschaftliche und historische Untersuchungen, die zeigen, dass dem Antagonismus von materialistischen und idealistischen Konzeptionen vom Menschen wie in einem System kommunizierender Röhren (Vorsicht: Metapher) mal mehr nach der einen, mal mehr nach der Seite der Vorrang eingeräumt wird [9]. Das heißt: Wie sich Menschen verstehen, hängt eben auch davon ab, in welcher dominanten Diskurslage – vorhin sprachen wir vom Horizont – sie sich vorfinden und welches Konzept mit welcher sozialen Praxis unterstützt und ‚eingeschrieben' wird. Dabei wird man davon ausgehen müssen, dass es in einer pluralen Gesellschaft wohl nie nur ein Konzept und nur eine Praxis geben wird, aber eben doch vorherrschende und solche, die weniger Aufmerksamkeit finden und Wirksamkeit entfalten.

Die Herausforderung besteht nun meines Erachtens darin, ob wir Menschen dieser ‚Formatierung' durch bestimmte (von uns selbst erstellte) Technik ansichtig werden oder nicht. Dabei können Metaphern helfen, sie können das aber auch verschleiern oder verschließen. In einem weiteren Schritt wäre darüberhinaus noch zu fragen, wie diese Rückwirkungen der Technik auf die Menschen bewertet werden. Hier sind wir dann mit ethischen Fragen konfrontiert, die umso überzeugender beraten werden können, je präziser die Konstellation sprachlich erfasst werden kann. Deshalb ist aus unserer Sicht eine solche Matrix hilfreich. Sie regt zunächst einmal an, die Differenziertheit von Übertragungen wahrzunehmen und so ein präziseres, weil vielschichtigeres Tableau möglicher Verstehensweisen der Menschen in Bezug auf x, y, ... zu gewinnen. Diese Analyse erlaubt es dann auch, die damit einhergehenden moralischen Bewertungen besser einordnen zu können und entsprechend in der ethischen Reflexion zielgenauer zu arbeiten.

Bruno Gransche: Hier noch einmal der Link zur Entwurfsversion unserer Matrix: https://www.brunogransche.de/publikationen#PosterundGrafiken. Eine Systematisierung solcher Übertragungen von Quelldomänen auf Zielkonzepte eröffnet einen konkreteren Blick auf das lebhafte Übertragungsgeschehen in unserer Sprache. Damit verbunden sind Einsichten, wie wir auf unbekannte Zieldomänen mittels bekannter Konzepte zugreifen und etwas in der Hinsicht von etwas Anderem, der Quelle, zu verstehen geben oder zu sehen lehren. Interessant ist dann ein zweiter Schritt, gewissermaßen ein Schritt zurück hinter die Systematisierung dieser Matrix, wenn einem in den Beispielen übergreifende Strukturen auffallen. So sieht man zum Beispiel, dass Technik und technizistische, technomorphe Vorstellungen sowie Menschen und anthropomorphe Vorstellungen sehr häufige Metaphernquellen darstellen. Wir haben also einen großen Metaphernreichtum, der uns nahelegt, andere Phänomene wie Natur, Technik, Tiere und Gottheiten in Hinsichten zu verstehen, wie wir sie auf Menschen anwenden. Genauso haben wir eine große Tradition darin, nicht-technische Dinge wie Natur, Leben und Menschen technizistisch, also in technischer Hinsicht zu begreifen und sie damit gemäß für Menschen als disponibel, nämlich für Eingriffe und Herstellungsprozesse offen zu suggerieren. Das wiederum legt eine Spur für Forschung und Entwicklung zur weiteren Eröffnung tatsächlicher technomorpher Zugriffmöglichkeiten von Natur und Menschen, wie beispielsweise über die Genetik oder der CRISPR/Cas Genschere. Im Übrigen ist die Genschere auch ein anachronistisch technizistischer Ausdruck für eine technische Zugriffweise auf Natürliches, die über die mechanische Schneidevorrichtung der Schere suggeriert wird.

Eine übergeordnete Frage und Forschungsgegenstand ist dann, welche Konsequenzen aus typischen Kombinationen von Quelldomäne und Zieldomäne entstehen. Was hat es für Implikationen, was hat es zu bedeuten, was folgt daraus, wenn wir verstärkt auf alle möglichen Zielkonzepte mit technomorphen, technizistischen Metaphern zugreifen, sie also wenngleich Nicht-Technik als etwas Technisches oder in technischer Hinsicht auffassen und denken? Was hat es für Konsequenzen, was ist damit ausgesagt, wenn wir auf künstliche Phänomene wie Technik in Form von physiomorphen, also naturförmigen Metaphern, zugreifen? Was hat die Physiomorphizität, die Naturförmigkeit von Metaphern, von künstlichen Zielbereichen, von allgemein aus der Natur sonst abgegrenzten Zielbereichen für Konsequenzen? Was bedeutet es, wenn wir etwas Nicht-Natürliches als Natürlich zu verstehen geben? Ethisch liegt hier das umstrittene Naturrechtsargument nicht fern, also die Idee, dass etwas, wenn es in der Natur der Fall ist, daraus auch eine normative Legitimität bezieht bzw. (häufiger genutzt), dass etwas angeblich ‚widernatürlich' sei, begründe auch dessen moralische Ablehnung. Was bedeutet es, wenn wir etwas Nicht-Menschliches als menschlich zu verstehen geben? Was folgt daraus, wenn wir etwas Menschliches als heroisch, halbgöttlich oder sogar göttlich als theomorph zu verstehen geben und so weiter? Die Hoffnung dieser Analyseperspektive ist es, übergreifende Muster identifizieren zu können, in die sich einzelne Metaphorisierungen als Exemplare, als Tokens von Types, einordnen lassen und somit im Kontext eines breiteren Verstehenshorizont analysiert werden können. So lässt sich beispielsweise bezüglich der Technik im Zuge der Kybernetik die Tendenz einer Biologisierung feststellen, die bei der künstlichen Intelligenz (die in der direkten Abfolge oder in Abgrenzung zur Kybernetik so bezeichnet wurde) dann zu einer Psychologisierung von Technik übergeht. Mit Psychologisierung ist auch eine Vergeistigung, eine gewisse Logizität dieser Technik impliziert. Es folgt daraus ein gewisser Psychologismus technischerseits und in der Folge werden passend zum Metapherngefüge auf KI-Seite, also IT-technische Systeme, psychische, psychologisierende Phänomene durch diese Metapher angeregt, wie entscheiden können, wahrnehmen können, etwas wollen, für psychologisch oder animierte Systeme prädestinierte Rollen einnehmen zu können, wie Berater, Tutoren, Assistenten, Gefährten und so weiter. So ist die größere Entwicklung der zunächst Biologisierung und Psychologisierung von Technikvorstellungen eine Art Großwetterlage, in der einzelne Wetter-Situationen gewissermaßen der Metaphorisierung von biomorphen und zoomorphen oder anthropomorphen Technikvorstellungen einzahlen bzw. miteinander einhergehen. Wichtig zu sehen ist, dass diese Tendenz als Fokus hier herausgestellt nicht die einzige ist, sondern sich gleichzeitig auch eine Technisierung des psychischen, des Lebens, der Tiere und der Menschen vollzieht, insofern etwa technomorphe Metaphern entsprechend auf Natur, Leben und Menschen übertragen werden. Analog dazu liefert die Matrix auch andere Kombinationen, die sich über die Sammlung einzelner Metaphern zu größeren Clustern zusammenstellen lassen, die dann Hinweise auf gewisse Verstehenshorizonte, semantische Großwetterlagen erlauben, mit denen wir aus unbekannten Phänomenen Sinn machen bzw. mit denen wir bekannte Phänomene in neuer Hinsicht sehen, lernen und zu verstehen geben.

Stefan Heuser: Könnte man Eure Matrix auch für die Kritik von Metaphorisierungen bzw. zur konstruktiven Arbeit an Metaphern zur Verbesserung ihrer Orientierungsleistung verwenden – und was wären die Kennzeichen eines kompetenten Umgangs mit Metaphern?

Bruno Gransche: Hier ergibt sich eine „Kultivierungsaufgabe“ wie sie Teil meines eingangs zitierten Vortragstitels war. Meines Erachtens stellt es eine wichtige Fähigkeit dar, sich im Geflecht der Metaphorisierungen so zurechtzufinden, dass für den Handlungsvollzug taugliche Orientierungen entstehen und nicht etwa ungeeignete Bedeutungen der Quelldomäne für das Verständnis der fraglichen Konzepte herangezogen werden. KI ist eben weder salzig noch haben KI-Systeme Selbstbewusstsein, Willen, Präferenzen usw. Von Kultivierung dieser Fähigkeit wäre zu sprechen, da die Sprachüblichkeiten und das kulturelle Geschehen dessen, was die Metaphern-Matrix in Auszügen fasst, nicht direkt (um)gestaltet werden können, sondern sich vielschichtige Eigendynamiken und Wechselwirkungen zeitigen. Dennoch wäre eine Metaphern-Literacy, eine Kritikfähigkeit der Übertragungen und das Verfügen über ein vielfältiges gepflegtes Metaphernrepertoire ein Zeichen der Kultiviertheit und wichtige Bedingung zur verantwortlichen Orientierung sowohl von Wissenschaft und Technikentwicklung, als auch von unserer lebensweltlichen Ausrichtung von konkreter Techniknutzung – und deren Menge und Stile – als auch allgemeiner unserer souveränen Positionierung in Bezug auf die metaphorisierten Konzepte wie Welt, Umwelt und Mitwelt, Natur, Leben und aller Arten von Wesen, göttlicher, tierischer, menschlicher und übermenschlicher.

Arne Manzeschke: Was Bruno die Metaphern-Literacy nennt, würde ich gerne so ausdeuten, dass die Matrix ein Instrument sein kann, um auf die vielschichtigen Verknüpfungsmöglichkeiten sprachlicher Äußerungen und ihre jeweiligen Bedeutungen aufmerksam zu werden. In dem Moment, in dem wir nicht mehr über eine starke Ontologie verfügen, die eine für uns durchsichtige Ordnung des Kosmos repräsentiert, wird es erkenntnismäßig entscheidend darauf ankommen, die Verknüpfungen, Verschiebungen, Überlappungen und Ausschlüsse, die metaphorisch hergestellt werden, möglichst genau zu verstehen. Möglichst genau heißt in diesem Fall aber nicht möglichst eindeutig, sondern gerade in den damit gegebenen Ungenauigkeiten, die erschließen, verschließen, aber auch verunklaren können.

Stefan Heuser: Vielen Dank Euch beiden für dieses Gespräch! Ich bin gespannt, wie Eure Arbeit an und mit dieser Matrix und Eure Forschung im Feld der Metaphern weitergeht.

Literatur

[1] Blumenberg H. Anthropologische Annäherung an die Rhetorik. In Ders. Wirklichkeiten, in denen wir leben. Stuttgart: Reclam, 1981, S. 104–136.

[2] Gransche B, Manzeschke A. Das bewegliche Heer der Künstlichen Intelligenz. Ein Technomythos als Summe menschlicher Relationen. In Künstliche Intelligenz, Mensch und Gesellschaft. Soziale

Dynamiken und gesellschaftliche Folgen einer technologischen Innovation, Heinlein M, Huchler, N (Ed.), Wiesbaden: Springer VS, 2024, S. 131–150.
[3] Manzeschke A, Gransche B. Bilder machen Menschen. Zur Bildermacht der Künstlichen Intellligenz. In Künstliche Intelligenz, Mensch und Gesellschaft. Soziale Dynamiken und gesellschaftliche Folgen einer technologischen Innovation, Heinlein M, Huchler N (Ed.), Wiesbaden: Springer VS, 2024, S. 109–130.
[4] Seising R. Es denkt nicht! Die vergessene Geschichte der KI. Frankfurt am Main: Büchergilde Gutenberg, 2021.
[5] Seising R (Ed.). Geschichten der Künstlichen Intelligenz in der Bundesrepublik Deutschland. Die Genese der KI-Forschung als Teilgebiet der bundesdeutschen Informatik. München: Deutsches Museum 2024.
[6] Suleyman M. The Coming Wave. Künstliche Intelligenz, Macht und das größte Dilemma des 21. Jahrhunderts. 1. Aufl. München: C. H. Beck, 2024.
[7] Blumenberg H. Arbeit am Mythos. 6. Aufl. Frankfurt a. Main: Suhrkamp, 2019.
[8] Deleuze G, Guatarri F. Rhizom. Berlin: Merve, 1977.
[9] Bammé A, Feuerstein G, Genth R, Holling E, Kahle R, Kempin P. Maschinen-Menschen. Mensch-Maschinen. Grundrisse einer sozialen Beziehung. 1. Aufl. Reinbek: Rowohlt, 1983.

Nicole C. Karafyllis

11 Nachruf auf Evelyn Fox Keller (1936–2023)

Am Frühabend des 8. Februar 2006 trat eine zierliche Dame mit grauem Pferdeschwanz an das Pult im Hörsaal der Goethe Universität Frankfurt am Main.[1] Dass sie fast 70 war, hätte niemand vermutet. Viele waren gekommen, um die Frau zu hören, die mit ihrer Biografie der Nobelpreisträgerin Barbara McClintock, lang unterschätzte Entdeckerin der „springenden Gene", mehr noch mit dem Bestseller *Liebe, Macht und Erkenntnis. Männliche oder weibliche Wissenschaft?* (1986, übersetzt von Bettina Blumenberg) die Feministische Epistemologie begründet hat. Die Frau, die an Joan Baez erinnerte, lieferte aber keine *Reflections on Gender and Science*, wie ihr Buch im Original hieß, sondern sprach genau über das, was im Programm stand. Ihr Thema waren Konzepte der Selbstorganisation, die aktuell als Anwärter zur Erklärung von Leben verhandelt werden. Dabei kamen neben Kant und Locke als Gewährsmännern für die ewige Verschiedenheit von Organismus und Maschine viele Physiker vor. Aber keine (andere) Frau, denn inhaltlich ergab es sich nicht. Zudem wurde die Vortragende von ihren Anhängern seit Jahren als Feminalistin fehlinterpretiert, als ob ihr Ziel eine weiblichere Wissenschaft sei. Mitnichten. Ihr Anspruch war eine erkenntniserweiterte Wissenschaft, in der die Kategorie Gender irgendwann keine Rolle mehr spielen werde. Die Erwartungen an jenem Abend wurden also trotz eines brillanten Vortrags tendenziell enttäuscht, was das Beste ist, was man von einer Erkenntnistheoretikerin sagen kann.

Die Referentin war Evelyn Fox Keller, seit 1992 Professorin für Philosophie und Wissenschaftsgeschichte am MIT in Cambridge/Massachusetts und mit internationalen Preisen hochdekoriert, darunter das MacArthur Fellowship. Wie ihr im Mai desselben Jahres verstorbener Altersgenosse Ian Hacking (1936–2023) hat sie die Wissenschaftsphilosophie und -geschichte ein halbes Jahrhundert geprägt. Beide bearbeiteten mit einer Mischung aus Realismus und Nominalismus Fragen der Objektkonstitution, d.h. wie Wissenschaftler ihren Untersuchungsgegenstand konzeptuell fassen, werten und konstellieren. Im Gegensatz zu Hacking tat Keller dies auch als praktizierende Naturwissenschaftlerin, die sich und ihr Feld dabei beobachtete. In der Wechselwirkung zwischen Wissenschaftlern und ihren Untersuchungsgegenständen entstehen teilsubjektivierte Objekte, in die individuelle Erwartungen und soziale Bedingungen eingeschrieben sind, darunter Geschlechterverhältnisse. Solche Objekte sind historisierbar und erlauben, die Produktion von Wissen als im Zwischenraum zwischen Subjekt und Objekt angesiedelt zu erzählen – nach Georg Simmel liegt dort der Hort der Kultur.

1 Im Rahmen der Ringvorlesung „Science in the Age of Extremes", organisiert von Moritz Epple.

https://doi.org/10.1515/9783112215685-011

1936 als jüngstes Kind russisch-jüdischer Immigranten in New York City geboren, wuchs Evelyn Fox im Stadtteil Queens in einer Arbeitersiedlung auf. Sie studierte Physik, spezialisierte sich auf Theoretische Physik und promovierte 1963 an der Harvard Universität bei dem Chemiker Matthew Meselson, der auch einen Bachelor in Philosophie hat. In jedem Schulbuch der Genetik steht das Meselson-Stahl-Experiment mit Nachweis der semikonservativen Replikation der DNA, wodurch das Doppelhelix-Modell von Watson/Crick auch für die Zellteilung plausibel wurde. Dabei bleibt ein DNA-Strang erhalten, der andere wird neu gebildet. 1961 entdeckte Meselson mit François Jacob und Sidney Brenner die Boten- bzw. Messenger-RNA, kurz mRNA. Sie ist Abschrift und Umschrift der DNA und Vorschrift für die Eiweißsynthese. Keller erlebt das goldene Zeitalter der Molekularbiologie, das imaginär von Codes und ihrer Entschlüsselung zehrte. Ihre Doktorarbeit zur unterschiedlichen Lichtempfindlichkeit der DNA-Stränge des Phagen-Lambda war experimenteller Natur, aber ihr Herz schlug für die Theoriearbeit. Sie verfolgte die These, dass die Komplexität des biologischen Lebens trotz aller molekularbiologischen Erkenntnisse nicht auf dessen Physik reduziert werden kann. Um diese zu prüfen, galt es aber zunächst, den mathematisch-physikalischen Gehalt hinter Metaphern wie „Schrittmacher", „Selbstorganisation" und „Gen" zu verstehen. So wurde Fox Keller zur Quereinsteigerin in die Philosophie und auch in die Biomathematik.

In den Geisteswissenschaften vollzog sich damals in den USA die sprachkritische Wende (linguistic turn), gesellschaftlich nahm die zweite Welle der Frauenbewegung an Fahrt auf. Aus diesen Fäden, anfangs verstärkt durch den der Psychoanalyse, wob Keller ihren Ansatz. Er thematisiert Denkstile in den Naturwissenschaften. Philosophisch zog Fox Keller u.a. Simmel, Benjamin, Kuhn, Feyerabend und zeitweise Piaget zu Rate gegen den damaligen wissenschaftstheoretischen Standard, dass „Wahrheit" die Übereinstimmung von Aussagesystemen mit Aussagesätzen meint. Dass naturwissenschaftliches Wissen nicht wertneutral ist, dass die Grenzen des Labors sprachlich durchlässig für das Alltägliche sind, ist heute ein Allgemeinplatz. Damals, noch vor der breiten Wiederentdeckung von Ludwik Flecks Lehre vom Denkstil (1935), musste die Idee spezifischer Wissenskulturen und ihrer möglichen Kohärenz erst begründet werden.

Begriffsanalysen waren der eine Strang von Kellers Forschungen. Der andere beschäftigte sich mit der Situation von Frauen in den Naturwissenschaften. Schon in ihrer akademischen Frühzeit unterrichtete sie parallel Physik und die noch jungen Women's Studies (Frauenforschungen). Forscherinnen („Women in Science") sah sie in der Physik der 1960er Jahre kaum und wenn, galten sie als schwierig. Fox Keller fragte sich: Hat diese personale Abwesenheit etwas damit zu tun, dass man auch über den Untersuchungsgegenstand allzu leicht – wie oben – sagt: „inhaltlich ergab es sich nicht", Frauen einzubeziehen? Nach Fox Keller spiegelt sich schon im Untersuchungsgegenstand eine bestimmte Geschlechterkonstruktion, ein „Gender of Science". Sie gehört zu seinem sozialen Gepräge. Dabei verschmelzen Maskulinitäts- und Objektivitätsideale in epistemischen Normen wie Rationalität, Einfachheit, Robustheit und

Verfügungsgewalt über Natur mittels apparativer Technik. Wenn Frauen überhaupt an Forschung beteiligt sind, werden laut Keller die Methoden der rationalen Handhabbarkeit des Untersuchungsobjekts zusammen erlernt mit Methoden der Ignoranz von Kolleginnen, weil man in einer Ideologie lebt, in der Frauen als weniger objektiv und rational gelten. Langfristig führen die durch Ausgrenzung aufrechterhaltenen Normen der Legitimation von wissenschaftlichem Wissen zu einer Aushöhlung der zugehörigen epistemischen Tugenden wie Neugierde, intellektuelle Demut und Aufgeschlossenheit für Alternativen.

Fox Keller begründete, dass man durch plurale Perspektivierung Wissenschaft besser im Sinne von wahrheitsgewisser machen kann. Mehr Forscherinnen verbesserten also die Wissenschaft insgesamt. Dieser Ansatz der Feministischen Epistemologie hat einen starken Einfluss auf die Science Studies und ihre Forderung nach Interdisziplinarität und Diversität gehabt. Poststrukturalistische Denker hingegen wollten Ideale wie Wahrheit und Ganzheit des Wissens dekonstruieren; natürlich auch die Heteronormativität von Geschlecht. So galten die Arbeiten Fox Kellers in entsprechenden Kreisen spätestens ab den Nuller Jahren als konservativ. Für sie stand fest, dass das Modell eines Objekts eine *reale* Entsprechung hat, die mehr oder weniger gut mit dem Modell korrespondiert. Nichts war ihr fremder als ein radikaler Konstruktivismus, selbst wenn sie schreibt, dass Objekte „gemacht" werden – aber als Untersuchungsgegenstände, nicht als Existenzen.

Fox Kellers hohe Reichweite lag nicht nur an den vierzehn Büchern, sondern an ihrem primären Forschungsobjekt: dem schillernden Begriff „Gen". In seinen Ausdeutungen als Code, Programm bis hin zum netzwerkenden Genom blieb sie ihm über die Jahrzehnte historisch-kritisch auf den Fersen. Dass man eine Verhaltensweise „in seiner DNA" habe, ist die alltagssprachliche Variante des molekulargenetischen Essenzialismus. Der sei Illusion, sagte Fox Keller, denn wie Gene bestimmte Krankheiten oder Verhaltensweisen verursachen, wüsste man nach wie vor nicht. Mit dem Abschluss des Human Genome Project sei, so ein berühmter ihrer Buchtitel, *Das Jahrhundert des Gens* vorbei (Rezension FAZ vom 23. Juli 2001). Gemeint waren mechanistische Vorstellungen des Erbguts wie die mehrfach nachgebesserte Ein-Gen-ein-Enzym-Hypothese und kybernetische Informationsmodelle. Optimistisch sah Fox Keller mit der Epigenetik eine Biologie des 21. Jahrhunderts auf dem Weg, die Relationen und Interaktionen höher schätzen werde als verdinglichte Einheiten wie Gene.

Keller arbeitete mit historischen Einzelstudien, die sie zu einer „Meditation" fügte. Mit ihren biomathematischen Artikeln zur Selbstorganisation von zellulären Schleimpilzen, auf der Suche nach dem Ursprung von Differenzierung, ist sie 1983 und 2006 sich selbst biographisches Objekt der Wissenschaftsgeschichtsschreibung. „Biographie statt Biologie!" war schon ein Kampfmotto der deutschen Lebensphilosophie um 1900. Fox Keller hat zur Beziehung der Antipoden gearbeitet. Dafür musste sie die Biologie als Strukturwissenschaft wie auch als hermeneutische Wissenschaft begreifen, letzteres in Form der Metaphernanalyse. Metaphern kanalisieren, wie Forscher ein Problem erfassen und welche Modelle sich zur Bearbeitung empfehlen. Das

Unbegriffene ist kreativ. Entwicklung etwa wird genetisch, aber auch embryologisch und morphologisch erklärt, wie Fox Keller in ihrem reifsten Buch *Making Sense of Life* (2002) zeigte. Auch das sogenannte Künstliche Leben (*Artificial Life*) bedarf zur Erklärung der Imitationsleistung der Metaphern aus dem und für das echte(n) Leben.

Evelyn Fox Keller starb am 22. September 2023 in einem Pflegeheim in Massachusetts. Ihre Autobiographie *Making Sense of my Life in Science: a Memoir* hat sie im Frühjahr noch fertiggestellt, bis zuletzt das Leben zwischen Subjekt und Objekt verhandelnd.

Autorinnen und Autoren

Jonathan Benecke, Wissenschaftlicher Mitarbeiter am Zentrum für erfolgreiches Lehren und Lernen (ZeLL) der Ostfalia Hochschule für angewandte Wissenschaften.

PD Dr. phil. Joachim Boldt, stellvertretender Direktor des Instituts für Ethik und Geschichte der Medizin der Universität Freiburg.

Prof. Dr. Stefan Dübel, Professor für Biotechnologie und Direktor der Abteilung für Biotechnologie, TU Braunschweig.

PD Dr. Bruno Gransche, Philosoph am Institut für Technikzukünfte ITZ am Karlsruher Institut für Technologie KIT.

Prof. Dr. Stefan Heuser, Professor für Systematische Theologie (Schwerpunkt Ethik), TU Braunschweig.

Prof. Dr. Nicole Karafyllis, Professorin für Philosophie, Schwerpunkt: Wissenschafts- und Technikphilosophie, TU Braunschweig.

Daniel Keck, Wissenschaftlicher Mitarbeiter am Institut für Evangelische Theologie, TU Braunschweig.

Prof. Dr. Arne Manzeschke, Professor für Ethik und Anthropologie, Leiter des Instituts für Pflegeforschung, Gerontologie und Ethik, Ev. Hochschule Nürnberg.

Dr. Domenico Schneider, Wissenschaftlicher Mitarbeiter am Institut für Philosophie, TU Braunschweig.

Prof. Dr. Hans G. Ulrich, em. Professor für Systematische Theologie/Ethik an der Friedrich-Alexander-Universität Erlangen-Nürnberg.

https://doi.org/10.1515/9783112215685-012

Index

https://doi.org/10.1515/9783112215685-013

www.ingramcontent.com/pod-product-compliance
Lightning Source LLC
Jackson TN
JSHW050218121225
95306JS00005B/16
* 9 7 8 3 1 1 9 1 4 5 1 2 1 *